Stockley's Drug Interc
Pocket Companion 20

D1758099

‹ is due for return on or before the last date shown below.

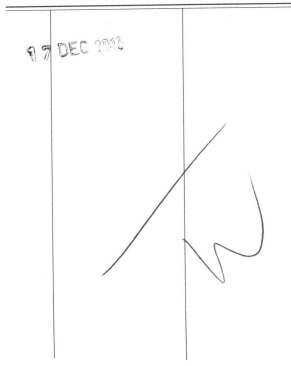

1 7 DEC 2012

Stockley's Drug Interactions Pocket Companion 2011

Editor
Karen Baxter, BSc, MSc, MRPharmS

Editorial Staff
Samuel Driver, BSc
Rebecca E Garner, BSc
Jennifer M Sharp, BPharm, DipClinPharm, MRPharmS

Based on data produced by the Stockley Editorial Team
Ian A Baxter BSc, PhD, MRPharmS
Mildred Davis, BA, BSc, PhD, MRPharmS
C Rhoda Lee, BPharm, PhD, MRPharmS
Alison Marshall, BPharm, DipClinPharm PG Cert-ClinEd, MRPharmS
Rosalind McLarney, BPharm, MSc, MRPharmS
Helen MN Neill, MPharm, MRPharmS, MPSNI
Rebecca Raymond, BSc, DipPharmPrac, MRPharmS
Julia Sawyer, BPharm, DipPharmPrac, MRPharmS

London · Chicago

Ph PP
Pharmaceutical Press

Published by Pharmaceutical Press

1 Lambeth High Street, London SE1 7JN, UK
1559 St. Paul Avenue, Gurnee, IL 60031, USA

© Pharmaceutical Press 2011

(**PhP**) is a trade mark of Pharmaceutical Press

Pharmaceutical Press is the publishing division of the Royal
Pharmaceutical Society

First published 2011

Typeset by Data Standards Ltd, Frome, Somerset
Printed in Italy by LEGO S.p.A.

ISBN 978 0 85369 977 4

A catalogue record for this book is available from the British Library

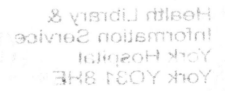

Contents

Preface

What is *Stockley's Drug Interactions Pocket Companion?*

Stockley's Drug Interactions is a reference work that provides concise, accurate, and clinically relevant information to healthcare professionals. Monographs are based on published sources including clinical studies, case reports, and systematic reviews, and are fully referenced. *Stockley's Drug Interactions Pocket Companion* has summarised this comprehensive work to create a small and conveniently-sized quick-reference text.

Stockley's Drug Interactions Pocket Companion provides the busy healthcare professional with quick and easy access to clinically relevant, evaluated and evidence-based information about drug interactions. As with the full reference work this publication attempts to answer the following questions:

- Are the drugs or substances in question known to interact or is the interaction only theoretical and speculative?
- If they do interact, how serious is it?
- Has it been described many times or only once
- Are all patients affected or only a few?
- Is it best to avoid some drug combinations altogether or can the interaction be accommodated in some way?
- What alternative and safer drugs can be used instead?

Coverage

Stockley's Drug Interactions Pocket Companion 2011 contains over 1500 interaction monographs pertaining to specific drugs or drug groups. Each monograph in *Stockley's Drug Interactions* was assessed by practising clinical pharmacists for its suitability for inclusion in the *Pocket Companion*. Broadly speaking interactions involving anaesthesia, the specialist use of multiple antiretrovirals, the specialist use of multiple antineoplastics or intravenous antineoplastics, and non-interactions were omitted. However, exceptions were made, particularly where there has been controversy over whether or not a drug interacts.

Monographs

Following the familiar format of the Stockley products, the information in this publication is organised into a brief summary of the evidence for the interaction and a description of how best to manage it. The information is based on the most recent quarterly update of *Stockley's Drug Interactions* at the time of going to press. This data is fully referenced and available at www.medicinescomplete.com. These references have not been included in the *Pocket Companion* to keep size to a minimum. Anyone interested in seeing our sources can consult *MedicinesComplete*, or the full reference work of *Stockley's Drug Interactions*.

Ratings

Each monograph has been assigned a rating symbol to offer guidance to the user on the clinical significance of the interaction. These ratings are the same as those used in *Stockley's Interaction Alerts*. The Alerts are rated using three separate categories:

- Action – This describes whether or not any action needs to be taken to accommodate the interaction. This category ranges from 'avoid' to 'no action needed'.
- Severity – This describes the likely effect of an unmanaged interaction on the patient. This category ranges from 'severe' to 'nothing expected'.
- Evidence – This describes the weight of evidence behind the interaction. This category ranges from 'extensive' to 'theoretical'.

These ratings are combined to produce one of four symbols:

❌ For interactions that have a life-threatening outcome, or where concurrent use is contraindicated by the manufacturers.

🔺 For interactions where concurrent use may result in a significant hazard to the patient and so dose adjustment or close monitoring is needed.

❓ For interactions where there is some doubt about the outcome of concurrent use, and therefore it may be necessary to give patients some guidance about possible adverse effects, and/or consider some monitoring.

✔ For interactions that are not considered to be of clinical significance, or where no interaction occurs.

We put a lot of thought in to the original design of these symbols, and have deliberately avoided a numerical or colour coding system as we did not want to imply any relationship between the symbols or colours. Instead we chose internationally recognisable symbols, which in testing were intuitively understood by our target audience of healthcare professionals.

Structure

Stockley's Drug Interactions Pocket Companion is structured alphabetically for ease of use, with International Nonproprietary Names (INNs) to identify drug names. Cross references to US Approved Names (USANs) are also included where drug names differ significantly. Consequently an interaction between aspirin and beta blockers will appear under A, and an interaction between beta blockers and digoxin will appear under B. We have only used drug groups where they are considered to be widely recognised, hence beta blockers is used, but alpha agonists is not. The drug groups we have used are as follows:

ACE inhibitors	Dopamine agonists	NSAIDs
Alpha blockers	Endothelin receptor	Opioids
Amfetamines	antagonists	Phosphodiesterase
Aminoglycosides	Ergot derivatives	type-5 inhibitors
Angiotensin II	Fibrates	Protease inhibitors
receptor antagonists	H_2-receptor	Proton pump
Antimuscarinics	antagonists	inhibitors
Antidiabetics	HRT	Quinolones
Antihistamines	5-HT_3-receptor	Salbutamol (Albuterol)
Antimuscarinics	antagonists	and related
Antipsychotics	Inotropes and	bronchodilators
Azoles	Vasopressors	SSRIs
Benzodiazepines	Low-molecular-weight	Statins
Beta blockers	heparins	Sulfonamides
Bisphosphonates	Macrolides	Tetracyclines
Calcium-channel	MAO-B inhibitors	Tricyclics
blockers	MAOIs	Triptans
Cephalosporins	Nasal decongestants	Vaccines
Contraceptives	Nitrates	Warfarin and other
Corticosteroids	NNRTIs	oral anticoagulants
Diuretics	NRTIs	

Acknowledgements

Aside from the editorial staff many other people have contributed to this publication and the Editor gratefully acknowledges the assistance and guidance they have provided. In particular, we would like to express our gratitude to Ithar Malik for his support in producing the final dataset, particularly the indexing, and to Tamsin Cousins who has handled the various aspects of the production of this book. Thanks are also due to Ivan Stockley, Sean Sweetman, and Robert Bolick for their support with this project.

Individual users of this product continue to take the time to provide us with feedback on the contents and structure of the data, and for that we are grateful. These comments are always useful to us in developing the products to better meet the needs of end-users.

Contact details

We are always very pleased to receive feedback from those using our products. Anyone wishing to comment can contact us at the following e-mail address: stockley@rpharms.com

Abbreviations

ACE	angiotensin-converting enzyme
ALT	alanine aminotransferase
AST	aspartate aminotransferase
AUC	area under the time–concentration curve
BPH	benign prostatic hyperplasia
bpm	beats per minute
CNS	central nervous system
CSF	cerebrospinal fluid
CSM	Committee on Safety of Medicines (UK) (now subsumed within the Commission on Human Medicines)
DMARD	disease modifying antirheumatic drug
ECG	electrocardiogram
e.g.	*exempli gratia* (for example)
FFPRHC	The UK Faculty of Family Planning and Reproductive Health Care
HIV	human immunodeficiency virus
HRT	hormone replacement therapy
i.e.	*id est* (that is)
INR	international normalised ratio
IUD	intra-uterine device
LFT	liver function test
MAO	monoamine oxidase
MAO-A	monoamine oxidase, type A
MAO-B	monoamine oxidase, type B
MAOI	monoamine oxidase inhibitor
mg	milligram(s)
MHRA	Medicines and Healthcare products Regulatory Agency (UK)
mL	millilitre(s)
mmHg	millimetre(s) of mercury
mol	mole
NNRTI	non-nucleoside reverse transcriptase inhibitor
NRTI	nucleoside reverse transcriptase inhibitor
NSAID	non-steroidal anti-inflammatory drug
pH	the negative logarithm of the hydrogen ion concentration
PPI	proton pump inhibitor
RNA	ribonucleic acid
SSRI	selective serotonin reuptake inhibitor
TSH	thyroid-stimulating hormone
UK	United Kingdom
US	United States of America
WHO	World Health Organization

About the Editor

Karen Baxter studied pharmacy at De Montfort University, Leicester, graduating in 1995 and then completing her pre-registration year in Yeovil, Somerset. She then moved to Derby where she was a resident pharmacist for 3 years, during which time she completed her Clinical Diploma and MSc. She then worked in a variety of clinical roles, before taking on an education and training role, during which time she undertook a joint appointment with the University of Derby, working on their postgraduate pharmacy programme. Karen started at the Pharmaceutical Press in 2001 as the Assistant Editor of *Stockley's Drug Interactions*, working under the guidance of Dr Ivan Stockley and the Martindale team. She became the Editor of *Stockley's Drug Interactions* in 2005.

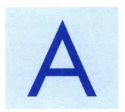

ACE inhibitors

Most ACE inhibitor interactions are pharmacodynamic, that is, interactions that result in an alteration in drug effects rather than drug disposition, so in most cases interactions of individual drugs will be applicable to the group as a whole. The ACE inhibitors do not appear to undergo interactions via cytochrome P450 isoenzymes.

ACE inhibitors + Allopurinol

Hypersensitivity, neutropenia and serious infection have occurred following the concurrent use of captopril and allopurinol. Other ACE inhibitors may interact similarly. Anaphylaxis and myocardial infarction occurred in one man taking enalapril with allopurinol. The combination of ACE inhibitors and allopurinol may increase the risk of leucopenia and serious infection.

Patients taking both drugs should be very closely monitored for any signs of hypersensitivity (e.g. skin reactions) or low white cell count (sore throat, fever etc.), especially if they have renal impairment. White blood cell counts should be monitored periodically (some suggest checking before starting allopurinol then every 2 weeks during the first 3 months of treatment, and periodically thereafter.

ACE inhibitors + Alpha blockers

The first-dose hypotensive effect seen with alpha blockers (particularly alfuzosin, prazosin and terazosin) is likely to be potentiated by ACE inhibitors. It is unclear whether there are real differences between the alpha blockers in their propensity to cause this first-dose effect. Note that the acute hypotensive reaction appears to be short-lived. In one small study tamsulosin did not have any clinically relevant effects on blood pressure that was already well controlled by enalapril.

Minimise the risk of hypotensive reactions by starting with a low dose of alpha blocker, preferably given at bedtime, and increase the dose slowly over a couple of weeks. It is recommended that the dose of the ACE inhibitor is reduced during initiation. If adding an ACE inhibitor to an alpha blocker, consider decreasing the dose of the alpha blocker and re-titrate as necessary. Patients should be warned to lie down and raise their legs if symptoms such as dizziness, fatigue or sweating develop, and to remain lying down until symptoms abate.

ACE inhibitors + **Antacids**

Fosinopril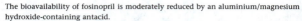

The bioavailability of fosinopril is moderately reduced by an aluminium/magnesium hydroxide-containing antacid.

> The manufacturers suggest separating fosinopril administration from that of antacids by at least 2 hours.

Other ACE inhibitors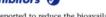

Antacids have been reported to reduce the bioavailability of some ACE inhibitors but this seems unlikely to be clinically important (except perhaps in the case of fosinopril, see above).

> The manufacturers of some ACE inhibitors warn that antacids may reduce their bioavailability, but there seems to be no evidence of a clinically significant interaction in practice.

ACE inhibitors + **Antidiabetics**

The concurrent use of ACE inhibitors and antidiabetics normally appears to be uneventful. However, hypoglycaemia, marked in some instances, has occurred in a small number of diabetics taking insulin or sulfonylureas with captopril, enalapril, lisinopril or perindopril. This has been attributed, but not proven, to be due to an interaction.

> This interaction is not established and remains the subject of considerable study and debate. It would be prudent to warn all patients taking insulin or oral antidiabetics who are just starting any ACE inhibitors that excessive hypoglycaemia has been seen very occasionally and unpredictably. It may be prudent to temporarily increase the frequency of blood glucose monitoring. Any problem seems easily resolved by reducing the sulfonylurea dose. The risk of an interaction appears low, and the use of ACE inhibitors in diabetes is considered beneficial.

ACE inhibitors + **Aspirin**

The antihypertensive efficacy of captopril and enalapril may be reduced by high-dose aspirin in about 50% of patients. Low-dose aspirin (less than or equal to 100 mg daily) appears to have little effect. It is unclear whether aspirin attenuates the benefits of ACE inhibitors in heart failure. The likelihood of an interaction may depend on disease state and its severity.

> For hypertension, no action is needed if antiplatelet dose aspirin is used. Suspect an interaction with analgesic dose aspirin if the ACE inhibitor seems less effective, or blood pressure control is erratic. Increase the ACE inhibitor dose or consider an alternative analgesic, but note that NSAIDs interact in the same way as high-dose aspirin. For heart failure it is generally advised that concurrent use is best avoided, unless a specific indication (e.g. coronary heart disease, stroke) exists.

ACE inhibitors + **Azathioprine**

Anaemia has been seen in kidney transplant patients given azathioprine with enalapril or captopril. Leucopenia occasionally occurs when captopril is given with azathioprine. Azathioprine is rapidly and extensively metabolised to mercaptopurine. Mercaptopurine is therefore expected to share the interactions of azathioprine.

The manufacturer of captopril recommends that it should be used with extreme caution in patients taking immunosuppressants, especially if there is renal impairment. They advise that differential white blood cell counts should be checked before starting captopril, then every 2 weeks in the first 3 months of captopril use, and periodically thereafter, although this is most likely to already be occurring or planned because of the azathioprine. Any effect seems likely to be a group interaction, and it would therefore seem prudent to consider monitoring with any ACE inhibitor.

ACE inhibitors + Ciclosporin (Cyclosporine)

Acute renal failure has developed in kidney transplant patients taking ciclosporin with enalapril. Oliguria was seen in another patient taking ciclosporin with captopril. There is a possible increased risk of hyperkalaemia when ACE inhibitors are given with ciclosporin, as both drugs may raise potassium levels. It is anticipated that all ACE inhibitors will interact similarly.

The incidence of renal failure appears to be low, nevertheless care and good monitoring are needed if ACE inhibitors and ciclosporin are used concurrently. Monitor potassium levels more closely in the initial weeks of concurrent use.

ACE inhibitors + Clonidine

ACE inhibitors may potentiate the antihypertensive effects of clonidine, and this can be clinically useful. However, limited evidence suggests that the effects of captopril may be delayed when patients are switched from clonidine. Note that sudden withdrawal of clonidine may cause rebound hypertension.

The general importance of this interaction is unknown, but be aware that it may occur.

ACE inhibitors + Co-trimoxazole

Two reports describe serious hyperkalaemia, apparently caused by the concurrent use of trimethoprim (given as co-trimoxazole) and enalapril or quinapril, in association with renal impairment.

Trimethoprim or ACE inhibitors alone can cause hyperkalaemia, particularly with other factors such as renal impairment. Monitor potassium levels if this combination is used in those with renal impairment. Note that co-trimoxazole is a combination preparation containing trimethoprim, and may therefore interact similarly. It has been suggested that patients with AIDS taking an ACE inhibitor for associated nephropathy should probably discontinue their ACE inhibitor during treatment with high-dose co-trimoxazole.

ACE inhibitors + Digoxin

No clinically significant interaction has been seen between digoxin and most ACE inhibitors. Some studies have found that serum digoxin levels rise by about 20% or more if captopril is used, but others have found no significant changes. It has been suggested that any interaction is likely to occur only in those patients who have pre-existing renal impairment.

> No action usually needed. In patients with renal impairment given digoxin and captopril it may be prudent to be alert for increased digoxin effects (e.g. bradycardia).

ACE inhibitors + Diuretics

Loop diuretics and Thiazides ❓

The use of ACE inhibitors with loop or thiazide diuretics is normally safe and effective, but first-dose hypotension (dizziness, fainting) can occur, particularly if the dose of diuretic is high (greater than furosemide 80 mg daily or equivalent) and often in association with predisposing conditions (heart failure, renovascular hypertension, haemodialysis, high levels of renin and angiotensin, low-sodium diet, dehydration, diarrhoea or vomiting, etc.). In addition, renal impairment, and even acute renal failure, have been reported, and diuretic-induced hypokalaemia may still occur when ACE inhibitors are used with potassium-depleting diuretics.

> First-dose hypotension is well established. In patients taking high-dose diuretics, ACE inhibitors should be initiated under close supervision. Consider temporarily stopping the diuretic or reducing its dose at least 24 hours before the ACE inhibitor is added. If this is not clinically appropriate the response to the first dose of the ACE inhibitor should be monitored for at least 2 hours, or until blood pressure has stabilised. ACE inhibitors should be started with a very low dose, even in patients at low risk (e.g. those with uncomplicated essential hypertension taking low-dose thiazides). All patients should be warned about what can happen, and advised to lie down if dizziness, lightheadedness or faintness occurs. Any marked hypotension is normally transient, but if problems persist it may be necessary to temporarily reduce the diuretic dose. Taking the first dose of the ACE inhibitor just before bedtime is also preferable. Severe reactions (e.g. renal impairment or hypokalaemia) are rare, and routine monitoring of the ACE inhibitor should suffice. However, if increases in urea and creatinine occur, a dose reduction and/or discontinuation of the diuretic and/or ACE inhibitor may be required.

Potassium-sparing diuretics ⚠

The use of ACE inhibitors with potassium-sparing diuretics, such as amiloride, eplerenone, spironolactone and triamterene, can result in hyperkalaemia, particularly in the presence of other risk factors (e.g. advanced age, diabetes, doses of spironolactone greater than 25 mg daily, and renal impairment).

> The concurrent use of ACE inhibitors and amiloride or triamterene is normally not advised, but if both drugs are appropriate potassium levels should be closely monitored. The presence of a loop or thiazide diuretic may not necessarily prevent hyperkalaemia. The combination of an ACE inhibitor and spironolactone or eplerenone is beneficial in some indications, but close monitoring of serum potassium and renal function is needed, especially with any changes in treatment or in the patient's clinical condition. It has been suggested that spironolactone should not be given with ACE inhibitors in those with a glomerular filtration rate of less than 30 mL/minute.

ACE inhibitors + **Epoetin**

Epoetin may cause hypertension and thereby reduce the effects of ACE inhibitors, and an additive hyperkalaemic effect is theoretically possible. ACE inhibitors appear to reduce the efficacy of epoetin, but any interaction may take many months to develop.

Blood pressure and electrolytes, particularly potassium, should be routinely monitored in those given epoetin. An increase in the ACE inhibitor dose appears to overcome any epoetin-induced increase in blood pressure; however, if blood pressure rises cannot be controlled or potassium levels rise, consider temporarily witholding the epoetin. The effect of ACE inhibitors on epoetin resistance is not established; it seems more likely to occur with concurrent use of high-dose ACE inhibitors and low-dose epoetin. As the epoetin dose is governed by response, no immediate intervention is necessary. If epoetin resistance occurs, consider increasing the epoetin dose.

ACE inhibitors + **Food**

Food reduces the absorption of imidapril and moexipril, and reduces the conversion of perindopril to its active metabolite, perindoprilat.

It is recommended that imidapril and perindopril should be taken before food. One US manufacturer suggests taking moexipril one hour before food, although the interaction is of doubtful clinical significance. Food has little or no clinically important effect on the absorption of captopril, cilazapril, enalapril, fosinopril, lisinopril, quinapril, ramipril, spirapril, and trandolapril.

ACE inhibitors + **Gold**

Peripheral vasodilatation (facial flushing, nausea, dizziness, and occasionally, hypotension) has occurred when some patients given gold with ACE inhibitors. Isolated cases of loss of consciousness, cardiovascular collapse and cerebrovascular accident have been reported. In some patients the reaction occurred soon after the start of the ACE inhibitor, while in others there appeared to be a lag time of several months or more.

The general importance of this interaction is unclear. It has been recommended that patients taking ACE inhibitors who require gold compounds should, if possible, be given aurothioglucose. If this is not available, a 50% reduction in the sodium aurothiomalate dose is recommended with the patient in the recumbent position, and under observation for 20 minutes following the next few injections.

ACE inhibitors + **Heparin**

An extensive review of the literature found that heparin (both unfractionated and low-molecular-weight heparins) and heparinoids inhibit the secretion of aldosterone, which can cause hyperkalaemia. This effect may be additive with the hyperkalaemic effects of the ACE inhibitors.

The CSM in the UK suggests that potassium should be measured in all patients with risk factors (e.g. renal impairment, diabetes mellitus, pre-existing acidosis and those taking potassium-sparing drugs) before starting heparin, and monitored regularly thereafter (at least every 4 days has been suggested) particularly in patients receiving heparin for more than 7 days.

A

ACE inhibitors + Herbal medicines or Dietary supplements

A patient taking lisinopril developed marked hypotension and became faint after taking garlic capsules.

This seems to be the first and only report of this reaction, so its general importance is small. However, bear it in mind in case of an unexpected response to treatment.

ACE inhibitors + Lithium

ACE inhibitors can raise lithium levels, and in some individuals 2- to 4-fold increases have occurred. Cases of lithium toxicity have been reported in patients given captopril, enalapril or lisinopril (and possibly perindopril). One analysis found an increased relative risk of 7.6 for lithium toxicity requiring hospitalisation in elderly patients newly started on an ACE inhibitor. Risk factors for this interaction seem to be poor renal function, heart failure, volume depletion, and increased age.

Adverse effects from concurrent use appear rare. Nevertheless, monitor for symptoms of lithium toxicity and consider monitoring lithium levels more frequently to avoid a potentially severe adverse interaction. As the onset of the interaction may be delayed, it has been advised that lithium levels should be monitored every week or every two weeks for several weeks. Patients taking lithium should be aware of the symptoms of lithium toxicity (e.g. increased nausea, weakness, fine tremor, drowsiness, lethargy) and told to immediately report them should they occur. This should be reinforced when they are given ACE inhibitors.

ACE inhibitors + Low-molecular-weight heparins

An extensive review of the literature found that heparin (both unfractionated and low-molecular-weight heparins) and heparinoids inhibit the secretion of aldosterone, which can cause hyperkalaemia. This effect may be additive with the hyperkalaemic effects of the ACE inhibitors.

The CSM in the UK suggests that potassium should be measured in all patients with risk factors (e.g. renal impairment, diabetes mellitus, pre-existing acidosis and those taking potassium-sparing drugs) before starting a low-molecular-weight heparin, and monitored regularly thereafter (at least every 4 days has been suggested) particularly in patients receiving a low-molecular-weight heparin for more than 7 days.

ACE inhibitors + NSAIDs

There is evidence that most NSAIDs (including the coxibs) can increase blood pressure in patients taking antihypertensives, including ACE inhibitors, although some studies have not found the increase to be clinically relevant. Indometacin appearing to have the most significant effect. The concurrent use of a NSAID and an ACE inhibitor may increase the risk of renal impairment, and rarely, hyperkalaemia.

Only some patients are affected. Consider increasing the frequency of blood pressure monitoring if an NSAID is started. Monitor renal function and electrolytes periodically.

ACE inhibitors + Potassium

ACE inhibitors can raise potassium levels. Hyperkalaemia is therefore possible if potassium supplements or potassium-containing salt substitutes are given, particularly in those patients where other risk factors are present, such as decreased renal function.

Monitor potassium levels, adjusting supplementation as necessary.

ACE inhibitors + Probenecid

Probenecid decreases the renal clearance of captopril and enalapril.

In general, these changes do not appear to result in a significant clinical effect, although it may be prudent to bear the possibility in mind in the case of any unexpected reductions in blood pressure in patients taking enalapril with probenecid. There is no information regarding other ACE inhibitors, but they would not be expected to interact any differently.

ACE inhibitors + Procainamide

The concurrent use of ACE inhibitors and procainamide possibly increases the risk of leucopenia, particularly in patients with renal impairment.

It is recommended that white cell counts are monitored before concurrent use, every 2 weeks during the first 3 months of concurrent use, and then periodically thereafter.

ACE inhibitors + Rifampicin (Rifampin)

An isolated report describes a rise in blood pressure in one hypertensive patient, which was attributed to an interaction between enalapril and rifampicin. Rifampicin may reduce the plasma levels of the active metabolites of imidapril and spirapril.

The general importance of these interactions is unknown, although they are expected to be minor), but bear them in mind in case of any unexpected elevations in blood pressure.

ACE inhibitors + Sirolimus

Oedema of the tongue, face, lips, neck and chest has been reported in patients taking sirolimus with enalapril or ramipril who had previously taken these ACE inhibitors without any adverse effects.

Caution should be used when either starting an ACE inhibitor in a patient already taking sirolimus or when starting sirolimus in a patient taking an ACE inhibitor. Higher doses of both drugs may pose a greater risk.

ACE inhibitors + Tacrolimus

Tacrolimus may cause nephrotoxicity and hyperkalaemia, which may be additive with the effects of the ACE inhibitors.

Consider the possible contribution of ACE inhibitors if nephrotoxicity or hyperkalaemia occur in a patient also taking tacrolimus.

A

ACE inhibitors + Tetracyclines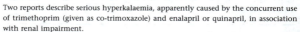

The absorption of oral tetracycline (and therefore probably most tetracyclines) is moderately reduced by the magnesium carbonate excipient in some quinapril formulations (e.g. *Accupro*). On this basis, the manufacturer of another quinapril preparation (*Quinil*), which contains magnesium oxide, predicts that it will interact similarly.

> The manufacturers recommend avoiding concurrent use. One possible way to accommodate this interaction (as with the interaction between tetracyclines and antacids) is to separate the doses as much as possible (2 to 3 hours should be sufficient).

ACE inhibitors + Trimethoprim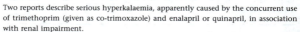

Two reports describe serious hyperkalaemia, apparently caused by the concurrent use of trimethoprim (given as co-trimoxazole) and enalapril or quinapril, in association with renal impairment.

> Trimethoprim or ACE inhibitors alone can cause hyperkalaemia, particularly with other factors such as renal impairment. Monitor potassium levels if this combination is used in those with renal impairment. It has been suggested that trimethoprim should probably be avoided in elderly patients with chronic renal impairment taking ACE inhibitors.

Acetazolamide

Note that although hypokalaemia may occur with acetazolamide it is said to be transient and rarely clinically significant.

Acetazolamide + Aspirin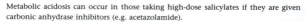

Metabolic acidosis can occur in those taking high-dose salicylates if they are given carbonic anhydrase inhibitors (e.g. acetazolamide).

> Carbonic anhydrase inhibitors should probably be avoided in those taking high-dose salicylates. If concurrent use is essential, the patient should be closely monitored for any evidence of toxicity (confusion, lethargy, hyperventilation, tinnitus) as the interaction may develop slowly and insidiously. In this context NSAIDs or paracetamol (acetaminophen) may be safer alternatives. It is not known whether eye drops interact similarly; there appear to be no reports of an interaction. No clinically relevant interaction would be expected with aspirin used in antiplatelet doses.

Acetazolamide + Carbamazepine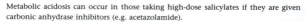

Rises in carbamazepine levels resulting in toxicity have been reported in a very small number of patients given acetazolamide.

> The general importance of this interaction is unknown, but it may be prudent to

monitor for indicators of carbamazepine toxicity (nausea, vomiting, ataxia, drowsiness) and take levels if necessary.

Acetazolamide + Ciclosporin (Cyclosporine)

There is some limited evidence that acetazolamide can cause a marked and rapid rise in ciclosporin levels (up to 6-fold in 72 hours), possibly accompanied by renal toxicity.

Ciclosporin levels and/or effects (e.g. on renal function) should be monitored as a matter of routine, but it may be prudent to increase monitoring if acetazolamide is started or stopped. Adjust the dose of ciclosporin as necessary.

Acetazolamide + Lithium

There is some evidence to suggest that the excretion of lithium can be increased by the short-term use of acetazolamide. However lithium *toxicity* occurred in one patient taking both drugs for a month.

The general importance of this interaction is unclear. Bear it in mind in case of an unexpected response to treatment.

Acetazolamide + Mexiletine

Large changes in urinary pH caused by the concurrent use of alkalinising drugs (such as acetazolamide) can, in some patients, have a marked effect on the plasma levels of mexiletine.

The effect does not appear to be predictable. There appear to be no reports of adverse interactions but if concurrent use is necessary, it should be closely monitored. The manufacturer of mexiletine recommends that concurrent use should be avoided.

Acetazolamide + Opioids

Theoretically, urinary alkalinisers such as acetazolamide may increase the effects of methadone.

The clinical significance of this interaction is unclear, but bear it in mind in case of an unexpected response to methadone.

Acetazolamide + Phenobarbital

Severe osteomalacia and rickets have been seen in a few patients taking phenobarbital or primidone with acetazolamide. A marked reduction in primidone levels with a loss in seizure control has also been described in a very small number of patients.

The general importance of this interaction is unknown. Concurrent use should be monitored for signs or symptoms of low levels of vitamin D or osteomalacia and for reduced primidone efficacy. Stop acetazolamide if possible should osteomalacia occur.

Acetazolamide + **Phenytoin**

Severe osteomalacia and rickets have been seen in a few patients taking phenytoin with acetazolamide. Rises in phenytoin levels have also been described in a very small number of patients. Fosphenytoin, a prodrug of phenytoin, may interact similarly.

> The clinical importance of this interaction is unknown. Concurrent use should be monitored for signs or symptoms of low levels of vitamin D, osteomalacia or phenytoin toxicity. Stop acetazolamide if possible should osteomalacia occur. Indicators of phenytoin toxicity include blurred vision, nystagmus, ataxia or drowsiness.

Acetazolamide + **Quinidine**

Large rises in urinary pH due to the concurrent use of acetazolamide could cause the retention of quinidine, which could lead to quinidine toxicity. Also note that hypokalaemia, which may rarely be caused by acetazolamide, can increase the toxicity of QT-prolonging drugs such as quinidine.

> Monitor the effects if acetazolamide is started or stopped and adjust the quinidine dose as necessary. Also consider monitoring potassium to ensure it is within the accepted range.

Aciclovir

Valaciclovir is a prodrug of aciclovir and therefore has the potential to interact similarly.

Aciclovir + **Ciclosporin (Cyclosporine)**

Aciclovir does not normally seem to affect ciclosporin levels or worsen renal function on concurrent use, but a very small number of cases of nephrotoxicity and increased ciclosporin levels have been reported. Valaciclovir, a prodrug of aciclovir, is expected to interact similarly.

> The handful of cases where problems have arisen clearly indicate that renal function should be closely monitored if both drugs are given. The manufacturers recommend that renal function is closely monitored if high doses of valaciclovir (more than 4 g daily) or aciclovir infusion are given with ciclosporin.

Aciclovir + **H$_2$-receptor antagonists**

Single-dose studies have found that cimetidine increases the AUC of valaciclovir and its metabolite, aciclovir, but this is thought unlikely to be clinically important.

> No action is generally needed. However, the manufacturers of valaciclovir recommend considering a non-interacting alternative to cimetidine if high-dose valaciclovir is used. A similar interaction seems possible with aciclovir.

Aciclovir + **Mycophenolate**

No clinically significant pharmacokinetic interaction appears to occur between aciclovir and mycophenolate. However, the manufacturers say that in renal impairment there may be competition for tubular secretion and increased concentrations of both drugs may occur. This is also possible with valaciclovir. A case report describes neutropenia in a patient taking valaciclovir with mycophenolate.

> Increased monitoring may be prudent in patients with reduced renal function. Neutropenia is a rare adverse effect of valaciclovir alone. Nevertheless, bear the possibility of an interaction in mind should neutropenia occur if mycophenolate is also given.

Aciclovir + **Probenecid**

Probenecid reduces the renal excretion of aciclovir and valaciclovir and therefore increases their plasma levels.

> Dose alterations are unlikely to be needed due to the wide therapeutic range of aciclovir and valaciclovir. However, the UK manufacturer states that caution is warranted if high-dose valaciclovir is given and recommends that alternatives to probenecid should be considered. Note that a clinically relevant interaction is more likely in those with reduced renal function.

Aciclovir + **Theophylline** ⚠

Preliminary evidence suggests that aciclovir can reduce the clearance of theophylline (and therefore possibly aminophylline) by about 30%. Evidence for valaciclovir appears to be lacking, although it would be expected to interact similarly.

> Evidence appears to be limited. Be alert for an increase in the adverse effects of theophylline (nausea, headache, tremor) if aciclovir or valaciclovir is added, and consider monitoring theophylline levels.

Acitretin

Acitretin + **Alcohol**

There is evidence that the consumption of alcohol may increase the serum levels of etretinate in patients taking acitretin.

> The clinical significance of this interaction is unknown, but it is suggested that it may have some bearing on the length of the period after acitretin treatment during which women are advised not to conceive.

Acitretin + **Contraceptives** ❓

There seems to be no evidence that the reliability of the oral combined hormonal

A

contraceptives is affected by acitretin, and they are the contraceptive method of choice with teratogenic drugs.

Combined hormonal contraceptives should be started one month before acitretin and continued for 2 years after stopping acitretin. In the US, it is standard practice to recommend that a second form of contraception, such as a barrier method, should also be used. This is because, even though hormonal methods of contraception are highly effective, they do, on rare occasions, fail. Note that progestogen-only oral contraceptives are not generally considered reliable enough for use with teratogenic drugs.

Acitretin + Food ❓

The absorption of acitretin is approximately doubled by food.

Acitretin should be taken with food or milk to maximise absorption.

Acitretin + Tetracyclines ✕

The development of 'pseudotumour cerebri' (benign intracranial hypertension) has been associated with the concurrent use of acitretin and tetracyclines.

The manufacturer of acitretin contraindicates its use with tetracyclines.

Acitretin + Vitamin A ⚠

A condition similar to vitamin A (retinol) overdose may occur if acitretin and vitamin A are given concurrently.

The manufacturers of acitretin states that high doses of vitamin A (more than 4000 to 5000 units daily, the recommended daily allowance) should be avoided.

Adenosine

Adenosine + Dipyridamole ✕

Dipyridamole markedly reduces the bolus dose of adenosine necessary to convert supraventricular tachycardia to sinus rhythm (by about 4-fold). Profound bradycardia occurred in a patient taking dipyridamole when an adenosine infusion was given for myocardial stress testing.

The manufacturers advise the avoidance of adenosine in patients taking dipyridamole. If adenosine must be used for supraventricular tachycardia in a patient taking dipyridamole, use an initial bolus dose of 0.5 to 1 mg. If adenosine is considered necessary for myocardial imaging in a patient taking dipyridamole, the dipyridamole should be stopped 24 hours before imaging, or the dose of adenosine should be greatly reduced. This may be insufficient for extended-release

A

dipyridamole preparations, and in this case it has been suggested that the dipyridamole will need to be stopped several days before the test.

Adenosine + **Theophylline**

Theophylline can inhibit the effects of adenosine infusions used in conjunction with radionuclide myocardial imaging. Theophylline may antagonise the effect of adenosine when used to treat supraventricular arrhythmias.

> Theophylline, aminophylline and other xanthines should be avoided for 24 hours before using an adenosine infusion for radionuclide myocardial imaging. Adenosine bolus injections for the termination of paroxysmal supraventricular tachycardia may still be effective in patients taking xanthines. The usual dose schedule should be followed. However, note that adenosine has induced bronchospasm and it has been suggested that adenosine should be avoided in patients with asthma, and used cautiously in those with obstructive pulmonary disease. Xanthines, such as intravenous aminophylline, may be used to terminate any persistent adverse effects of adenosine infusions given for myocardial imaging.

Albendazole

Albendazole + **Carbamazepine**

Carbamazepine approximately halves the levels of albendazole.

> For systemic infections it may be necessary to increase the albendazole dose. Monitor the outcome of concurrent use. This interaction is of no importance in the treatment of intestinal worm infections.

Albendazole + **Food**

Giving albendazole with a meal (especially fatty meals) markedly increases the levels of its active metabolite.

> Albendazole absorption is poor, and if it is being used for systemic infections, it is advisable to take it with a meal.

Albendazole + **Phenobarbital**

Phenobarbital (and therefore probably primidone) approximately halves the levels of albendazole.

> For systemic infections it may be necessary to increase the albendazole dose. Monitor the outcome of concurrent use. This interaction is of no importance in the treatment of intestinal worm infections.

A

Albendazole + Phenytoin

Phenytoin approximately halves the levels of albendazole. Fosphenytoin, a prodrug of phenytoin, may interact similarly.

> For systemic infections it may be necessary to increase the albendazole dose. Monitor the outcome of concurrent use. This interaction is of no importance in the treatment of intestinal worm infections.

Alcohol

Probably the most common drug interaction of all occurs if alcohol is drunk by those taking other drugs that have CNS depressant activity, the result being even further CNS depression. Blood-alcohol levels well within the legal driving limit may, in the presence of other CNS depressants, be equivalent to blood-alcohol levels at or above the legal limit in terms of worsened driving and other skills. A less common interaction that can occur between alcohol and some drugs, chemicals, and fungi is the flushing reaction. This is exploited in the case of disulfiram (*Antabuse*) as an alcohol deterrent. However, it can occur unexpectedly with some other drugs and can be both unpleasant and possibly frightening, but it is not usually dangerous. See also antihypertensives, page 89, for general comments about hypertension and alcohol consumption.

Alcohol + Alpha blockers

Alpha blockers may enhance the hypotensive effect of alcohol in subjects susceptible to the alcohol flush syndrome. This appears to be rare in whites and blacks, but more common in Orientals. The levels of both indoramin and alcohol may be raised by concurrent use, which could lead to increased drowsiness.

> The general significance of the hypotensive effects are unclear, but it may be prudent to warn susceptible patients when they start treatment. The degree of impairment caused by drinking alcohol whilst taking indoramin will depend on the individual patient. However, warn all patients of the potential effects, and counsel against driving or undertaking other skilled tasks. See also antihypertensives, page 89, for general comments about hypertension and alcohol consumption.

Alcohol + Amfetamines

Dexamfetamine, and related drugs such as ecstasy, may reduce the deleterious effects of alcohol (such as sedation), but some impairment still occurs making it unsafe to drive. Tests with metamfetamine suggest that it increases the feeling of intoxication caused by alcohol. Alcohol may increase the cardiac adverse effects of amfetamines.

> The effects of this interaction are not clear, but as some psychomotor impairment occurs warn all patients of the potential effects, and counsel against driving or undertaking other skilled tasks. Information about an increase in cardiac toxicity with the combination of amfetamines and alcohol is limited, and no general conclusions can be drawn.

Alcohol + **Antidiabetics**

Diabetics managed with insulin, oral antidiabetics, or diet alone need not abstain from alcohol, but they should drink only in moderation and accompanied by food. However, alcohol makes the signs of hypoglycaemia less clear, and delayed hypoglycaemia can occur. The CNS depressant effects of alcohol in association with hypoglycaemia can make driving or the operation of dangerous machinery much more hazardous. Metformin does not carry the same risk of lactic acidosis seen with phenformin and it is suggested by the British Diabetic Association that one or two drinks a day are unlikely to be harmful to those taking metformin. A flushing reaction is common in patients taking chlorpropamide who drink alcohol, but is rare with other sulfonylureas.

> Diabetics are advised not to exceed 2 drinks (for women) or 3 drinks (for men) daily and limit the intake of drinks with high-carbohydrate content (e.g. sweet sherries, liqueurs, low alcohol wines). Diabetics should not drink on an empty stomach and they should know that the warning signs of hypoglycaemia may possibly be obscured by the effects of the alcohol and that the hypoglycaemic effects of alcohol may occur several hours after drinking. Driving or handling dangerous machinery should be avoided because the CNS depressant effects of alcohol in association with hypoglycaemia can be particularly hazardous. The chlorpropamide-alcohol interaction (flushing reaction) is very well documented, but of minimal importance. It is a nuisance and possibly socially embarrassing but normally requires no treatment. Patients should be warned.

Alcohol + **Antihistamines**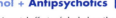

Some antihistamines cause drowsiness, which can be increased by alcohol. The detrimental effects of alcohol on driving skills are considerably increased by the use of the older more sedative antihistamines (e.g. chlorphenamine, diphenhydramine, hydroxyzine) and appear to be minimal or absent with the newer non-sedating antihistamines (e.g. cetirizine, loratadine). Note that some of the more sedative antihistamines are common ingredients of cough, cold and influenza remedies.

> The degree of impairment will depend on the individual patient. However, warn all patients taking sedating antihistamines of the potential effects, and counsel against driving or undertaking other skilled tasks. The incidence of sedation varies with the non-sedating antihistamine and depends on the individual patient. Therefore patients should be advised to be alert to the possibility of drowsiness if they have not taken the drug before. Any drowsiness would be apparent after the first few doses. Note that the manufacturer of cetirizine suggests avoiding excessive amounts of alcohol.

Alcohol + **Antipsychotics**

The detrimental effects of alcohol on the skills related to driving are greatly increased by chlorpromazine, increased by flupentixol, sulpiride, and thioridazine, and possibly increased by olanzapine, prochlorperazine and quetiapine. Any interaction with amisulpride, haloperidol, or tiapride seems to be mild; nevertheless, all antipsychotic drugs that cause drowsiness have the potential to enhance the effects of alcohol. The postural hypotension seen with antipsychotics is likely to be worsened by alcohol. There is some evidence that drinking can precipitate extrapyramidal adverse effects in patients taking antipsychotics.

The degree of sedation will depend on the antipsychotic given and the individual patient. However, warn all patients of the potential effects, and counsel against driving or undertaking other skilled tasks. It has been suggested that patients should routinely be advised to abstain from alcohol during antipsychotic treatment in order to avoid potentiating extrapyramidal adverse effects, although note that cases of a problem seem rare. Patients should also be warned about postural hypotension and counselled on how to manage it (i.e. lay down, raise the legs, and on recovering to get up slowly).

Alcohol + Apomorphine ❓

Apomorphine may increase the effects of alcohol. The hypotensive adverse effects of apomorphine may possibly be increased and sexual performance may be reduced by alcohol.

Concurrent use of alcohol with sublingual apomorphine need not be avoided, but warn patients they may feel dizzy if they drink, and to sit or lie down if this occurs. One US manufacturer of subcutaneous apomorphine advises avoiding alcohol.

Alcohol + Aspirin ✔️

Aspirin 3 g daily for a period of 3 to 5 days induces an average blood loss of about 5 mL. Some increased loss undoubtedly occurs with alcohol, but it seems to be quite small and unlikely to be of much importance in most healthy individuals taking moderate doses of aspirin and drinking moderate amounts of alcohol. However, people who consume at least 3 or more alcoholic drinks daily and who regularly take more than 325 mg of aspirin have been shown to have a high risk of bleeding. Chronic and/or gross overuse of aspirin and alcohol may result in gastric ulceration. Other salicylates would be expected to have similar effects to aspirin.

This interaction is only likely to be of significance where high doses of aspirin or other oral salicylates are given to heavy drinkers.

Alcohol + Azoles ⚠️

A few cases of disulfiram-like reactions (nausea, vomiting, facial flushing) have been seen in patients who drank alcohol while taking ketoconazole.

The incidence of this reaction appears to be very low and its importance is probably small. Reactions of this kind are usually more unpleasant than serious. Nevertheless, the manufacturer of ketoconazole advises avoiding alcohol.

Alcohol + Benzodiazepines ⚠️

Benzodiazepine and related hypno-sedatives increase the CNS depressant effects of alcohol to some extent. Alcohol modestly affects the pharmacokinetics of some benzodiazepines, and may increase aggression or amnesia, and/or reduce their anxiolytic effects.

The deterioration in the skills related to driving (as a result of the increased CNS depression that may occur) will depend on the individual patient, the particular drug in question, its dose and the amounts of alcohol taken. The risk is heightened because the patient may be unaware of being affected. Some benzodiazepines used at night for sedation are still present in appreciable amounts the next day and therefore may continue to interact. Anyone taking any of these drugs should be warned that their usual response to alcohol may be greater than expected, and their ability to drive a car, or carry out any other tasks requiring alertness, may be impaired.

Alcohol + Beta blockers

The effects of atenolol and metoprolol do not appear to be changed by alcohol. Some preliminary evidence suggests that the detrimental effects of alcohol and atenolol (with chlortalidone) or propranolol are additive on the performance of some psychomotor tests. There is some evidence that alcohol modestly reduces the haemodynamic effects of propranolol and that the blood pressure-lowering effects of sotalol appear to be increased by alcohol.

The clinical significance of these minor effects is undetermined, but they seem unlikely to be of great importance. See also antihypertensives, page 89, for general comments about antihypertensives and alcohol consumption.

Alcohol + Bupropion

The concurrent use of bupropion and alcohol does not appear to affect the pharmacokinetics of either drug; however, adverse neuropsychiatric events or reduced alcohol tolerance has been reported on concurrent use. The risk of seizures with bupropion may be increased with both the excessive use and abrupt withdrawal of alcohol.

The manufacturers of bupropion recommend that the consumption of alcohol should be minimised or avoided. However, it seems unlikely that moderate consumption of alcohol (within recommended limits) would be a problem. Note that bupropion is contraindicated during abrupt withdrawal from alcohol.

Alcohol + Buspirone

The use of buspirone with alcohol may cause drowsiness and weakness, although it does not appear to impair the performance of a number of psychomotor tests.

The degree of impairment will depend on the individual patient. However, warn all patients of the potential effects, and counsel against driving or undertaking other skilled tasks (such as driving or handling dangerous machinery). The UK manufacturer advises avoiding concurrent use until they are certain that buspirone does not adversely affect them. The evidence would appear to support this suggestion.

Alcohol + Calcium-channel blockers

Felodipine, Diltiazem or Nifedipine

Alcohol may increase the AUC of felodipine by 77% and nifedipine by 54%. This

A

resulted in an increase in heart rate in patients taking felodipine but no effects were noted in patients taking nifedipine. The manufacturers of one prolonged-release diltiazem preparation (*Adizem*) warns that alcohol may increase the rate of diltiazem release.

Information about these interactions is limited. Their clinical significance is uncertain, but probably small. Note that the manufacturer of the prolonged-release diltiazem preparation (*Adizem*) suggests that alcohol should not be taken at the same time as this preparation. See also antihypertensives, page 89, for general comments about antihypertensives and alcohol consumption.

Verapamil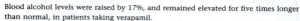

Blood alcohol levels were raised by 17%, and remained elevated for five times longer than normal, in patients taking verapamil.

Information about this interaction is limited and unconfirmed. An alcohol concentration rise of almost 17% is quite small, but it could be enough to raise legal blood levels to illegal levels if driving. Moreover, the intoxicant effects of alcohol may persist for a much longer period of time. Warn patients of these potential effects, and counsel against driving or undertaking other skilled tasks. See also antihypertensives, page 89, for general comments about antihypertensives and alcohol consumption.

Alcohol + Carbamazepine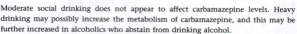

Moderate social drinking does not appear to affect carbamazepine levels. Heavy drinking may possibly increase the metabolism of carbamazepine, and this may be further increased in alcoholics who abstain from drinking alcohol.

No action needed for moderate social drinking. However, note that the sedative effects of antiepileptics may be additive with those of alcohol. The risk of seizures may be increased in heavy drinkers on tapering or stopping alcohol.

Alcohol + Cephalosporins ▲

Disulfiram-like reactions have been seen in patients taking cefamandole, cefmenoxime, cefoperazone, and possibly cefonicid after drinking alcohol or following an injection of alcohol. This is not a general reaction of the cephalosporins, but is confined to those with particular chemical structures. Due to their structure ceforanide, cefotiam, and cefpiramide also present a risk. Other cephalosporins are not expected to interact.

The reaction appears normally to be more embarrassing or unpleasant and frightening than serious, with the symptoms subsiding spontaneously after a few hours. Treatment is not usually needed although two elderly patients needed treatment for hypotension. Patients taking the interacting cephalosporins should be advised to avoid alcohol during treatment and for up to 3 days (7 days in the presence of renal or hepatic impairment) after treatment is finished.

Alcohol + Ciclosporin (Cyclosporine)

An isolated report describes a marked increase in ciclosporin levels in a patient after an episode of binge drinking, but a subsequent study found that moderate single doses of alcohol in other patients had no such effect. Red wine (350 mL) appears to decrease ciclosporin bioavailability.

It seems that alcohol in moderation will not affect ciclosporin levels, although greater care should be taken with red wine. However, note that the study with red wine was in patients taking the old *Sandimmun* preparation orally, which is known to have greater fluctuations in bioavailability than the *Neoral* preparation. Note that patients may be advised to avoid alcohol if they are taking ciclosporin after transplantation.

Alcohol + Contraceptives

The detrimental effects of alcohol may be reduced to some extent in women taking hormonal contraceptives, but blood alcohol levels do not seem to be altered.

No action is needed in those taking contraceptives.

Alcohol + Disulfiram ✗

The ingestion of alcohol while taking disulfiram will result in flushing and fullness of the face and neck, tachycardia, breathlessness, giddiness and hypotension, nausea, and vomiting. A mild flushing reaction of the skin may possibly occur in particularly sensitive individuals if alcohol is applied to the skin or if the vapour is inhaled. Note that some products (e.g. *Norvir oral solution*) are formulated with alcohol and, although the volume of alcohol taken with the dose is likely to be small, may still provoke this reaction.

This interaction is exploited therapeutically to deter alcoholics from drinking. Patients should also be warned about the exposure to alcohol from some unexpected sources such as foods, cosmetics, medicinal remedies, and solvents. Disulfiram is eliminated slowly from the body and therefore exposure to alcohol may produce unpleasant symptoms up to 14 days after taking the last dose of disulfiram.

Alcohol + Duloxetine

No important psychomotor interaction normally appears to occur between duloxetine and alcohol. However, additive effects (e.g. drowsiness) are considered possible.

The degree of impairment will depend on the individual patient. However, warn all patients of the potential effects, and counsel against driving or undertaking other skilled tasks. Note that the US manufacturer states that duloxetine should ordinarily not be prescribed for patients with substantial alcohol use as severe liver injury may result.

Alcohol + Food

Food (particularly milk) may reduce the absorption of alcohol. Foods rich in serotonin (e.g. bananas, pineapples) taken with alcohol may produce adverse effects such as diarrhoea and headache. A disulfiram-like reaction can occur if alcohol is taken up to 24 hours after eating the smooth ink(y) cap fungus (*Coprinus atramentarius*) or certain other edible fungi.

> No action is generally needed, although whether the interaction with food leading to reduced alcohol absorption can be regarded as advantageous or undesirable is a moot point. The intensity of the disulfiram-like reaction depends upon the quantity of fungus and alcohol consumed, and the time interval between them. However, reports of this reaction in the medical literature are few and far between. Treatment does not normally appear to be necessary.

Alcohol + Furazolidone

A disulfiram-like reaction may occur in patients taking furazolidone if they drink alcohol. One report suggests that about 1 in 5 patients may be affected.

> Reactions of this kind appear to be more unpleasant and possibly frightening than serious, and normally need no treatment. Nevertheless, patients should be warned about what may happen if they drink.

Alcohol + Griseofulvin

An isolated case report describes a very severe disulfiram-like reaction when a man taking griseofulvin drank a can of beer. Other isolated reports describe flushing and tachycardia, or increased alcohol effects when patients taking griseofulvin consumed alcohol.

> The documentation is extremely sparse, which would seem to suggest that adverse interactions between alcohol and griseofulvin are uncommon. Concurrent use need not be avoided, but it may be prudent to warn all patients of the potential effects, and counsel against driving or undertaking other skilled tasks.

Alcohol + H$_2$-receptor antagonists

Although some studies have found that blood alcohol levels can be slightly raised and possibly remain elevated for longer than usual in patients taking H$_2$-receptor antagonists, other studies report that no significant interaction occurs. Hypoglycaemia, which can occur following alcohol intake, may be enhanced by H$_2$-receptor antagonists.

> Extensive reviews of the data have concluded that the interaction is not, in general, clinically significant. There are insufficient grounds to justify any general warning regarding alcohol and H$_2$-receptor antagonists, but note that many of the conditions for which H$_2$-receptor antagonists are used may be made worse by alcohol, so restriction of alcohol intake may be needed.

Alcohol + **Herbal medicines or Dietary supplements**

Ginseng ✓

Panax ginseng (Asian ginseng) increases the clearance of alcohol and lowers blood alcohol levels.

> The clinical significance of this interaction is unclear.

Kava ⚠

There is some evidence that kava may worsen the CNS depressant effects of alcohol.

> The effects of this interaction are not clear, but as some psychomotor impairment occurs warn all patients of the potential effects, and counsel against driving or undertaking other skilled tasks. The use of kava is restricted in the UK because of reports of idiosyncratic hepatotoxicity.

Liv.52

Liv.52, an Ayurvedic herbal remedy, appears to reduce the hangover symptoms after drinking. However it also raises the blood alcohol levels of moderate drinkers (by about 30%) for the first few hours after drinking.

> Increases of up to 30% may be enough to raise the blood alcohol from legal to illegal levels when driving. Moderate drinkers should be warned.

Alcohol + **HRT** ✓

Acute ingestion of alcohol markedly increases the levels of circulating estradiol in women using oral HRT. A smaller increase occurs with transdermal HRT. In addition, regular alcohol intake (as low as 1 to 2 drinks per day) appears to modestly increase the risk of some types of breast cancer in women receiving HRT. Estradiol does not affect blood alcohol levels.

> It has been suggested that women taking HRT should limit their alcohol intake (about one drink or less per day has been proposed), but more study is needed to confirm any interaction and its importance.

Alcohol + **Hyoscine (Scopolamine)** ✓

Although additive CNS effects are possible, a study found no adverse interaction appears to occur if patients using transdermal hyoscine (*Scopoderm TTS*) drink alcohol. Hyoscine butylbromide may delay peak alcohol levels, but the clinical significance of this is unclear.

> In general, the manufacturers of several hyoscine hydrobromide preparations suggest that alcohol should be avoided, although note that hyoscine butylbromide and hyoscine methobromide do not readily pass the blood-brain barrier, and would not be expected to cause additive adverse effects with alcohol.

A

Alcohol + Isoniazid ❓

Isoniazid slightly increases the hazards of driving after drinking alcohol. Isoniazid-induced hepatitis may also possibly be increased, and the effects of isoniazid are possibly reduced, by alcohol.

There appear to be some extra risks for patients taking isoniazid who drink, but the effect does not appear to be large. Patients should nevertheless be warned about the potential psychomotor adverse effects. The clinical significance of the other effects are unclear, but it may be prudent to limit alcohol intake whilst taking isoniazid.

Alcohol + Leflunomide ✖

The UK manufacturers state that the concurrent use of alcohol and leflunomide has the potential to cause additive hepatotoxic effects. However, one study suggested that self-reported alcohol consumption had no significant influence on ALT levels.

The manufacturers recommend that alcohol should be avoided by patients taking leflunomide, whereas the British Society for Rheumatology guidelines make a practical recommendation, suggesting that alcohol intake should be limited to 4 to 8 units a week.

Alcohol + Levamisole ❓

There is some evidence that a disulfiram-like reaction can occur if patients taking levamisole drink alcohol.

The clinical significance of this interaction is not known. The reaction, when it occurs, normally seems to be more unpleasant and possibly frightening than serious. Symptoms usually resolve in a few hours, and it usually requires no treatment. It would seem prudent to warn patients of the possibility.

Alcohol + Lithium ❓

Some limited evidence suggests that the use of lithium with alcohol may impair the performance of skills related to driving, without affecting blood-alcohol levels.

Information is limited, but patients should be warned of the potential psychomotor adverse effects, and counselled against driving or undertaking other skilled tasks.

Alcohol + Macrolides ❓

Alcohol can cause a moderate reduction in the absorption of erythromycin ethylsuccinate. There is some evidence that intravenous erythromycin can raise blood alcohol levels but the extent and the practical importance of this (e.g. on driving ability) is unknown.

The extent to which this reduced absorption might alter the antibacterial effects of erythromycin is uncertain, but it seems likely to be small.

Alcohol + MAOIs

Patients taking non-selective MAOIs can suffer a serious hypertensive reaction if they drink some beers, lagers or wines, including low-alcohol drinks, but apparently not spirits; however, this is a reaction to the tyramine content rather than the alcohol. The hypotensive adverse effects of the MAOIs may be exaggerated in a few patients by alcohol and they may experience dizziness and faintness after drinking relatively modest amounts.

Avoid tyramine-rich drinks and counsel patients on the possible response to alcohol. Patients taking MAOIs should also be warned of the possibility of orthostatic hypotension and fainting if they drink alcohol. They should be advised not to stand up too quickly, and to remain sitting or lying if they experience dizziness or faintness.

Alcohol + Maprotiline ?

Maprotiline can cause drowsiness and impair the ability to drive or handle other dangerous machinery, particularly during the first few days of treatment. This impairment may be increased by alcohol.

Patients should be warned that their usual response to alcohol may be greater than expected, and their ability to drive a car, or carry out any other tasks requiring alertness, may be impaired.

Alcohol + Methotrexate ✖

There is some inconclusive evidence to suggest that the consumption of alcohol may increase the risk of methotrexate-induced hepatic cirrhosis and fibrosis.

The manufacturers of methotrexate advise the avoidance of drugs, including alcohol, which have hepatotoxic potential. It is not clear whether moderate drinking poses a significant risk.

Alcohol + Methylphenidate ✖

Alcohol may increase methylphenidate levels and exacerbate some of its CNS effects.

The manufacturer recommends that alcohol should be avoided in those taking methylphenidate. Also, methylphenidate should be given cautiously to patients with a history of drug dependence or alcoholism because of its potential for abuse.

Alcohol + Metoclopramide ?

There is some evidence to suggest that metoclopramide can increase the rate of absorption of alcohol, raise maximum blood alcohol levels, and possibly increase alcohol-related sedation.

At the risk of being over-cautious, warn all patients of the potential adverse effects, and counsel against driving or undertaking other skilled tasks.

A

Alcohol + Metronidazole

A disulfiram-like reaction has occurred in a few patients taking oral metronidazole who drank alcohol. There is one report of its occurrence when metronidazole was applied as a vaginal insert, and another when metronidazole was given intravenously. The interaction is alleged to occur with all other 5-nitroimidazoles (e.g. tinidazole).

This interaction has been extensively studied but it remains slightly controversial because the incidence has been reported as between 0 and 100%. Because of its unpredictability all patients given metronidazole should be warned what may happen if they drink alcohol. Alcohol should be avoided for 24 to 48 hours (72 hours for extended-release preparations) after metronidazole is stopped, and for 72 hours after tinidazole is stopped. The reaction, when it occurs, normally seems to be more unpleasant and possibly frightening than serious, and usually requires no treatment, although rarely fatalities have occurred.

Alcohol + Mianserin

Mianserin can cause drowsiness and impair the ability to drive or handle other dangerous machinery, particularly during the first few days of treatment. This impairment may be increased by alcohol.

The degree of impairment will depend on the individual patient. Patients should be warned that their usual response to alcohol may be greater than expected, and their ability to drive a car, or carry out any other tasks requiring alertness, may be impaired.

Alcohol + Mirtazapine

The sedative effects of mirtazapine may be increased by alcohol.

The manufacturers advise against concurrent use. Patients should be warned that their usual response to alcohol may be greater than expected, and their ability to drive a car, or carry out any other tasks requiring alertness, may be impaired.

Alcohol + Nitrates

Patients who take glyceryl trinitrate (nitroglycerin) and drink alcohol may feel faint and dizzy because of an increased susceptibility to postural hypotension. Consider also, antihypertensives, page 89.

The consumption of alcohol should not stop patients from using glyceryl trinitrate (nitroglycerin), but they should be warned of the possible effects and told what to do if they feel faint and dizzy (i.e. lie down, and to remain lying down until symptoms abate).

Alcohol + NSAIDs

Indometacin and Phenylbutazone

The skills related to driving are impaired by indometacin and phenylbutazone.

Additive sedation occurs if patients drink while taking phenylbutazone, but this does not appear to occur with indometacin. See also Miscellaneous NSAIDs, below.

> The degree of impairment will depend on the individual patient. However, warn all patients of the potential effects, and counsel against driving or undertaking other skilled tasks.

Miscellaneous NSAIDs

NSAIDs may increase the risk of gastrointestinal haemorrhage associated with alcohol, and a few isolated reports attribute acute renal failure to the acute excessive consumption of alcohol in patients taking NSAIDs.

> Serious problems seem rare. Concurrent use need not be avoided but be aware that there are some risks and these are increased in heavy drinkers.

Alcohol + Opioids

The opioid analgesics can enhance the CNS depressant effects of alcohol, which has been fatal in some cases. The CNS depressant effects of alcohol are modestly increased by normal therapeutic doses of dextropropoxyphene (propoxyphene), but in deliberate suicidal overdose the CNS depressant effects appear to be additive, and can be fatal. A single case report describes a fatality due to the combined CNS depressant effects of hydromorphone and alcohol. Alcohol has been associated with rapid release of hydromorphone and morphine from extended-release preparations, which could result in potentially fatal doses.

> The degree of impairment and/or sedation will depend on the individual patient, the opioid dose used and the amount of alcohol consumed. However, warn all patients of the potential effects, and with larger doses counsel against driving or undertaking other skilled tasks.

Alcohol + Paracetamol (Acetaminophen)

Many case reports describe severe liver damage, fatal in some instances, in some alcoholics and persistent heavy drinkers who take only moderate doses of paracetamol. However, controlled studies have found no association between alcoholism and paracetamol-induced hepatotoxicity. There is controversy about the use of paracetamol in alcoholics. Some consider standard therapeutic doses can be used, whereas others recommend the dose of paracetamol should be reduced, or paracetamol avoided. Occasional and moderate drinkers do not seem to be at any extra risk.

> There seems to be no way of identifying those alcoholics at risk. The combination need not be avoided, but caution patients against long-term regular use without close monitoring.

Alcohol + Phenobarbital

Moderate social drinking does not appear to cause a clinically significant alteration in phenobarbital levels, and does not appear to cause changes in the control of epilepsy. Alcohol and the barbiturates are CNS depressants, which together can have additive and possibly even synergistic effects. Activities requiring alertness and good co-ordination, such as driving a car or handling other potentially dangerous machinery, can be made more difficult and more hazardous. Alcohol may also continue to interact the next day if the barbiturate has hangover effects.

> The degree of impairment will depend on the individual patient. Patients should be warned that their usual response to alcohol may be greater than expected, and their ability to drive a car, or carry out any other tasks requiring alertness, may be impaired.

Alcohol + Phenytoin

Chronic heavy drinking reduces serum phenytoin levels so that above average doses of phenytoin may be needed to maintain adequate levels. Acute alcohol intake may possibly increase phenytoin levels, but moderate social drinking appears to have little clinical effect in those taking phenytoin. Fosphenytoin, a prodrug of phenytoin, may interact similarly.

> Monitor heavy drinkers for decreased phenytoin effects, as they may need above-average doses of phenytoin to maintain adequate serum levels. However, be aware that patients with liver impairment usually need lower doses of phenytoin, so the picture may be more complicated.

Alcohol + Pimecrolimus

Alcohol intolerance (moderate to severe facial flushing) and application site erythema have been reported rarely with pimecrolimus cream.

> Patients should be warned of the possibility of a flushing reaction with alcohol, although the incidence of this reaction seems to be rare.

Alcohol + Pregabalin

No clinically relevant pharmacokinetic interaction occurs between pregabalin and alcohol, and concurrent use does not appear to have a clinically important effect on respiration. However, the manufacturers suggest that pregabalin may potentiate the effects of alcohol.

> The degree of impairment will depend on the individual patient. Patients should be warned that their usual response to alcohol may be greater than expected, and their ability to drive a car, or carry out any other tasks requiring alertness, may be impaired.

Alcohol + Reboxetine

A study found that reboxetine does not effect cognitive or psychomotor function, and there is no interaction with alcohol.

> No action needed, but note that as reboxetine has CNS effects the manufacturers say that patients should be cautioned if operating machinery or driving.

Alcohol + SSRIs

Citalopram, escitalopram, fluoxetine, paroxetine and sertraline have no significant pharmacokinetic interaction with alcohol, but some modest increase in sedation may possibly occur with fluvoxamine and paroxetine.

> Although no interaction has clearly been demonstrated, most manufacturers of SSRIs suggest that concurrent use with alcohol is not advisable. This is presumably because both drugs act on the CNS and also because of the risk of alcohol abuse in depressed patients.

Alcohol + Tacrolimus

Alcohol may cause facial flushing or skin erythema in patients using tacrolimus ointment. This reaction appears to be fairly common and has also occurred with medicines formulated with alcohol.

> Patients should be warned of the possibility of a flushing reaction with alcohol and that alcohol may need to be avoided if flushing occurs.

Alcohol + Tetracyclines

Doxycycline levels may fall below minimum therapeutic concentrations in alcoholic patients, but tetracycline is not affected. There is nothing to suggest that moderate amounts of alcohol have a clinically relevant effect on the levels of any tetracycline in non-alcoholic subjects.

> One possible solution is to give alcoholic subjects double the dose of doxycycline. Alternatively tetracycline may be a suitable non-interacting alternative. There is nothing to suggest that moderate or even occasional heavy drinking has a clinically relevant effect on any of the tetracyclines in non-alcoholic subjects.

Alcohol + Tizanidine

Sedation occurs in up to 50% of patients taking tizanidine; these effects may be additive with alcohol. Additive hypotensive effects also considered possible, see antihypertensives, page 89. Alcohol modestly increases tizanidine levels, which may enhance these effects.

> The degree of impairment will depend on the individual patient. However, warn all patients of the potential adverse effects, and counsel against driving or undertaking other skilled tasks, and to sit or lie down if they become dizzy or faint.

Alcohol + Trazodone

Trazodone can make driving or handling other dangerous machinery more hazardous, particularly during the first few days of treatment, and further impairment may occur with alcohol.

> The degree of impairment will depend on the individual patient. However, warn all patients of the potential effects, and counsel against driving or undertaking other skilled tasks.

A

Alcohol + Tricyclics ❓

The ability to drive, handle dangerous machinery, or do other tasks requiring complex psychomotor skills may be impaired by amitriptyline, and to a lesser extent by doxepin, particularly during the first few days of treatment. This impairment is increased by alcohol. Amoxapine, clomipramine, desipramine, imipramine, and nortriptyline appear to interact with alcohol only minimally. Specific information about other tricyclic antidepressants appears to be lacking. There is also evidence that alcoholics (without liver disease) may need larger doses of desipramine and imipramine to control depression. However, the toxicity of some tricyclics may be increased by alcohol, and in alcoholics with liver disease.

Although an interaction has not been clearly demonstrated with all the tricyclic antidepressants some caution is warranted as they all have some sedative effects. The degree of impairment will depend on the individual patient. However, warn all patients of the potential effects, and counsel against driving or undertaking other skilled tasks. In addition some prescribers may feel it appropriate to offer further precautionary advice, because during the first 1 to 2 weeks of treatment many tricyclics (without alcohol) may temporarily impair the skills related to driving, although the effects of the interaction diminish during continued treatment. Also be aware that alcoholic patients (without liver disease) may need higher doses of imipramine (possibly doubled) and desipramine to control depression, and if long-term abstinence is achieved the doses may then eventually need to be reduced. Information about other tricyclics seems to be lacking.

Alcohol + Venlafaxine ❓

No important psychomotor interaction normally appears to occur between alcohol and venlafaxine in therapeutic doses. However, additive sedative effects are considered possible.

The manufacturers state that patients should be advised to avoid alcohol while taking venlafaxine. Nevertheless, it may be prudent to warn all patients of the potential effects, and counsel against driving or undertaking other skilled tasks. The degree of impairment will depend on the individual patient.

Alcohol + Warfarin and other oral anticoagulants

The effects of anticoagulants such as warfarin are unlikely to be changed in those with normal liver function who drink small or moderate amounts of alcohol: one large study showed no relationship between raised INR and alcohol consumption. However, heavy drinkers or patients with some liver disease may show considerable fluctuations in their prothrombin times when they drink alcohol. Some sources also say that the indanedione phenindione may interact with alcohol, but there seems no direct evidence available to support this prediction.

Patients should be counselled about appropriate alcohol consumption when they start anticoagulant therapy.

Aliskiren

Aliskiren + **Amiodarone**

Ketoconazole increases the plasma levels of aliskiren by 80%. The manufacturers predict that amiodarone will interact similarly.

> Monitor concurrent use for aliskiren adverse effects such as diarrhoea, dyspepsia and hypotension. Adjust the aliskiren dose as necessary. Note that doses twice the usual recommended dose of aliskiren have been safely used in clinical studies.

Aliskiren + **Azoles**

Ketoconazole increases the plasma levels of aliskiren by 80%. The manufacturers predict that itraconazole will interact similarly.

> Monitor concurrent use for aliskiren adverse effects such as diarrhoea, dyspepsia and hypotension. Adjust the aliskiren dose as necessary. Note that doses twice the usual recommended dose of aliskiren have been safely used in clinical studies.

Aliskiren + **Calcium-channel blockers**

Verapamil

Verapamil doubled the exposure to aliskiren in one study. Aliskiren does not affect verapamil pharmacokinetics.

> It has been suggested that no initial aliskiren dose adjustment is required with verapamil; however, it would be prudent to ensure that the blood pressure-lowering effects of aliskiren do not become excessive. Note that the UK manufacturer of aliskiren contraindicates concurrent use of verapamil; however, this contraindication was issued before this study was published.

Other calcium-channel blockers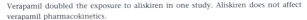

The use of aliskiren with calcium-channel blockers is expected to result in additive blood pressure-lowering effects.

> This is likely to be a desirable interaction. No action is needed unless the reduction in blood pressure becomes excessive.

Aliskiren + **Ciclosporin (Cyclosporine)**

Ciclosporin increases the maximum plasma levels and AUC of aliskiren by 2.5-fold and 5-fold, respectively.

> The manufacturers contraindicate concurrent use.

A

Aliskiren + Diuretics

Loop diuretics

Aliskiren reduces the plasma levels of furosemide by about 50%. Additive hypotensive effects are likely when aliskiren is given with any diuretic, see antihypertensives, page 89.

> The effects of furosemide may be reduced. Monitor blood pressure and/or disease control, and adjust the doses/treatment accordingly.

Potassium-sparing diuretics

Based on experience with the use of other substances that affect the renin-angiotensin system, the concurrent use of potassium-sparing diuretics and aliskiren may lead to increases in serum potassium. Additive hypotensive effects are likely when aliskiren is given with any diuretic, see antihypertensives, page 89.

> Monitor potassium levels and adjust treatment as necessary.

Aliskiren + Food

A high-fat meal reduces the plasma levels of aliskiren by about 85%.

> The manufacturer advises taking aliskiren with a light meal, preferably at the same time each day.

Aliskiren + Herbal medicines or Dietary supplements

Rifampicin reduces the levels of aliskiren and reduces its effects on plasma renin activity. The manufacturers of aliskiren predict that St John's wort may interact similarly.

> Monitor concurrent use for a reduced effect on blood pressure and increase the dose of aliskiren if necessary.

Aliskiren + Macrolides

Ketoconazole increases the plasma levels of aliskiren by 80%. The manufacturers predict that some macrolides (clarithromycin, erythromycin and telithromycin) will interact similarly.

> Monitor concurrent use for aliskiren adverse effects such as diarrhoea, dyspepsia and hypotension. Adjust the aliskiren dose as necessary. Note that doses twice the usual recommended dose of aliskiren have been safely used in clinical studies.

Aliskiren + NSAIDs

NSAIDs may reduce the antihypertensive effects of aliskiren. In dehydrated or elderly patients with some renal impairment, the concurrent use of aliskiren and NSAIDs may result in further deterioration of renal function and possible renal failure.

> Monitor the outcome of concurrent use, and consider monitoring renal function.

Aliskiren + Quinidine

Ciclosporin, a potent inhibitor of P-glycoprotein causes a 5-fold increases in the exposure to aliskiren. Quinidine is predicted to interact similarly.

> The manufacturers contraindicate concurrent use.

Aliskiren + Rifampicin (Rifampin)

Rifampicin reduces the maximum level and AUC of aliskiren by 39% and 56%, respectively. Plasma renin activity was 61% greater during rifampicin use, suggesting that rifampicin reduces the effects of aliskiren on renin activity.

> Monitor concurrent use for a reduced effect on blood pressure and increase the dose of aliskiren if necessary.

Aliskiren + Statins

Atorvastatin increases the AUC and maximum plasma level of aliskiren by about 50%.

> Monitor concurrent use for aliskiren adverse effects such as diarrhoea, dyspepsia and hypotension. Adjust the aliskiren dose as necessary. Note that doses twice the usual recommended dose of aliskiren have been safely used in clinical studies.

Allopurinol

Allopurinol + Antidiabetics

Allopurinol adversely affected glycaemic control in a patient with type 2 diabetes receiving insulin. Marked hypoglycaemia and coma occurred in one patient taking gliclazide and allopurinol. Allopurinol causes an increase in the half-life of chlorpropamide, and a minor decrease in the half-life of tolbutamide.

> More study is needed to find out whether any of these interactions has general clinical importance, but it seems unlikely.

Allopurinol + Azathioprine

The haematological effects of azathioprine and mercaptopurine are markedly increased by the concurrent use of allopurinol.

> The dose of azathioprine or mercaptopurine should be reduced by two-thirds to

A

three-quarters to minimise the risk of toxicity. Despite taking these precautions toxicity may still be seen and very close haematological monitoring is advisable if concurrent use is necessary.

Allopurinol + Capecitabine

The activity of capecitabine is predicted to be decreased by allopurinol.

The UK manufacturers of capecitabine say that allopurinol should be avoided.

Allopurinol + Carbamazepine ⚠

There is some evidence to suggest that high-dose allopurinol (15 mg/kg or 600 mg daily) can gradually raise serum carbamazepine levels by about one-third. It appears that allopurinol 300 mg daily has no effect on carbamazepine levels.

This interaction may take weeks or months to develop. Warn patients taking high-dose allopurinol to monitor for indicators of carbamazepine toxicity, which include nausea, vomiting, ataxia and drowsiness. Monitor carbamazepine levels as necessary.

Allopurinol + Ciclosporin (Cyclosporine) ❓

Isolated cases of markedly raised ciclosporin levels have been reported in patients given allopurinol (100 or 200 mg). However, two clinical studies found a trend towards lower ciclosporin levels with low-dose allopurinol (e.g. 25 mg).

This interaction is unconfirmed and of uncertain clinical significance. There is insufficient evidence to recommend increased monitoring, but be aware of the potential for an interaction in case of an unexpected response to treatment.

Allopurinol + Diuretics ❓

The thiazide diuretics may increase the incidence of hypersensitivity reactions (rash, vasculitis, hepatitis, eosinophilia, progressive renal impairment) in patients taking allopurinol, especially in the presence of renal impairment.

The clinical significance of this interaction is unclear but some caution is warranted, particularly if the patient has renal impairment. Remember that thiazides can cause hyperuricaemia.

Allopurinol + NRTIs

Allopurinol increases didanosine absorption (69% rise in the maximum serum levels with normal renal function, over 2-fold in the presence of renal impairment). In some patients the dose of didanosine has been halved without the loss of antiviral efficacy.

The manufacturers contraindicate concurrent use and advise that patients requiring allopurinol should be changed from didanosine to an alternative antiretroviral regimen.

A

Allopurinol + Penicillins

The incidence of skin rashes among those taking either ampicillin or amoxicillin is increased by allopurinol.

> There would seem to be no strong reason for avoiding concurrent use, but prescribers should recognise that the development of a rash is by no means unusual. Whether this also occurs with penicillins other than ampicillin or amoxicillin is uncertain, but it does not seem to have been reported.

Allopurinol + Phenytoin

A case report describes phenytoin toxicity in a boy given allopurinol. Another study found raised phenytoin levels in 2 of 18 patients given allopurinol.

> Although information is limited, it appears that allopurinol may raise phenytoin levels in some patients. It would therefore be prudent to monitor for phenytoin toxicity when allopurinol, particularly in high doses, is added. Indicators of phenytoin toxicity include blurred vision, nystagmus, ataxia or drowsiness.

Allopurinol + Probenecid

Probenecid appears to increase the renal excretion of the active metabolite of allopurinol, while allopurinol is thought to inhibit the metabolism of probenecid. Theoretically, the concurrent use of allopurinol and probenecid could lead to uric acid precipitation in the kidneys.

> The clinical significance of these interactions appears to be minimal. Nevertheless, the UK manufacturer of allopurinol recommends any reduction in efficacy should be assessed in each case. For allopurinol injection, the US manufacturer recommends a high urinary output of at least 2 litres daily, and the maintenance of neutral or slightly alkaline urine, to help prevent renal precipitation of urates.

Allopurinol + Pyrazinamide

Allopurinol is expected to increase the levels of pyrazinoic acid (an active metabolite of pyrazinamide), and increase its hyperuricaemic effect.

> Allopurinol is unlikely to be an effective treatment for pyrazinamide-induced hyperuricaemia, and may exacerbate the situation. Note that pyrazinamide should be used with caution or is contraindicated in patients with a history of gout. If hyperuricaemia accompanied by gouty arthritis (without liver dysfunction) occurs, pyrazinamide should be stopped.

Allopurinol + Theophylline

Allopurinol may modestly increase theophylline levels, but not all studies have found this effect. It seems likely that aminophylline may interact similarly.

> Watch for symptoms of raised theophylline levels (headache, nausea, tremor). Consider monitoring theophylline levels, especially with high doses of allopurinol.

A

Allopurinol + Warfarin and other oral anticoagulants ⚠️

Most patients taking coumarins with allopurinol do not develop an adverse interaction, but excessive hypoprothrombinaemia and bleeding can occur quite unpredictably in a few individuals. The interaction has only been reported with warfarin and phenprocoumon, but it would be prudent to apply the same precautions with any coumarin.

> An interaction between allopurinol and the coumarins is not established; however, bear it in mind when using both drugs. Consider increasing the frequency of INR monitoring during the initial stages of concurrent use.

Alpha blockers

Alpha blockers + Angiotensin II receptor antagonists ❓

The first-dose hypotensive effect seen with alpha blockers (particularly alfuzosin, prazosin and terazosin) is likely to be potentiated by angiotensin II receptor antagonists.

> Acute hypotension (dizziness, fainting) sometimes occurs unpredictably with the first dose of some alpha blockers (particularly alfuzosin, prazosin and terazosin), and this may be exaggerated by the angiotensin II receptor antagonists. Minimise the risk by starting with a low dose of alpha blocker, preferably given at bedtime, and increase the dose slowly over a couple of weeks. If adding an angiotensin II receptor antagonist to an alpha blocker, consider decreasing the dose of the alpha blocker and re-titrate as necessary. Patients should be warned to lie down and raise their legs if symptoms such as dizziness, fatigue or sweating develop, and to remain lying down until symptoms abate.

Alpha blockers + Azoles

Alfuzosin, Silodosin and Tamsulosin ❌

Ketoconazole, a potent inhibitor of CYP3A4, increases the AUC of alfuzosin (as a modified-release preparation) and silodosin 3.2-fold. Tamsulosin is predicted to be similarly affected. Itraconazole would be expected to interact with these alpha blockers in the same way as ketoconazole.

> The manufacturers of these alpha blockers contraindicate or advise against the concurrent use of potent inhibitors of CYP3A4, such as ketoconazole and itraconazole. However, if concurrent use is essential, it would seem prudent to use the minimum dose of the alpha blocker and titrate as necessary, monitoring for adverse effects, particularly first-dose hypotension. The risks are likely to be greater in patients also taking other antihypertensives.

Doxazosin

Doxazosin is primarily metabolised by CYP3A4. The US manufacturer therefore predicts that inhibitors of CYP3A4 (they name ketoconazole, itraconazole and voriconazole) may inhibit the metabolism of doxazosin.

The clinical relevance of this prediction is unclear as other pathways are involved in doxazosin metabolism, but until more is known some caution seems prudent. If concurrent use is undertaken be aware that the adverse effects of doxazosin (e.g. dizziness, headache, postural hypotension) may be increased.

Alpha blockers + Beta blockers

The risk of first-dose hypotension with prazosin (resulting in dizziness or even fainting) is higher if the patient is already taking a beta blocker. This is likely to be true of other alpha blockers, particularly alfuzosin and terazosin, although it is unclear whether there are real differences between the alpha blockers in their propensity to cause this first dose effect. Alpha blockers and beta blockers may be combined for additional lowering of blood pressure in patients with hypertension.

It is recommended that those already taking beta blockers should have the dose reduced to a maintenance dose and begin with a low-dose of an alpha blocker, with the first dose taken just before going to bed. They should also be warned about the possibility of postural hypotension and how to manage it (i.e. lay down, raise the legs, and get up slowly when recovered). Similarly, when adding a beta blocker to an alpha blocker, it may be prudent to decrease the dose of the alpha blocker and re-titrate as necessary to achieve adequate blood pressure control.

Alpha blockers + Calcium-channel blockers

Diltiazem and Verapamil ⚠

Verapamil may increase the AUC of prazosin and terazosin, and may also increase the adverse effects related to tamsulosin. The concurrent use of diltiazem and alfuzosin can raise the levels of both drugs. The manufacturer of silodosin predicts that diltiazem and verapamil, may inhibit the metabolism of silodosin, leading to an increase its levels and effects.

It seems likely that any pharmacokinetic interaction between the alpha blockers and the calcium-channel blockers will be accounted for by the dose titration that is recommended when starting concurrent use, see under Other calcium-channel blockers, below.

Other calcium-channel blockers

Blood pressure may fall sharply when calcium-channel blockers are first given to patients already taking alpha blockers (particularly alfuzosin, prazosin, bunazosin and terazosin), and vice versa. Alpha blockers and calcium-channel blockers may be combined for additional blood pressure-lowering in patients with hypertension.

It is recommended that patients already taking calcium-channel blockers should have the dose reduced and start with a low-dose of alpha blocker, with the first dose taken just before going to bed. Caution should also be exercised when calcium-channel blockers are added to established alpha blocker therapy. Patients should also be warned about the possibility of postural hypotension and how to manage it (i.e. lay down, raise the legs, and get up slowly when recovered).

Alpha blockers + Ciclosporin (Cyclosporine)

Prazosin ⚠

Preliminary studies show that prazosin causes a small reduction in the glomerular filtration rate of kidney transplant patients taking ciclosporin.

> There would seem to be no strong reasons for totally avoiding prazosin in patients taking ciclosporin, but the authors of the report point out that the fall in glomerular filtration rate makes prazosin a less attractive antihypertensive.

Silodosin ✗

Ciclosporin is predicted to raise silodosin levels by inhibiting P-glycoprotein.

> Concurrent use is not recommended; however, if both drugs are given it would seem prudent to be alert for any evidence of silodosin adverse effects (e.g. dizziness, diarrhoea and orthostatic hypotension). If these become troublesome consider reducing the dose of silodosin or withdrawing the drug as necessary.

Alpha blockers + Clonidine ?

There is evidence that prazosin can reduce the antihypertensive effects of clonidine, whereas some other evidence suggests that this does not occur.

> No action needed unless hypotension becomes excessive. If the combination of prazosin and clonidine is less effective than expected consider an interaction as the cause.

Alpha blockers + Digoxin ?

A 60% rise in digoxin levels occurred over 3 days in one study when prazosin was also given. Another study found the opposite effect. Clinical experience suggests that any interaction is rare.

> No action is usually need when prazosin is given with digoxin, although consider an interaction if adverse effects, such as bradycardia, or evidence of a reduction in effect, occur. Alfuzosin, doxazosin, silodosin, tamsulosin and terazosin appear not to interact with digoxin.

Alpha blockers + Diuretics ?

As would be expected, the use of an alpha blocker with a diuretic may result in an additive hypotensive effect, but aside from first-dose hypotension, this usually seems to be a beneficial interaction in patients with hypertension. The effects in patients with congestive heart failure may be more severe.

> As postural hypotension is a possibility, warn patients to lie down if symptoms

such as dizziness, fatigue or sweating develop, and to remain lying down until they abate completely. A dose reduction and then re-titration may be necessary in some patients. In particular, patients with congestive heart failure, who have had large doses of diuretics, should start prazosin treatment at the lowest dose.

Alpha blockers + H₂-receptor antagonists

No clinically important interaction occurs between cimetidine and alfuzosin, doxazosin, or tamsulosin.

> No action needed. However, note that because tamsulosin levels are slightly raised the US manufacturers state that caution should be used, particularly with tamsulosin doses greater than 400 micrograms. In practice this probably means being aware that an increase in the adverse effects of tamsulosin (e.g. dizziness, headache, postural hypotension) might occur as a result of this interaction.

Alpha blockers + Macrolides

Silodosin

Ketoconazole increases the maximum plasma levels and AUC of silodosin 3.8-fold and 3.2-fold, respectively. Clarithromycin is predicted to interact similarly, whereas erythromycin is predicted to interact to a lesser extent.

> The US manufacturer contraindicates the concurrent use of silodosin and clarithromycin. If silodosin is given with a macrolide it would be prudent to monitor for silodosin adverse effects (e.g. dizziness, diarrhoea, orthostatic hypotension).

Doxazosin or Tamsulosin

Doxazosin is metabolised by CYP3A4. The US manufacturer predicts that clarithromycin and telithromycin, both CYP3A4 inhibitors, may inhibit doxazosin metabolism. Tamsulosin is extensively metabolised (mainly by CYP2D6 and CYP3A4). The US manufacturer therefore suggests that it should be used with caution with CYP3A4 inhibitors (they name erythromycin), particularly at doses higher than 400 micrograms.

> The clinical relevance of this prediction is unclear. If concurrent use is undertaken be aware that the adverse effects of doxazosin or tamsulosin (e.g. dizziness, headache, postural hypotension) may be increased.

Alpha blockers + MAOIs

Indoramin ✕

The manufacturers of indoramin predict that the effects of noradrenaline (norepinephrine) may be potentiated by concurrent use, resulting in raised blood pressure. However, the pharmacology of these drugs suggests just the opposite, namely that hypotension is the more likely outcome. The manufacturers are not aware of any reported interactions between indoramin and MAOIs.

> The manufacturers contraindicate concurrent use.

A

Other alpha blockers ❓

Both the MAOIs and the alpha blockers have hypotensive effects, which may be additive.

No action needed, but be aware that hypotension is a possibility if any alpha blocker is given with an MAOI.

Alpha blockers + NSAIDs ❓

Indometacin reduces the blood pressure-lowering effects of prazosin in some individuals. Other alpha blockers do not appear to interact with NSAIDs, including indometacin.

If indometacin is added to established treatment with prazosin, be alert for a reduced antihypertensive response. It is not known exactly what happens in patients taking both drugs long-term, but note that with other interactions between antihypertensives and NSAIDs the effects seem to be modest.

Alpha blockers + Phosphodiesterase type-5 inhibitors ⚠️

Postural hypotension may occur with higher doses of sildenafil, tadalafil or vardenafil given at the same time as doxazosin or terazosin. It seems likely that this effect will occur with most alpha blockers, although it is seen less frequently with modified-release alfuzosin and tamsulosin.

Patients should be stable on an alpha blocker before a phosphodiesterase type-5 inhibitor is started, and the lowest starting dose of the phosphodiesterase inhibitor (e.g. sildenafil 25 mg) should be considered. If an alpha blocker is required in a patient already taking a phosphodiesterase type-5 inhibitor, additional caution is required and the alpha blocker should be started at the lowest dose. Patients should be advised what to do if they develop postural hypotension (i.e. lay down, raise the legs and, when recovered, get up slowly).

Alpha blockers + Protease inhibitors
Alfuzosin and Silodosin ✖️

Ketoconazole increases the AUC of alfuzosin (modified-release preparation) and silodosin levels 3.2-fold. The protease inhibitors are predicted to interact similarly (the manufacturers of silodosin name ritonavir only) and in theory, this may lead to serious hypotension.

The US manufacturers contraindicate the use of alfuzosin with the protease inhibitors. Similarly, the US manufacturer of silodosin contraindicates the use of ritonavir. However, if concurrent use is essential, it would seem prudent to use the minimum dose of the alpha blocker and titrate as necessary, monitoring for adverse effects, particularly first-dose hypotension. The risks are likely to be greater in patients also taking other antihypertensives.

A

Doxazosin

Doxazosin is metabolised by CYP3A4 and the US manufacturer predicts that ritonavir, a CYP3A4 inhibitor, may inhibit its metabolism.

> The clinical relevance of this prediction is unclear. If concurrent use is undertaken be aware that the adverse effects of doxazosin (e.g. dizziness, headache, postural hypotension) may be increased.

Alpha blockers + **SSRIs**

Tamsulosin is extensively metabolised (mainly by CYP2D6 and CYP3A4). The US manufacturers therefore suggest that inhibitors of CYP2D6 (e.g. fluoxetine, parox-etine) may raise tamsulosin levels.

> The clinical relevance of these predictions is unclear, but until more is known some caution seems prudent. If concurrent use is undertaken be aware that the effects of tamsulosin (dizziness, headache, postural hypotension) may be increased. The US manufacturers advise caution, particularly at doses higher than 400 micrograms.

Alpha blockers + **Terbinafine**

Tamsulosin is extensively metabolised (mainly by CYP2D6 and CYP3A4). The US manufacturers therefore suggest that inhibitors of CYP2D6 (e.g. terbinafine) may raise tamsulosin levels.

> The clinical relevance of these predictions is unclear, but until more is known some caution seems prudent. If concurrent use is undertaken be aware that the effects of tamsulosin (dizziness, headache, postural hypotension) may be increased. The US manufacturers advise caution, particularly at doses higher than 400 micrograms.

Amantadine

Amantadine + **Bupropion**

The manufacturer of bupropion states that limited clinical data suggests a higher incidence of undesirable effects (nausea, vomiting, excitement, restlessness, postural tremor) in patients also given amantadine.

> Patients taking amantadine should be given small initial doses of bupropion, which are increased gradually. Good monitoring is advisable.

Amantadine + Dopamine agonists

The manufacturers of pramipexole predict that its clearance will be reduced by amantadine.

> The clinical significance of this is uncertain, and there appear to be no reports of any adverse interactions. The manufacturers suggest a reduction of the pramipexole dose should be considered in patients taking amantadine.

Amfetamines

Amfetamines + Atomoxetine

The use of atomoxetine in patients taking amfetamines may lead to adverse effects, such as psychosis and movement disorders. The effects of the amfetamines on mood and blood pressure may be reduced.

> If both drugs are given, be aware that adverse CNS effects may develop, and consider reducing the doses or stopping one of the drugs should this occur.

Amfetamines + Furazolidone

The pressor responses to dexamfetamine in 4 hypertensive patients were increased 2- to 3-fold after 6 days of furazolidone use, and after 13 days they had increased by about 10-fold. Furazolidone has MAO-inhibitory activity, after 5 to 10 days of use, which is about equivalent to that of the non-selective MAOIs.

> The concurrent use of furazolidone with amfetamines may be expected to result in a potentially serious rise in blood pressure and should therefore be avoided.

Amfetamines + Guanethidine

When hypertensive patients taking guanethidine were given single doses of dexamfetamine or metamfetamine, the hypotensive effects of the guanethidine were completely abolished, and in some instances the blood pressures rose higher than before treatment with the guanethidine. Other amfetamines would be expected to interact similarly.

> Concurrent use should be avoided.

Amfetamines + Inotropes and Vasopressors

The manufacturers of amfetamine, dexamfetamine and lisdexamfetamine state that amfetamines enhance the adrenergic effects of noradrenaline (norepinephrine). This may result in increased vasoconstriction, and could enhance the pressor effects of

A

noradrenaline. Other inotropes and vasopressors with adrenergic actions may be similarly affected, but this does not appear to be specifically mentioned.

> As the effects of these inotropes and vasopressors on blood pressure are likely to be closely monitored, any interaction should be picked up by routine monitoring.

Amfetamines + MAOIs

The concurrent use of amfetamines and non-selective MAOIs can result in a potentially fatal hypertensive crisis and/or serotonin syndrome, page 454.

> Concurrent use is contraindicated. It would seem prudent to also avoid the use of an amfetamine for 14 days after an MAOI has been taken.

Amfetamines + Moclobemide

The concurrent use of an amfetamine and an MAOI can result in a potentially fatal hypertensive crisis and/or serotonin syndrome. Moclobemide may interact with the amfetamines similarly.

> It may be prudent to avoid the concurrent use of moclobemide and an amfetamine.

Amfetamines + Protease inhibitors

An HIV-positive man taking ritonavir and saquinavir died after also taking metamfetamine and amyl nitrate. Toxicology reported extremely high metamfetamine levels, which were attributed to an interaction with ritonavir. Evidence is limited, but ritonavir and tipranavir are expected to raise the levels of the amfetamines (by inhibiting CYP2D6). Haemolytic anaemia has also been reported in a patient taking metamfetamine with indinavir.

> Patients should be made aware of the additional potential risks of using amfetamines with ritonavir and tipranavir (deaths have occurred). Some recommend that patients taking ritonavir should avoid amfetamines. It would seem prudent to reduce the amfetamine dose.

Amfetamines + SSRIs

There may be an increased risk of serotonin syndrome and neurotoxic reactions if amfetamines or related drugs are given with SSRIs. Fluoxetine and paroxetine may inhibit the metabolism of the amfetamines; toxicity has been reported.

> Be alert for evidence of amfetamine adverse effects if fluoxetine and paroxetine are also given. The general significance of the case reports describing serotonin syndrome, page 454 and neurotoxicity is unknown, but bear it in mind in case of an unexpected response to treatment.

A

Amfetamines + **Tricyclics**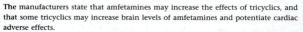

The manufacturers state that amfetamines may increase the effects of tricyclics, and that some tricyclics may increase brain levels of amfetamines and potentiate cardiac adverse effects.

> The clinical relevance of these warnings is unclear. It may be prudent to consider the risks of combining an amfetamine with a tricyclic in patients with pre-existing cardiovascular disorders.

Amfetamines + **Venlafaxine**

An isolated case of serotonin syndrome, page 454, has been attributed to the concurrent use of dexamfetamine and venlafaxine.

> The clinical significance of this interaction is unknown, but bear it in mind in case of an unexpected response to treatment.

Aminoglutethimide

Aminoglutethimide + **Corticosteroids**

The effects of dexamethasone can be reduced or abolished by aminoglutethimide. Other synthetic corticosteroids are predicted to interact in the same way as dexamethasone, but this needs confirmation.

> Monitor the outcome of concurrent use of aminoglutethimide and the corticosteroids. Doubling the dexamethasone dose has proven effective in some cases, although greater increases have been needed. Hydrocortisone is routinely given with aminoglutethimide without problem, and so may provide an alternative in some cases.

Aminoglutethimide + **Medroxyprogesterone**

Aminoglutethimide reduces the plasma levels of oral medroxyprogesterone by at least half.

> Monitor the outcome of concurrent use. It has been suggested that to achieve adequate plasma medroxyprogesterone acetate levels in breast cancer therapy (above 100 nanograms/mL) a daily dose of 800 mg of *Provera* is probably necessary in the presence of aminoglutethimide 125 or 250 mg twice daily. This is double the usual recommended dose of this preparation.

Aminoglutethimide + **Tamoxifen**

Aminoglutethimide markedly increases the clearance of tamoxifen and reduces its levels. Tamoxifen does not appear to affect aminoglutethimide levels.

> Theoretically, the combination of an oestrogen antagonist such as tamoxifen and

an aromatase inhibitor should provide additional benefit in the treatment of hormone-dependent cancers, however, no clinical studies have yet found this to be so. This interaction may partly explain this. It may be preferable to use these drugs sequentially rather than concurrently.

Aminoglutethimide + Theophylline

Aminoglutethimide increases theophylline clearance by almost 50% in some patients, but it is not known whether this results in a clinically relevant decrease in the effects of theophylline. Aminophylline would be expected to be similarly affected.

Monitor the effects and, if necessary, take theophylline levels. Increase the theophylline or aminophylline dose accordingly.

Aminoglutethimide + Warfarin and other oral anticoagulants

Aminoglutethimide increases the clearance of warfarin: higher doses seem to have a greater effect, and up to 4-fold increases in the warfarin dose have been needed. The effects of the interaction seem to develop over 14 days, and the interaction may persist for 2 weeks after aminoglutethimide is stopped. Similar effects have been seen with acenocoumarol.

Monitor the INR and adjust the anticoagulant dose accordingly if aminoglutethimide is started or stopped. Information about other coumarins is generally lacking but it would seem prudent to use the same precautions with any of them.

Aminoglycosides

The aminoglycosides are known to be nephrotoxic and many of their interactions occur as a result of this effect. Due to the number of known interactions with other nephrotoxic drugs (for examples see amphotericin B, below, and ciclosporin, page 44), many manufacturers of other drugs with nephrotoxic effects advise caution on their concurrent use. It is advisable to monitor renal function in patients taking aminoglycosides, and it may be prudent to increase the frequency of this monitoring in patients taking other nephrotoxic drugs.

Aminoglycosides + Amphotericin B

A number of patients developed nephrotoxicity, which was attributed to amphotericin B. Raised gentamicin or amikacin levels, without significant changes in creatinine, were seen in children also given amphotericin B.

Aminoglycosides are nephrotoxic and it is generally recommended that they should be avoided with other nephrotoxic drugs (such as amphotericin B, particularly the conventional formulation). However, if concurrent use is essential it may be prudent to increase the renal function and drug level monitoring that is advised during the use of an aminoglycoside.

A

Aminoglycosides + Bisphosphonates

Severe hypocalcaemia has been reported in three patients given sodium clodronate when they were also given netilmicin or amikacin. Theoretically, additive calcium lowering effects could occur with any bisphosphonate and aminoglycoside combination.

> If bisphosphonates are given with aminoglycosides, caution and close monitoring of calcium and magnesium levels has been advised. The renal loss of calcium and magnesium can continue for weeks after aminoglycosides are stopped, and bisphosphonates can also persist in bone for weeks. This means that the interaction is potentially possible whether the drugs are given concurrently or sequentially.

Aminoglycosides + Ciclosporin (Cyclosporine)

Nephrotoxicity is increased in some patients by the concurrent use of ciclosporin and amikacin, gentamicin or tobramycin. This interaction would be expected with all systemic aminoglycosides.

> The concurrent use of ciclosporin and aminoglycosides should only be undertaken if the clinical benefit outweighs the risk of renal damage. Close monitoring of renal function and aminoglycoside levels is required.

Aminoglycosides + Digoxin

Digoxin levels have been reported to be increased (more than doubled) by the concurrent use of gentamicin in patients with congestive cardiac failure and diabetes.

> This interaction seems rare. Patients should be monitored for signs of digoxin toxicity if gentamicin is given, especially those with diabetes or impaired renal function. Initially, checking pulse rate is probably adequate. There seems to be no information about other parenteral aminoglycosides. Consider also neomycin, page 260.

Aminoglycosides + Diuretics

Etacrynic acid

The concurrent use of aminoglycosides and etacrynic acid should be avoided because their damaging actions on the ear can be additive. The intravenous use of etacrynic acid and renal impairment are additional causative factors. Even sequential use may not be safe, and the effects may be irreversible.

> Avoid concurrent use. Other loop diuretics appear to be safer.

Other loop diuretics

Although some patients have developed nephrotoxicity and/or ototoxicity while taking furosemide and an aminoglycoside, it has not been established that this was as a result of an interaction. It has been suggested that any interaction may be more likely to occur if high-dose infusions of furosemide are used.

> As there is some uncertainty about the safety of concurrent us, increased monitoring (e.g. of renal function) would seem appropriate, particularly if high

doses of furosemide are given. The same precautions would seem to be appropriate with other loop diuretics (although see *Etacrynic acid*, above).

Aminoglycosides + NRTIs

The aminoglycosides are known to be nephrotoxic and many of their interactions occur as a result of this effect. Due to the number of known interactions with other nephrotoxic drugs (for examples see amphotericin B, page 43, and ciclosporin, page 44), many manufacturers of other drugs with nephrotoxic effects, including adefovir and tenofovir, caution concurrent use.

> Renal function should be routinely monitored in patients given aminoglycosides, and if the concurrent use of adefovir or tenofovir is necessary, it may be prudent to increase the frequency of this monitoring: the manufacturers of tenofovir advise that renal function should be monitored at least weekly.

Aminoglycosides + NSAIDs

Some reports claim that gentamicin and amikacin levels may be raised by indometacin, and that amikacin levels may be raised by ibuprofen lysine, when given to premature babies to treat patent ductus arteriosus, whereas others have not found an interaction.

> Concurrent use should be closely monitored (e.g. renal function, aminoglycoside levels) because of the toxicity that is associated with raised aminoglycoside levels. It has been suggested that the aminoglycoside dose should be reduced before giving indometacin. It has also been suggested that the dose interval of amikacin should be increased by at least 6 to 8 hours if ibuprofen lysine is also given during the first days of life. Other aminoglycosides possibly behave similarly. This interaction does not seem to have been studied in adults.

Aminoglycosides + Penicillins

A reduction in aminoglycoside levels can occur if aminoglycosides and penicillins are given together to patients with severe renal impairment. Carbenicillin, piperacillin and ticarcillin have been implicated with both gentamicin and tobramycin. No interaction of importance appears to occur either with intravenous aminoglycoside and penicillins in those with normal renal function.

> In patients with renal impairment it has been recommended that the penicillin dose should be adjusted according to renal function, and the levels of both antibacterials closely monitored. However, note that antibacterial inactivation can continue in the assay sample, and rapid assay is probably necessary. There would seem to be no reason for avoiding concurrent use in patients with normal renal function because no significant *in vivo* inactivation appears to occur. Moreover there is good clinical evidence that concurrent use is valuable, especially in the treatment of *Pseudomonas* infections. Consider also neomycin, page 393.

Aminoglycosides + Tacrolimus

The aminoglycosides are known to be nephrotoxic and many of their interactions

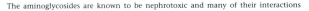

occur as a result of this effect. Due to the number of known interactions with other nephrotoxic drugs (for examples see amphotericin B, page 43, and ciclosporin, page 44), many manufacturers of other drugs with nephrotoxic effects, including tacrolimus, advise caution on their concurrent use.

> It is advisable to monitor renal function in patients taking aminoglycosides, and it may be prudent to increase the frequency of this monitoring in patients taking other nephrotoxic drugs.

Aminoglycosides + Vancomycin

The nephrotoxicity of the aminoglycosides appears to be potentiated by vancomycin.

> Concurrent use is therapeutically useful, but the risk of increased nephrotoxicity should be borne in mind. Therapeutic drug monitoring and regular assessment of renal function is warranted.

Amiodarone

Note that amiodarone has a long half-life (25 to 100 days) so that interactions may occur for some time after amiodarone has been withdrawn.

Amiodarone + Beta blockers

Hypotension, bradycardia, ventricular fibrillation and asystole have been seen in a few patients given amiodarone with propranolol, metoprolol or sotalol (for sotalol, see also drugs that prolong the QT interval, page 277). Amiodarone raises metoprolol levels, and may raise the levels of other beta blockers metabolised by CYP2D6, which may contribute to both the beneficial and adverse effects reported. However, analysis of clinical studies suggests that the combination of amiodarone and beta blockers can be beneficial.

> The concurrent use of beta blockers and amiodarone is not uncommon and may be therapeutically useful. However, it should be undertaken with caution and an appreciation of the potential adverse effects, especially with sotalol. Monitor for bradycardia, adjusting the doses or stopping one drug if the heart rate becomes too slow.

Amiodarone + Calcium-channel blockers

Increased cardiac depressant effects (potentiation of negative chronotropic properties and conduction slowing effects) would be expected if amiodarone is given with diltiazem or verapamil. One case of sinus arrest and serious hypotension has been reported in a woman taking diltiazem with amiodarone.

> It is advised that amiodarone should be avoided or used with caution with diltiazem or verapamil because cardiodepression may occur. Note that diltiazem has been used for rate control in patients developing postoperative atrial

fibrillation despite the use of prophylactic amiodarone. There do not appear to be any reports of adverse effects attributed to the use of amiodarone with the dihydropyridine class of calcium-channel blockers (e.g. nifedipine), which typically have little or no negative inotropic activity at usual doses.

Amiodarone + Chloroquine

Some UK manufacturers of amiodarone and chloroquine suggest that concurrent use may increase the risk of torsade de pointes. Chloroquine may cause arrhythmias and ECG changes when used alone, particularly in high doses and for prolonged periods; however, chloroquine is not generally considered a high risk for causing cardiovascular toxicity, especially when given at the correct dose and administered appropriately.

Some (but not all) UK manufacturers of amiodarone and chloroquine contraindicate concurrent use, whereas the US manufacturers do not include any warnings about this theoretical interaction.

Amiodarone + Ciclosporin (Cyclosporine)

Ciclosporin levels can be increased by amiodarone and nephrotoxicity has occurred as a result. Increased amiodarone levels and pulmonary toxicity have been reported in patients stopping amiodarone and starting ciclosporin.

Ciclosporin levels and/or effects (e.g. on renal function) should be monitored as a matter of routine, but it may be prudent to increase monitoring if amiodarone is started or stopped. Adjust the dose of ciclosporin as necessary. The significance of the increase in amiodarone levels and the occurrence of pulmonary toxicity is unclear but bear these reports in mind in case of unexpected effects.

Amiodarone + Colestyramine and related drugs

Colestyramine appears to reduce amiodarone levels by about 50%.

Because amiodarone undergoes some enterohepatic recirculation, separating the doses may only minimise the interaction. Monitor for decreased amiodarone effects if colestyramine is started, and adjust the amiodarone dose as necessary, or consider an alternative to colestyramine.

Amiodarone + Co-trimoxazole

Some UK manufacturers of amiodarone state that co-trimoxazole (trimethoprim with sulfamethoxazole) prolongs the QT interval and increases the risk of torsade de pointes; however co-trimoxazole is not generally associated with causing significant QT interval prolongation and torsade de pointes.

One UK manufacturer contraindicates concurrent use. However, the US manufacturers and other UK manufacturers make no mention of any possible interaction.

A

Amiodarone + Digoxin

Digoxin levels can be approximately doubled by amiodarone. Some individuals may show even greater increases. Digitalis toxicity is likely to occur if the dose of digoxin is not reduced appropriately.

> The interaction occurs in most patients and is clearly evident after a few days but may take 4 weeks to fully develop. Reduce the digoxin dose by between one-third to one-half initially and monitor digoxin levels. Further adjustment of the digoxin dose may be needed after a week or two, and possibly a month or more depending on digoxin levels. Particular care is needed in children, who may show much larger rises in digoxin levels.

Amiodarone + Disopyramide

The QT interval prolonging effects are increased when disopyramide and amiodarone are used together (see drugs that prolong the QT interval, page 277, for a general discussion of QT prolongation).

> The UK manufacturer contraindicates concurrent use. If concurrent use is essential, the dose of disopyramide should be reduced by 30 to 50% several days after starting amiodarone. The continued need for disopyramide should be monitored, and withdrawal attempted if possible. If disopyramide is added to amiodarone, the initial dose of disopyramide should be about half of the usual recommended dose. Close monitoring is essential.

Amiodarone + Diuretics

Mild to moderate inhibitors of CYP3A4 (such as amiodarone) may increase the AUC of eplerenone up to threefold, which increases the risk of hyperkalaemia.

> It is generally recommended that the dose of eplerenone should not exceed 25 mg daily in patients taking amiodarone.

Amiodarone + Donepezil

The risk of adverse effects, including bradycardia, may be increased if a centrally-acting anticholinesterase is given with amiodarone.

> Be alert for bradycardia if amiodarone is given with donepezil.

Amiodarone + Flecainide

Flecainide levels are increased by about 50% by amiodarone. An isolated report describes torsade de pointes in a patient taking amiodarone with flecainide.

> Reduce the flecainide dose by one-third to one-half if amiodarone is added and monitor for flecainide adverse effects (dizziness, nausea, and tremor). The interaction may take 2 weeks or more to develop fully.

A

Amiodarone + **Galantamine**

The risk of adverse effects, including bradycardia, may be increased if a centrally-acting anticholinesterase is given with amiodarone.

Be alert for bradycardia if amiodarone is given with galantamine.

Amiodarone + **Grapefruit juice**

Grapefruit juice appears to completely inhibit the metabolism of amiodarone to its major active metabolite, increases the AUC of amiodarone by 50% and increases its peak level by 84%, which may lead to toxicity. However, the effect of amiodarone on the PR and QTc intervals is apparently *decreased*, possibly due to reduced levels of the active metabolite.

Further study is needed. In the meantime, it may be prudent to suggest to patients that they avoid grapefruit juice.

Amiodarone + **H$_2$-receptor antagonists**

Cimetidine possibly causes a modest rise in amiodarone levels in some patients.

Information seems to be limited to one study but this interaction may be clinically important in some patients. Be alert for amiodarone adverse effects (e.g. bradycardia, taste disturbances, tremor, nausea).

Amiodarone + **Levothyroxine**

Patients taking levothyroxine for hypothyroidism may develop elevated levels of thyroid-stimulating hormone or overt hypothyroidism when also given amiodarone.

The manufacturer of amiodarone contraindicates its use in patients with evidence or a history of thyroid dysfunction and recommends thyroid function tests in all patients before starting amiodarone. Close monitoring of thyroid function is required if amiodarone is given with levothyroxine. Note that levothyroxine has been given to correct hypothyroidism induced by amiodarone.

Amiodarone + **Lidocaine**

Isolated reports describe a seizure in a man taking lidocaine about 2 days after he started to take amiodarone, and sinoatrial arrest in another man with sick sinus syndrome who was given both drugs. There is conflicting evidence as to whether or not amiodarone affects the pharmacokinetics of lidocaine.

Careful monitoring is required if both drugs are used. The manufacturers of topical lidocaine also advise caution, especially if large amounts of lidocaine are applied.

Amiodarone + **Lithium**

Hypothyroidism developed very rapidly in 2 patients taking amiodarone when lithium was started.

Note that lithium has been tried for the treatment of amiodarone-induced hyperthyroidism, and regular monitoring of thyroid status is recommended throughout amiodarone treatment. Lithium has rarely been associated with QT prolongation, and consequently the UK manufacturer of amiodarone contraindicates its concurrent use (see drugs that prolong the QT interval, page 277, for a general discussion of QT prolongation).

Amiodarone + Phenytoin

Phenytoin levels can be raised by amiodarone, markedly so in some individuals (4-fold **rise** reported) and phenytoin toxicity may occur. Amiodarone levels are reduced by phenytoin.

Monitor phenytoin levels and for phenytoin adverse effects (e.g. blurred vision, nystagmus, ataxia or drowsiness), and adjust the phenytoin dose if necessary. A 25 to 30% reduction in the phenytoin dose has been recommended for those taking 2 to 4 mg/kg daily, but it should be remembered that small alterations in phenytoin dose may result in a large change in phenytoin levels, as phenytoin kinetics are non-linear. The clinical significance of the effects on amiodarone are unclear.

Amiodarone + Procainamide

The QT interval prolonging effects are increased when procainamide and amiodarone **are** used together (see drugs that prolong the QT interval, page 277, for a general discussion of QT prolongation). Amiodarone increases the levels of procainamide and **its** metabolite by 60% and 30%, respectively.

Concurrent use should generally be avoided due to the QT prolonging effects of the combination. If the two drugs are considered essential, the ECG should be closely monitored and the dose of procainamide may need to be reduced by 20 to 50%. Levels should be monitored where possible, and patients observed closely for adverse effects.

Amiodarone + Protease inhibitors

A rise in amiodarone levels of about 50% has been seen in a patient given indinavir. **Other** protease inhibitors would be expected to interact similarly.

The concurrent use of amiodarone with a protease inhibitor is generally contraindicated. However, in the UK the exception is ritonavir-boosted atazanavir, and in the US, caution and increased monitoring, including taking amiodarone levels, is recommended with amprenavir, atazanavir, ritonavir-boosted darunavir, fosamprenavir, and ritonavir-boosted lopinavir.

Amiodarone + Quinidine ⊗

The QT interval prolonging effects of quinidine and amiodarone are increased when **they** are used together, and torsade de pointes has occurred (see drugs that prolong the QT interval, page 277, for a general discussion of QT prolongation). Quinidine levels **can** be increased by about 30% by amiodarone, although larger increases have been reported in some individuals.

Concurrent use is generally contraindicated due to the QT prolonging effects of the combination. If the two drugs are considered essential, the dose of quinidine may need to be reduced by 30 to 50%. Levels should be monitored where possible. The QT interval on the ECG should also be monitored and patients observed closely for quinidine-related adverse effects.

Amiodarone + Rivastigmine

The risk of adverse effects, including bradycardia, may be increased if a centrally-acting anticholinesterase is given with amiodarone.

Be alert for bradycardia if amiodarone is given with rivastigmine.

Amiodarone + Statins ⚠

There is some evidence of a high incidence of myopathy when amiodarone is given with high doses of simvastatin or possibly atorvastatin. Rarely, cases of myopathy and rhabdomyolysis have been reported in patients taking this combination. Lovastatin is expected to interact similarly.

The dose of simvastatin should not exceed 20 mg daily in patients taking amiodarone unless the clinical benefit is likely to outweigh the increased risk of myopathy and rhabdomyolysis. The manufacturer of lovastatin suggests a maximum dose of 40 mg daily in the presence of amiodarone. Lipid levels should be monitored to ensure that the lowest dose necessary of atorvastatin is used. All patients taking statins should be warned to report promptly any unexplained muscle aches, tenderness, cramps, stiffness or weakness.

Amiodarone + Tacrine

The risk of adverse effects, including bradycardia, may be increased if a centrally-acting anticholinesterase is given with amiodarone.

Be alert for bradycardia if amiodarone is given with tacrine.

Amiodarone + Warfarin and other oral anticoagulants ⚠

The anticoagulant effects of warfarin, phenprocoumon and acenocoumarol are increased by amiodarone in most patients and bleeding may occur. The extent of the interaction appears to be dependent on the dose of amiodarone, with higher doses having a greater effect. The interaction starts within a few days and is usually maximal by 2 to 7 weeks.

The dose of warfarin and phenprocoumon should be reduced by one- to two-thirds if amiodarone is added, and the dose of acenocoumarol should be reduced by between about 30 and 50%. However, these suggested reductions are only broad generalisations and individual patients may need more or less. The INR (or prothrombin times) should be very closely monitored both during and following treatment. One study advises weekly monitoring for the first 4 weeks of concurrent use. Some sources say that the metabolism of the indanedione phenindione is inhibited by amiodarone, but this appears to be an extrapolation from the known interaction with warfarin. There seems to be no clinical evidence available to support this prediction.

Amphotericin B

See also drugs that prolong the QT interval, page 277, as QT-prolongation can be exacerbated by hypokalaemia, which is a common adverse effect of amphotericin B. The renal toxicity of amphotericin B may be associated with sodium depletion.

Amphotericin B + Azoles

There is some clinical evidence to suggest that amphotericin B given with either itraconazole, ketoconazole or miconazole may possibly be less effective than amphotericin B given alone, and the adverse effects may be greater.

Despite extensive *in vitro* and *animal* data, it is not entirely clear whether or not azoles inhibit the efficacy of amphotericin B. Until more is known combined treatment should be limited to specific cases and the outcome should be very well monitored, being alert for a reduced antifungal response, or increasing LFTs.

Amphotericin B + Ciclosporin (Cyclosporine)

The risk of nephrotoxicity appears to be increased if ciclosporin is given with amphotericin B. Limited evidence suggests that liposomal amphotericin B (*AmBisome*) does not increase nephrotoxicity or hepatotoxicity when given to infants taking ciclosporin. Ciclosporin levels may be increased or decreased by amphotericin B.

It has been suggested that if amphotericin B must be given, withholding ciclosporin until the serum level is less than about 150 nanograms/mL may be a means of decreasing renal toxicity without losing the immunosuppressive effect. The reports supporting a lack of significant nephrotoxicity all used liposomal amphotericin, which would seem to suggest that, in patients taking ciclosporin, these formulations are advisable. Monitor both ciclosporin levels and renal function carefully on concurrent use.

Amphotericin B + Corticosteroids

Amphotericin B and corticosteroids can cause potassium loss and salt and water retention, which can have adverse effects on cardiac function.

Monitor electrolytes (especially potassium, which should be closely monitored in any patient taking amphotericin B) and fluid balance if amphotericin B is given with corticosteroids. The elderly would seem to be particularly at risk. Note that the renal toxicity of amphotericin B may be associated with sodium depletion.

Amphotericin B + Digoxin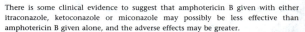

Amphotericin B causes potassium loss which could lead to the development of digitalis toxicity.

Potassium levels should be monitored when amphotericin B is given, but extra care is needed in those taking digoxin. Supplement potassium or prevent its loss as appropriate.

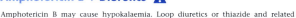

Amphotericin B + Diuretics

Amphotericin B may cause hypokalaemia. Loop diuretics or thiazide and related diuretics increase the risk of hypokalaemia when given with amphotericin.

Potassium should be monitored closely on concurrent use, with levels adjusted accordingly.

Amphotericin B + Flucytosine

For some fungal infections the combination of flucytosine with amphotericin B may be more effective than flucytosine alone, but increased flucytosine toxicity may also occur.

For some systemic fungal infections concurrent use is specifically recommended. Nevertheless, flucytosine levels and renal function should be very closely monitored when the drugs are given.

Amphotericin B + NRTIs

Tenofovir and amphotericin B are known to be nephrotoxic and this effect may be additive on concurrent use. Drugs that affect renal function, such as amphotericin B, may theoretically reduce adefovir excretion.

Monitor renal function on the concurrent use of adefovir or tenofovir and amphotericin B: the manufacturers of tenofovir specifically advise monitoring renal function at least weekly.

Amphotericin B + Pentamidine

There is evidence that acute renal failure and electrolyte disturbances (e.g. hypomagnesaemia) may develop in patients taking amphotericin B if they are also given parenteral pentamidine: both drugs are known to be nephrotoxic. See also drugs that prolong the QT interval, page 277.

Increased monitoring of renal function and electrolytes would be appropriate if both drugs are given: daily monitoring is recommended with parenteral pentamidine. It may be prudent to use liposomal amphotericin B rather than conventional amphotericin B to reduce the risk of renal impairment. No interaction seems to occur when pentamidine is given by inhalation, probably because the serum levels achieved are low.

Amphotericin B + Salbutamol (Albuterol) and related bronchodilators

Beta$_2$ agonists, such as salbutamol and terbutaline, can cause hypokalaemia. This can be increased by other potassium-depleting drugs such as amphotericin B. In severe cases the risk of serious cardiac arrhythmias could be increased.

The CSM in the UK advises monitoring potassium in severe asthma, because of the probability of multiple potassium-depleting drugs being used, and because some

A

conditions predispose these patients to hypokalaemia (e.g. hypoxia). Consider monitoring based on the severity of the patient's condition, and the number of potassium-depleting drugs used.

Amphotericin B + Tacrolimus

Both amphotericin B and tacrolimus may cause renal failure and this may be additive on concurrent use: cases of nephrotoxicity have been reported.

Renal function should be monitored when either drug is used alone, but it may be prudent to increase the frequency of this monitoring if both drugs are given.

Amphotericin B + Vancomycin

The risk of nephrotoxicity with vancomycin may possibly be increased if it is given with other drugs with similar nephrotoxic effects, such as amphotericin B.

There seems to be no direct evidence to support the existence of an interaction, and some evidence suggesting that no interaction occurs. Even so, the general warning issued by the manufacturers to monitor carefully is a reasonable precaution, given the known adverse effects of these drugs.

Anastrozole

Anastrozole + HRT

HRT would be expected to diminish the effects of anastrozole.

Some information suggests that there need not be a complete restriction on their concurrent use, but this needs confirmation. Until then, concurrent use should be avoided; it is contraindicated by the manufacturers.

Angiotensin II receptor antagonists

Most angiotensin II receptor antagonist interactions are pharmacodynamic, that is, interactions that result in an alteration in drug effects rather than drug disposition, so in most cases interactions of individual drugs will be applicable to the group as a whole.

Angiotensin II receptor antagonists + Antidiabetics

No clinically relevant pharmacokinetic interactions occur between glibenclamide

A

(glyburide) and candesartan, telmisartan or valsartan, or between tolbutamide and irbesartan. Losartan and possibly eprosartan may reduce awareness of hypoglycaemic symptoms.

> The symptoms of hypoglycaemia may be reduced by losartan and possibly other angiotensin II receptor antagonists. Further study is needed to establish this interaction, but note that this is similar to the effect of ACE inhibitors, page 2.

Angiotensin II receptor antagonists + Aspirin

Low-dose aspirin does not appear to affect the antihypertensive efficacy of losartan and would therefore not be expected to alter the effects of other angiotensin II receptor antagonists. High-dose aspirin does not appear to have been studied.

> No action needed if low-dose aspirin is used. Suspect an interaction with high-dose aspirin if the angiotensin II receptor antagonist seems less effective or blood pressure control is erratic. Consider an alternative analgesic, but note that NSAIDs may also affect blood pressure control.

Angiotensin II receptor antagonists + Azoles

Fluconazole decreases the metabolism of irbesartan and reduces the conversion of losartan to its active metabolite, although no significant changes in the hypotensive effect of losartan were noted.

> No clinically significant interaction appears to occur between the angiotensin II receptor antagonists and the azoles; however, bear the pharmacokinetic interaction between losartan and fluconazole in mind in case of any unexplained reduction in the antihypertensive effects of losartan.

Angiotensin II receptor antagonists + Ciclosporin (Cyclosporine)

Studies have found no significant changes in renal function in patients taking ciclosporin with candesartan or losartan. There is a possible increased risk of hyperkalaemia if angiotensin II receptor antagonists are given with ciclosporin, as both drugs may raise potassium levels.

> Although renal failure has not been reported on concurrent use, note that cases have occurred with ACE inhibitors, page 3. Monitor potassium levels more closely in the initial weeks of concurrent use.

Angiotensin II receptor antagonists + Digoxin

Telmisartan may increase digoxin trough and peak levels by 13% and 50%, respectively.

> The small increase in the trough levels suggests that the dose of digoxin need not automatically be reduced when telmisartan is started, but consideration should be given to monitoring for digoxin adverse effects such as bradycardia, taking digoxin levels if necessary. Candesartan, eprosartan, irbesartan, losartan, olmesartan, and valsartan appear not to affect digoxin levels.

A

Angiotensin II receptor antagonists + Diuretics

Loop diuretics ❓

Symptomatic hypotension may occur if an angiotensin II receptor antagonist is started in patients taking high-dose diuretics. Potassium levels may be either increased, decreased or not affected.

> Concurrent use is generally well tolerated and may be clinically beneficial. Monitor blood pressure and potassium levels initially. In patients with heart failure or those who are volume or sodium depleted, it has been recommended that the dose of diuretic or angiotensin II receptor antagonist be reduced to begin with, to avoid hypotension.

Potassium-sparing diuretics ⚠️

There is an increased risk of hyperkalaemia if angiotensin II receptor antagonists are given with potassium-sparing diuretics (such as amiloride, triamterene or the aldosterone antagonists eplerenone, spironolactone), particularly if other risk factors (such as advanced age, dose of spironolactone greater than 25 mg, reduced renal function and type II diabetes) are also present.

> The concurrent use of amiloride or triamterene and an angiotensin II receptor antagonist is not usually recommended and should be avoided in patients with moderate or severe renal impairment, whereas the concurrent use of an angiotensin II receptor antagonists with an aldosterone antagonist such as spironolactone may be useful in heart failure. If any of these potassium-sparing diuretics is given with an angiotensin II receptor antagonist increased monitoring of potassium levels is required.

Thiazide diuretics ❓

Symptomatic hypotension may occur if an angiotensin II receptor antagonist is started in a patient taking high-dose diuretics. Potassium levels may be either increased, decreased or not affected by the concurrent use of these drugs. No clinically relevant pharmacokinetic interactions appear to occur between candesartan, eprosartan, irbesartan, losartan, olmesartan, telmisartan or valsartan, and hydrochlorothiazide, although the bioavailability of hydrochlorothiazide may be modestly reduced.

> Concurrent use is generally well tolerated and may be clinically beneficial. Monitor blood pressure and potassium levels initially. In patients with heart failure or those who are volume or sodium depleted, it has been recommended that the dose of diuretic or angiotensin II receptor antagonist be reduced to avoid hypotension.

Angiotensin II receptor antagonists + Epoetin ❓

Epoetin may cause hypertension and thereby reduce the effects of angiotensin II receptor antagonists. An additive hyperkalaemic effect is theoretically possible. In one study, patients taking losartan needed higher epoetin doses to achieve similar haemoglobin levels to those in patients not taking losartan.

> Blood pressure and electrolytes, particularly potassium, should be routinely monitored in patients given epoetin. If blood pressure rises cannot be controlled or potassium levels rise, consider temporarily withholding the epoetin. Note that the manufacturers contraindicate epoetin in uncontrolled hypertension. The

clinical relevance of the effect of losartan on epoetin efficacy is unclear; however, as the epoetin dose is titrated to effect, no immediate intervention is necessary.

Angiotensin II receptor antagonists + **Food**

Food increases the bioavailability of eprosartan and losartan, slightly reduces the bioavailability of telmisartan, and modestly reduces the AUC of valsartan. Food appears to have little or no effect on the bioavailability of candesartan, irbesartan, or olmesartan.

None of these changes is likely to be clinically important. The UK manufacturer recommends that eprosartan is given with food, but the US manufacturer suggests that the interaction is not clinically significant.

Angiotensin II receptor antagonists + **Heparin**

An extensive review of the literature found that heparin (both unfractionated and low-molecular-weight heparins) and heparinoids inhibit the secretion of aldosterone, which can cause hyperkalaemia. This may be additive with the hyperkalaemic effects of angiotensin II receptor antagonists.

The CSM in the UK suggests that potassium should be measured in all patients with risk factors (renal impairment, diabetes mellitus, pre-existing acidosis and those taking potassium-sparing drugs) before starting heparin, and monitored regularly thereafter (at least every 4 days has been suggested).

Angiotensin II receptor antagonists + **Lithium**

Case reports describe lithium toxicity in patients given candesartan, losartan, valsartan and possibly irbesartan. Other angiotensin II receptor antagonists would be expected to interact similarly. The risk of lithium toxicity would be expected to increase when risk factors such as advanced age, renal impairment, heart failure and volume depletion are also present.

Even though the interaction appears rare, patients should have their lithium levels monitored to avoid a potentially severe adverse interaction. The development of the interaction may be delayed (up to 7 weeks seen) so that weekly monitoring of lithium levels for several weeks has been advised. Patients taking lithium should be aware of the symptoms of lithium toxicity, page 355 and told to immediately report them should they occur. This should be reinforced when they are given angiotensin II receptor antagonists. Note that some manufacturers do not recommend concurrent use.

Angiotensin II receptor antagonists + Low-molecular-weight heparins

An extensive review of the literature found that heparin (both unfractionated and low-molecular-weight heparins) and heparinoids inhibit the secretion of aldosterone, which can cause hyperkalaemia. This may be additive with the hyperkalaemic effects of angiotensin II receptor antagonists.

The CSM in the UK suggests that potassium should be measured in all patients with

A

risk factors (renal impairment, diabetes mellitus, pre-existing acidosis and those taking potassium-sparing drugs) before starting a low-molecular-weight heparin and monitored regularly thereafter (at least every 4 days has been suggested).

Angiotensin II receptor antagonists + NSAIDs

Indometacin may attenuate the antihypertensive effect of losartan, valsartan, or other angiotensin II receptor antagonists, although only some patients are affected. Other NSAIDs may interact similarly. No clinically relevant pharmacokinetic interactions occur between telmisartan and ibuprofen or between valsartan and indometacin. The combination of an NSAID and angiotensin II receptor antagonist can increase the risk of renal impairment and hyperkalaemia.

Patients taking angiotensin II receptor antagonists who require indometacin and probably other NSAIDs should be monitored for alterations in blood pressure control. Poor renal perfusion may increase the risk of renal failure if angiotensin II receptor antagonists are given with NSAIDs and so regular hydration of the patient and monitoring of renal function is recommended.

Angiotensin II receptor antagonists + Potassium

There is an increased risk of hyperkalaemia if angiotensin II receptor antagonists are given with potassium supplements or potassium-containing salt substitutes, particularly in those patients where other risk factors (such as advanced age, reduced renal function, and type II diabetes) are present.

If concurrent use is necessary, monitor potassium levels, adjusting supplementation as necessary.

Angiotensin II receptor antagonists + Rifampicin (Rifampin)

Rifampicin reduces the levels of the active metabolite of losartan and therefore diminishes its blood pressure-lowering effects. In theory, irbesartan and possibly candesartan may also be affected.

This interaction is by no means established, but monitor the effects of concurrent use on blood pressure. Consider raising the losartan dose or using an alternative to losartan if problems occur.

Angiotensin II receptor antagonists + Tacrolimus

Candesartan and losartan do not affect the pharmacokinetics of tacrolimus. Concurrent use with angiotensin II receptor antagonists may increase the risk of developing hyperkalaemia and/or nephrotoxicity in those taking tacrolimus.

Consider the possible contribution of angiotensin II receptor antagonists should hyperkalaemia and/or nephrotoxicity occur.

Antacids

Antacids + **Antihistamines**

An aluminium/magnesium hydroxide-containing antacid reduced the AUC of fexofenadine by about 40% in one study.

> Although the clinical significance of this effect has not been assessed it is recommended that administration is separated by 2 hours.

Antacids + **Antipsychotics**

Antacids containing aluminium/magnesium hydroxide or magnesium trisilicate can reduce the urinary excretion of chlorpromazine by up to 45%. Similarly, an aluminium/magnesium hydroxide antacid reduced the absorption of sulpiride. Anecdotal evidence suggests a possible interaction between haloperidol and aluminium hydroxide-containing antacids. *In vitro* studies suggest that this interaction may possibly also occur with other antacids and phenothiazines.

> The clinical importance of these interactions are not established, but it would seem reasonable to separating the doses of chlorpromazine or sulpiride and aluminium/magnesium hydroxide antacids by 2 to 3 hours to minimise any interaction. Similarly, consider separating the doses if an interaction between haloperidol and antacids is suspected.

Antacids + **Aspirin**

The salicylate concentrations of patients taking large doses of aspirin or other salicylates as anti-inflammatory drugs can be reduced to subtherapeutic levels by aluminium/magnesium hydroxide or sodium bicarbonate antacids.

> Care should be taken to monitor salicylate levels if any antacid is started or stopped in patients where the control of salicylate levels is critical. Probably of little importance with small or one-off doses of aspirin. Note that antacids may also increase the rate of absorption of aspirin given as enteric-coated tablets.

Antacids + **Azoles**

The absorption of ketoconazole and itraconazole capsules is markedly reduced by antacids.

> Advise patients to take antacids not less than 2 to 3 hours before or after ketoconazole and at least 2 hours after itraconazole capsules. Monitor the effects to confirm that these azoles are effective. The absorption of fluconazole, itraconazole solution and posaconazole does not appear to be significantly affected by antacids, so these azoles may be suitable alternatives.

Antacids + **Bisphosphonates**

The oral absorption of bisphosphonates is significantly reduced by aluminium/magnesium hydroxide and other antacids containing metallic tri- and divalent ions.

> Bisphosphonates should be prevented from coming into contact with antacids (containing aluminium, bismuth, calcium, magnesium). Recommendations on the timing of administration of bisphosphonates in relation to food and other drugs varies. Alendronate should be taken (after an overnight fast) at least 30 minutes before antacids, clodronate should probably be taken at least 1 hour before or after antacids, ibandronate should be taken (after at least a 6 hour fast) at least 30 minutes to 1 hour before antacids, risedronate should be taken at least 30 minutes before the first dose of antacid in the morning and at least 2 hours from any further doses of antacids during the rest of the day, and etidronate and tiludronate should be taken at least 2 hours apart from antacids.

Antacids + **Cephalosporins**

Cefpodoxime

Aluminium/magnesium hydroxide has been shown to reduce the bioavailability of cefpodoxime proxetil by about 40%. Sodium bicarbonate and aluminium hydroxide alone seem to have similar effects.

> It has been recommended that cefpodoxime is given at least 2 hours apart from antacids.

Other cephalosporins

Aluminium/magnesium hydroxide reduced the AUC of a modified-release preparation of cefaclor by 18%, but this reduction is small and considered unlikely to be clinically important.

> No action needed.

Antacids + **Chloroquine**

In a small study magnesium trisilicate reduced the AUC of chloroquine by about 20%. Related *in vitro* studies found that the absorption of chloroquine was also moderately decreased by magnesium trisilicate, calcium carbonate and gerdiga. Gerdiga is a clay-based antacid containing hydrated silicates, and various carbonates and bicarbonates. Hydroxychloroquine is predicted to interact like chloroquine.

> The clinical significance of this reduction is unclear, but one way to minimise any possible effect on chloroquine absorption is to separate the doses from the antacids by at least 2 to 3 hours. One manufacturer recommends that the chloroquine dose should be separated from antacids by at least 4 hours. Hydroxychloroquine should be given 4 hours before or after antacids.

Antacids + **Corticosteroids**

The absorption of prednisone can be reduced by up to 40% by large (60 mL) doses of aluminium/magnesium hydroxide antacids; small doses (20 or 30 mL) of antacid do

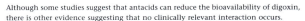

not appear to interact. Prednisolone probably behaves similarly. Dexamethasone absorption is reduced by about 75% by magnesium trisilicate.

Some manufacturers of dexamethasone suggest that the doses of antacid should be separated as far as possible from the dexamethasone. In other similar antacid interactions 2 to 3 hours is usually sufficient. The manufacturers of deflazacort also issue a similar warning. It would seem prudent to follow this advice for large doses of antacid and any corticosteroid. Concurrent use should be monitored to confirm that the therapeutic response is adequate.

Antacids + Digoxin

Antacids

Although some studies suggest that antacids can reduce the bioavailability of digoxin, there is other evidence suggesting that no clinically relevant interaction occurs.

A clinically relevant interaction seems unlikely, although it may be worth bearing in mind if, on rare occasions, a patient seems to experience an interaction. In this situation, consider separating the dosing by 2 to 3 hours, as this minimises other absorption interactions with antacids.

Calcium

The effects of digitalis glycosides might be increased by rises in blood calcium levels, and in two cases the concurrent use of intravenous calcium and digoxin resulted in fatal arrhythmias. This seems to be the only direct clinical evidence of a serious adverse interaction, although there is plenty of less direct evidence that an interaction is possible.

Intravenous calcium should be avoided in patients taking digoxin. If that is not possible, it has been suggested that it should be given slowly or only in small amounts in order to avoid transient high serum calcium levels.

Antacids + Dipyridamole

The effective disintegration, dissolution and eventual absorption of dipyridamole in tablet or suspension form depends upon having a low pH in the stomach. Drugs that raise the gastric pH (such as the antacids) are expected to reduce the bioavailability of dipyridamole.

The clinical significance of this possible interaction is unknown. Note that modified-release preparations of dipyridamole (that are buffered) do not appear to be affected. For other preparations, consider separating the dosing of dipyridamole tablets or suspension and antacids by 2 to 3 hours, as this minimises other absorption interactions with antacids.

Antacids + Diuretics

Hypercalcaemia and possibly metabolic alkalosis can develop in patients given large amounts of calcium (with or without high doses of vitamin D) if they are also given thiazide diuretics, which can reduce the urinary excretion of calcium.

Consider monitoring calcium levels in those given a thiazide and a calcium supplement or large amounts of calcium antacids regularly. Patients taking thiazides should be warned about the ingestion of very large amounts of calcium carbonate (readily available without prescription). This interaction is unlikely to be of importance in patients taking occasional calcium e.g. in antacids.

Antacids + **Enteral feeds**

Aluminium-containing antacids can interact with high-protein liquid enteral feeds (in enteral or nasogastric tubes) within the oesophagus to produce an obstructive plug (a bezoar).

It has been suggested that if an antacid is needed, it should be given some time after the nutrients, and the tube should be vigorously flushed beforehand.

Antacids + **Ethambutol**

Both aluminium hydroxide and aluminium/magnesium hydroxide can cause a small reduction in the absorption of ethambutol (e.g. AUC decreased by 10%) in some patients.

The reduction in absorption is generally small and variable, and it seems doubtful if it will have a significant effect on the treatment of tuberculosis. However, the US manufacturer suggests that aluminium hydroxide-containing antacids should not be taken until 4 hours after a dose of ethambutol.

Antacids + **Fibrates**

Antacids (aluminium hydroxide, aluminium magnesium silica hydrate) reduced gemfibrozil maximum levels by about 50 to 70% in one study. More study is needed to confirm these findings.

It has been suggested that gemfibrozil should be given 1 to 2 hours before antacids.

Antacids + **Gabapentin**

An aluminium/magnesium hydroxide antacid given with or 2 hours after gabapentin reduced its bioavailability by about 20%. When the antacid was given 2 hours before gabapentin, the bioavailability was reduced by about 10%.

These small changes are unlikely to be of clinical importance. However, the manufacturer recommends that gabapentin is taken about 2 hours after aluminium/magnesium-containing antacids.

Antacids + **Iron**

Calcium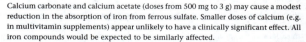

Calcium carbonate and calcium acetate (doses from 500 mg to 3 g) may cause a modest reduction in the absorption of iron from ferrous sulfate. Smaller doses of calcium (e.g. in multivitamin supplements) appear unlikely to have a clinically significant effect. All iron compounds would be expected to be similarly affected.

Monitor the response to iron in patients taking large doses of calcium. It may be prudent to separate the administration of iron preparations and calcium as much as possible to avoid admixture in the gut. Bear it in mind in case of a reduced response to iron.

Iron

The absorption of iron and the expected haematological response can be reduced by the concurrent use of antacids (sodium bicarbonate, calcium carbonate, aluminium/magnesium hydroxide, magnesium trisilicate). However, information is limited and difficult to assess.

As a general precaution, separate the administration of iron compounds and antacids as much as possible to avoid admixture in the gut. Note that separating the dosing by 2 to 3 hours minimises other absorption interactions with antacids.

Antacids + Isoniazid

The absorption of isoniazid is modestly reduced by aluminium hydroxide (about 25%), less so by magaldrate, and not affected by aluminium/magnesium hydroxide tablets or didanosine chewable tablets (formulated with an antacid buffer).

The clinical importance of the modest reductions in isoniazid levels is uncertain, but it is likely to be small.

Antacids + Levodopa

Antacids do not appear to interact significantly with immediate-release levodopa, but they may reduce the bioavailability of modified-release preparations of levodopa (e.g. *Madopar CR*).

Concurrent use need not be avoided with standard preparations. With modified-release preparations it would seem advisable to separate administration (2 to 3 hours is usually enough in other similar situations). The outcome should be monitored.

Antacids + Levothyroxine ⚠

A few reports describe reduced levothyroxine effects in patients given aluminium/magnesium-containing antacids. The efficacy of levothyroxine can also be reduced by the concurrent use of calcium carbonate, whereas limited evidence suggests that calcium acetate might not interact.

The general importance of the interaction with aluminium/magnesium-containing antacids is not known, but be alert for the need to increase the levothyroxine dose in any patient given antacids. With calcium carbonate, the mean reduction in the absorption of levothyroxine is quite small, but some individuals can experience a clinically important effect. The cautious approach would be to advise all patients to separate the doses by at least 4 hours.

Antacids + Lithium

The ingestion of marked amounts of sodium can prevent the establishment or maintenance of adequate lithium levels. Conversely, dietary salt restriction can cause lithium levels to rise to toxic concentrations if the lithium dose is not reduced appropriately.

Warn patients not to take non-prescription antacids or urinary alkalinisers without first seeking informed advice. Sodium bicarbonate comes in various guises and disguises e.g. Alka-Seltzer (55.8%), *Andrews Salts* (22.6%), Eno (46.4%), *Jaap's Health Salts* (21.3%), or Peptac (28.8%). Substantial amounts of sodium also occur in some urinary alkalinising agents (e.g. *Citralka*, *Citravescent*). An antacid containing aluminium/magnesium hydroxide with simeticone has been found to have no effect on the bioavailability of lithium carbonate, and so antacids of this type may be suitable alternatives.

Antacids + Macrolides

Aluminium/magnesium hydroxide antacids may reduce the peak levels of azithromycin but the overall absorption was unchanged.

It is suggested that azithromycin should not be given at the same time as antacids, but should be taken at least 1 hour before or 2 hours after.

Antacids + Mexiletine

Large changes in urinary pH caused by the concurrent use of alkalinising drugs such as sodium bicarbonate can, in some patients, have a marked effect on mexiletine levels.

The effect does not appear to be predictable. The UK manufacturer of mexiletine recommends that concurrent use should be avoided.

Antacids + Mycophenolate

Aluminium/magnesium hydroxide antacids modestly reduce the AUC of mycophenolate.

The US manufacturer says that aluminium/magnesium antacids can be used in patients taking mycophenolate, but that they should not be given simultaneously. With many other antacid interactions, a 2 to 3 hour separation is usually sufficient to avoid an interaction. One UK manufacturer advises against long-term use of antacids with mycophenolate. It would seem prudent to check that the immunosuppressant effects of mycophenolate remain adequate.

Antacids + NNRTIs

When delavirdine was given 10 minutes after an antacid (type and dose not stated) delavirdine maximum levels were reduced by about 50%.

The manufacturer of delavirdine recommends separating administration by at least one hour.

A

Antacids + **NSAIDs**

Diflunisal

Antacids containing aluminium with or without magnesium can reduce the absorption of diflunisal by up to 40%, but no important interaction occurs if food is taken at the same time. Magnesium hydroxide can increase the rate of diflunisal absorption, which may improve the onset of analgesia.

> If diflunisal is taken with or after food as advised, it appears that this interaction should have little clinical relevance.

Other NSAIDs

Studies have shown that antacids have no clinically significant effect on the pharmacokinetics of azapropazone, celecoxib, dexketoprofen, diclofenac, etodolac, etoricoxib, ibuprofen, indometacin, flurbiprofen, ketoprofen, ketorolac, lornoxicam, mefenamic acid, meloxicam, metamizole, nabumetone, piroxicam, sulindac, tenoxicam, tolfenamic acid, or tolmetin. The rate of absorption of some of these NSAIDs is moderately affected by antacids, which may affect the onset of analgesia. However, if NSAIDs are taken after food, as recommended, these effects are unlikely to be clinically significant.

> No action needed.

Antacids + **Penicillamine**

The absorption of penicillamine can be reduced by 30 to 40% by antacids containing aluminium/magnesium hydroxide.

> For maximal absorption separate administration. A separation of 2 to 3 hours is usually sufficient with other similar interactions. Note that sodium bicarbonate does not appear to interact to a clinically significant extent.

Antacids + **Phenytoin**

Some, but not all studies have shown that antacids (containing aluminium, calcium or magnesium) do not usually interact to a clinically relevant extent with phenytoin. However, in some instances antacids have reduced phenytoin serum levels and this may have been responsible for loss of seizure control in some patients.

> A clinically relevant interaction does not appear to occur in most patients. However, if there is any sign that phenytoin levels are being reduced, separating the doses by 2 to 3 hours may minimise the effects. In this situation monitor concurrent use to ensure phenytoin remains effective.

Antacids + **Proguanil**

The bioavailability of proguanil was reduced by almost two-thirds by magnesium trisilicate. Other antacids, such as those containing aluminium, may interact similarly.

> The clinical significance of this reduction is unclear, but one way to minimise any possible effect is to separate the doses by at least 2 to 3 hours.

A

Antacids + **Protease inhibitors**

Drugs that increase gastric pH (such as the H_2-receptor antagonists) reduce atazanavir levels: and antacids would be expected to interact similarly. Tipranavir levels are decreased by up to 30% by antacids (containing aluminium/magnesium hydroxide). Amprenavir may be similarly affected.

> The manufacturers of atazanavir recommend that it should be given 2 hours before or one hour after buffered medicinal products. This would include didanosine buffered tablets and antacids. The manufacturer of amprenavir recommended that it should not be given within one hour of antacids. The manufacturer of tipranavir recommends that it should not be given within 2 hours of antacids.

Antacids + **Proton pump inhibitors**

Aluminium/magnesium-containing antacids may cause a slight 13% reduction in the bioavailability of lansoprazole, but no interaction was seen when the lansoprazole was given one hour after the antacid.

> This interaction is not expected to be clinically significant. However the UK manufacturers recommend separating administration by one hour, although this seems overly cautious.

Antacids + **Quinidine**

Large rises in urinary pH due to the concurrent use of some antacids (such as sodium bicarbonate) can cause the retention of quinidine, which could lead to toxicity, but there seems to be only one case on record of an adverse interaction (with aluminium/magnesium hydroxide).

> It is difficult to predict which antacids, if any, are likely to interact (although note that aluminium hydroxide alone does not appear to interact). Monitor the effects if drugs that can markedly change urinary pH are started or stopped. Adjust the quinidine dose as necessary.

Antacids + **Quinolones**

The levels of many of the quinolones can be reduced by aluminium/magnesium antacids. Calcium compounds interact to a lesser extent, and bismuth compounds only minimally.

> As a very broad rule-of-thumb, the quinolones should be taken at least 2 hours before and not less than 4 to 6 hours after aluminium/magnesium antacids. The only obvious exception is fleroxacin, which appears to interact minimally. The interaction with calcium compounds is variable, and some quinolones may not interact (levofloxacin, lomefloxacin, moxifloxacin or ofloxacin), but in the absence of direct information a 2-hour separation errs on the side of caution. The interaction with bismuth is minimal and no action is likely to be needed. The H_2-receptor antagonists and the proton pump inhibitors do not interact and may therefore be suitable alternatives.

A

Antacids + **Rifampicin (Rifampin)**

The absorption of rifampicin can be reduced up to about one-third by antacids.

If antacids are given it would be prudent to be alert for any evidence that rifampicin is less effective than expected. The US manufacturers advise giving rifampicin one hour before antacids.

Antacids + **Statins**

Rosuvastatin

The bioavailability of rosuvastatin is halved by aluminium/magnesium-containing antacids, but to a lesser extent when the doses were separated by 2 hours. The clinical significance of this reduction is uncertain.

Separate the doses of rosuvastatin and antacids by at least 2 hours.

Other statins

Aluminium/magnesium hydroxide antacids cause a moderate reduction in the bioavailability of atorvastatin and pravastatin, but this does not appear to reduce their lipid-lowering efficacy.

No action needed.

Antacids + **Strontium**

Aluminium/magnesium hydroxide slightly reduces the absorption of strontium ranelate (AUC decreased by 20 to 25%) if given with or 2 hours before strontium, but not when given 2 hours after strontium. Calcium reduces the bioavailability of strontium ranelate by about 60 to 70%.

Antacids should be taken 2 hours after strontium ranelate. However, because it is also recommended that strontium is taken at bedtime, the manufacturers say that if this dosing interval is impractical, concurrent intake is acceptable. For calcium preparations administration should be separated by 2 hours.

Antacids + **Tetracyclines**

The levels and therefore the therapeutic effectiveness of the tetracyclines can be markedly reduced or even abolished by antacids containing aluminium, bismuth, calcium or magnesium. Other antacids, such as sodium bicarbonate, may also reduce the bioavailability of some tetracyclines. Even intravenous doxycycline levels can be reduced by antacids. Note that interactions with antacids within formulations may also occur, such as didanosine tablets.

As a general rule aluminium, bismuth, calcium or magnesium-containing antacids should not be given at the same time as the tetracyclines. If they must be used, patients should be advised to separate the doses by 2 to 3 hours or more, to prevent their admixture in the gut. This also applies to quinapril formulations containing substantial quantities of magnesium (such as *Accupro*), although the interaction is less pronounced, and buffered didanosine tablets formulated with antacids.

H$_2$-receptor antagonists do not interact, and they may therefore be a suitable alternative.

Antacids + Zinc

Calcium (either as the carbonate or the citrate) reduces the AUC of zinc by up to 80%.

The clinical importance of this interaction is unknown, but it would seem prudent to separate the administration of zinc and calcium. Note that separating the doses by 2 to 3 hours minimises other absorption interactions with antacids.

Antidiabetics

Antidiabetics + Antidiabetics

Pioglitazone and rosiglitazone may cause fluid retention and peripheral oedema, which can worsen or cause heart failure. There is evidence that the incidence of these effects is higher when pioglitazone or rosiglitazone are combined with insulin, sulfonylureas or saxagliptin. In addition, there may be an increased risk of myocardial ischaemia when rosiglitazone is used with insulin. The incidence of hypoglycaemia may also be increased on concurrent use.

In October 2007 the European Medicines Agency concluded that the combination of rosiglitazone and insulin should only be used in exceptional cases and under close supervision. In the UK and US concurrent use is contraindicated or not advised. If both drugs are given, close monitoring is warrantedIf oedema occurs in a patient taking a thiazolidinedione it has been recommended that the possible causes be assessed, and that if symptoms and signs suggest congestive heart failure, a dose change and temporary or permanent discontinuance of the thiazolidinedione should be considered. The UK manufacturer advises that when rosiglitazone is used with a sulfonylurea, the dose of rosiglitazone should be increased to 8 mg daily only with caution, assessing the risk of fluid retention. Bear in mind the possibility of an increased risk of peripheral oedema if saxagliptin is added to thiazolidinedione therapy.

Antidiabetics + Antihistamines

The concurrent use of biguanides (e.g. metformin) and ketotifen appears to be well tolerated, but a fall in the number of platelets has been seen in one study in patients taking the combination.

The general importance of this report is uncertain. The manufacturers contraindicate concurrent use until the effect is explained.

Antidiabetics + Antipsychotics

Chlorpromazine may raise blood glucose levels, particularly in daily doses of 100 mg or more (incidence of hyperglycaemia is about 25%). Smaller chlorpromazine doses of 50 to 70 mg daily do not appear to cause hyperglycaemia. Other classical antipsychotics may also affect diabetic control (haloperidol, zuclopenthixol and a number of phenothiazines have been implicated) and the atypical antipsychotics, clozapine, olanzapine and risperidone, are also associated with an increased risk of glucose intolerance. One epidemiological study found evidence of an association between antipsychotic drug use and worsening of metabolic control and another found an increased risk of hospitalisation for hyperglycaemia, especially in the first month of use of the antipsychotic.

Increases in the dose requirements of the antidiabetic should be anticipated during concurrent use. It would seem prudent to increase monitoring of glycaemic control, particularly when starting or stopping any classical or atypical antipsychotic in a patient with diabetes.

Antidiabetics + Aprepitant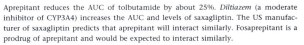

Aprepitant reduces the AUC of tolbutamide by about 25%. *Diltiazem* (a moderate inhibitor of CYP3A4) increases the AUC and levels of saxagliptin. The US manufacturer of saxagliptin predicts that aprepitant will interact similarly. Fosaprepitant is a prodrug of aprepitant and would be expected to interact similarly.

As the clinical relevance of this reduction in tolbutamide has not been assessed the manufacturer advises caution, but changes of this magnitude are rarely clinically significant. No dose adjustment of saxagliptin is expected to be needed. However, bear the potential for an increase in the effects of saxagliptin in mind. Consider monitoring blood sugars more closely and reduce the dose of saxagliptin if clinically indicated.

Antidiabetics + Aspirin ❓

Analgesic doses of aspirin and other salicylates can lower blood glucose levels, but small analgesic doses do not normally have an adverse effect on patients taking antidiabetics. Large doses of salicylates may have a more significant effect.

It may be prudent to increase monitoring of blood glucose levels during the initial use of large doses of aspirin or salicylates, and adjust the antidiabetic dose accordingly. Small antiplatelet doses of aspirin are unlikely to cause a problem.

Antidiabetics + Azoles

Fluconazole ❓

Fluconazole normally appears not to affect the diabetic control of most patients taking sulfonylureas, but isolated reports describe hypoglycaemic coma and aggressive behaviour following concurrent use. There is some evidence that the blood-glucose-lowering effects of both glipizide and glibenclamide (glyburide) may be modestly increased by fluconazole. Fluconazole may cause marked increases in plasma levels of glimepiride, but the significance of this is unclear. Nateglinide plasma levels may also be increased by fluconazole, but this did not potentiate the blood-glucose lowering effects of low-dose nateglinide.

There is no reason to avoid the concurrent use of fluconazole and these sulfonylureas but warn patients to report any unexpected changes in blood glucose levels. A greater blood-glucose lowering effect may possibly occur with

A

higher doses of nateglinide in clinical practice. Monitor the outcome of concurrent use on blood glucose levels and adjust the antidiabetic treatment accordingly.

Itraconazole

Itraconazole causes modest increases in repaglinide and nateglinide levels, but in one study this did not affect the control of blood glucose levels. Ketoconazole, a potent CYP3A4 inhibitor, increases saxagliptin levels. Itraconazole is predicted to interact similarly.

> Consider monitoring blood glucose levels on concurrent use. The US manufacturer of saxagliptin recommends that the dose of saxagliptin should be limited to 2.5 mg daily.

Ketoconazole

Ketoconazole increases the blood glucose-lowering effects of tolbutamide in healthy subjects, modestly increases the AUC of rosiglitazone and pioglitazone and has more marked effects on the AUC of saxagliptan.

> It may be prudent to increase the frequency of blood glucose monitoring if any of these antidiabetics is given with ketoconazole. Adjust the antidiabetic medication accordingly. Note that the US manufacturer recommends that the dose of saxagliptin should be limited to 2.5 mg daily.

Miconazole

Hypoglycaemia has been seen in a few diabetics taking tolbutamide, glibenclamide (glyburide) or gliclazide when they were given oral miconazole.

> Concurrent use of oral miconazole should be monitored and the dose of the sulfonylurea reduced if necessary. Warn patients to report any unexpected changes in blood glucose levels. Miconazole oral gel (which may be sufficiently absorbed to potentially have systemic effects) may interact similarly.

Posaconazole ❓

Posaconazole slightly enhanced the blood glucose-lowering effects of glipizide in healthy subjects.

> The clinical significance of this interaction is unclear, but it may be prudent to warn patients to report any unexpected changes in blood glucose levels.

Voriconazole

The manufacturers of voriconazole predict that it may raise the levels of the sulfonylureas, and hypoglycaemia may result.

> Until more is known careful monitoring of blood glucose is advisable during concurrent use.

Antidiabetics + Beta blockers ❓

In diabetics using insulin, the normal rise in blood sugar in response to hypoglycaemia may be impaired by propranolol, but serious and severe hypoglycaemia (sometimes accompanied by an increase in blood pressure) seems rare. Other beta blockers normally interact to a lesser extent or not at all. The blood glucose-lowering effects of sulfonylureas may possibly be reduced by beta blockers. Be aware that in the presence of beta blockers some of the familiar warning signs of hypoglycaemia may not occur.

Monitor the effects of concurrent use well, avoid the non-selective beta blockers where possible, and check for any evidence that the dose of the antidiabetic needs some adjustment. Warn all patients that some of the normal premonitory signs of a hypoglycaemic attack may not appear, in particular tachycardia and tremor, whereas hunger, irritability and nausea may be unaffected, and sweating may even be increased.

Antidiabetics + Calcium-channel blockers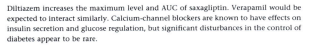

Diltiazem increases the maximum level and AUC of saxagliptin. Verapamil would be expected to interact similarly. Calcium-channel blockers are known to have effects on insulin secretion and glucose regulation, but significant disturbances in the control of diabetes appear to be rare.

The US manufacturer does not recommend any initial dose adjustment of saxagliptin. However, bear the potential for an increase in its effects in mind: consider monitoring blood sugars more closely with concurrent use and reduce the dose of saxagliptin if necessary. No particular precautions normally seem to be necessary with other antidiabetics, but bear the potential for interaction in mind if the control of diabetes seems unusually difficult.

Antidiabetics + Carbamazepine

Repaglinide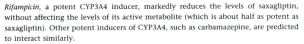

Rifampicin (*rifampin*), an inducer of CYP2C8 and CYP3A4, reduces the levels of repaglinide, and the manufacturers state that they cannot exclude the possibility that other enzyme inducers, such as carbamazepine, may interact similarly.

It would seem prudent to increase blood glucose level monitoring when carbamazepine is started to ensure that repaglinide is still effective and adjust the antidiabetic treatment accordingly.

Saxagliptin

Rifampicin, a potent CYP3A4 inducer, markedly reduces the levels of saxagliptin, without affecting the levels of its active metabolite (which is about half as potent as saxagliptin). Other potent inducers of CYP3A4, such as carbamazepine, are predicted to interact similarly.

The US manufacturer considers that no dose adjustment of saxagliptin is needed as dipeptidylpeptidase-4 inhibitory activity was unaffected. However, as it cannot be ruled out that carbamazepine might reduce the blood-glucose lowering effect of saxagliptin the UK manufacturer advises caution. Bear this interaction in mind should any reduced saxagliptin effects occur.

A

Antidiabetics + **Chloramphenicol**

The blood glucose-lowering effects of tolbutamide and chlorpropamide can be increased by chloramphenicol and acute hypoglycaemia can occur. Other sulfonylureas are often predicted to interact similarly, but there does not seem to be any direct evidence of this.

> An increased blood glucose-lowering effect should be expected if both drugs are given but few patients experience a severe effect. Monitor concurrent use carefully and reduce the dose of the sulfonylurea as necessary. No interaction would be expected with topical chloramphenicol because the systemic absorption is likely to be small.

Antidiabetics + **Ciclosporin (Cyclosporine)**

Some preliminary evidence suggests that glibenclamide (glyburide) can raise serum ciclosporin levels to a moderate extent. Glipizide caused about a 2-fold increase in ciclosporin levels in 2 patients, but no change was noted in a study. Ciclosporin increased repaglinide bioavailability in one study. Repaglinide had no effect on ciclosporin levels in another study.

> These interactions are unconfirmed, and of uncertain clinical significance. There is insufficient evidence to generally recommend increased monitoring, but be aware of the potential for an interaction with the sulfonylureas if ciclosporin levels are unexpectedly raised. The possibility of increased hypoglycaemia should be borne in mind if ciclosporin is added to established repaglinide therapy, and patients should be warned. Note that the UK manufacturer of repaglinide suggests avoiding the concurrent use of ciclosporin, but recommends close monitoring if it is necessary. Note that ciclosporin may rarely cause hyperglycaemia, and therefore interfere with diabetic control. However, the effect is rare, and does not justify an increase in monitoring all patients.

Antidiabetics + **Clonidine**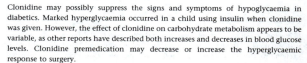

Clonidine may possibly suppress the signs and symptoms of hypoglycaemia in diabetics. Marked hyperglycaemia occurred in a child using insulin when clonidine was given. However, the effect of clonidine on carbohydrate metabolism appears to be variable, as other reports have described both increases and decreases in blood glucose levels. Clonidine premedication may decrease or increase the hyperglycaemic response to surgery.

> The general importance of this interaction is unclear. It would seem prudent to warn all patients that some of the normal premonitory signs of hypoglycaemia may not appear. Suspect an interaction if disturbances in the control of diabetes occur in patients given clonidine. Monitor blood glucose levels closely if clonidine is used as a premedication before surgery.

Antidiabetics + **Colestyramine and related drugs**

Acarbose

Colestyramine may enhance the antidiabetic effects of acarbose, and a rebound effect may occur if both drugs are stopped at the same time.

> The clinical importance of the effects of colestyramine on acarbose in diabetics is uncertain, but some care seems appropriate. It would seem prudent to increase blood-glucose monitoring if concurrent use is started or stopped and adjust the antidiabetic treatment accordingly.

Chlorpropamide or Tolbutamide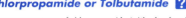

The concurrent use of chlorpropamide (with phenformin) or tolbutamide inhibited the normal hypocholesterolaemic effects of colestipol in 12 diabetic patients.

> Colestipol may not be suitable for lowering the blood cholesterol levels of diabetics taking chlorpropamide or tolbutamide, but more study is needed.

Glibenclamide

Colesevelam reduced the AUC of glibenclamide by 32% when taking at the same time. The AUC was still reduced by 20% when it was taken one hour before colesevelam. No significant interaction occurred when it was taken 4 hours before colesevelam.

> The manufacturers recommend that glibenclamide is taken at least 4 hours before colesevelam.

Glipizide

The absorption of glipizide may be reduced by about 30% if it is taken at the same time as colestyramine.

> It has been suggested that glipizide should be taken 1 to 2 hours before colestyramine, but this may only be partially effective because glipizide may undergo some enterohepatic recirculation.

Antidiabetics + **Contraceptives**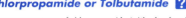

Some women may require small increases or decreases in their dose of antidiabetic while taking hormonal contraceptives, but it is unusual for the control of diabetes to be seriously disturbed.

> Routine monitoring should be adequate to detect any interaction as the effects seem to be gradual. However, note that occasionally severe disturbances in control do occur. Irrespective of diabetic control, hormonal contraceptives should be used with caution in patients with diabetes because of the increased risk of arterial disease: the lowest-strength combined oral contraceptive preparations (20 micrograms of oestrogen) is advised and this may minimise the adverse effect on diabetic control. The choice of progestogen may also be important, with levonorgestrel having the most detrimental effect.

Antidiabetics + **Corticosteroids**

Corticosteroids with glucocorticoid (hyperglycaemic) activity oppose the blood glucose-lowering effects of the antidiabetics. Significant hyperglycaemia has been seen with systemic corticosteroids, and in cases with inhaled corticosteroids or high-potency topical corticosteroids.

> It would seem prudent to increase blood glucose monitoring when a corticosteroid is started and adjust the antidiabetic treatment accordingly. Routine monitoring of local corticosteroids appears over-cautious, but be aware that isolated cases of hyperglycaemia have been reported.

Antidiabetics + **Co-trimoxazole**

Occasionally and unpredictably acute hypoglycaemia has occurred in patients given various sulfonylureas and co-trimoxazole, although pharmacokinetic studies have not established an interaction. Note that co-trimoxazole alone may rarely cause hypoglycaemia. See also trimethoprim, page 84, for its effects on repaglinide and rosiglitazone.

> Information is limited and serious adverse effects appear to be rare. Nevertheless, the cautious approach would be to increase blood glucose monitoring in diabetics taking co-trimoxazole and warn the patient that increased blood glucose-lowering effects, sometimes excessive, are a possibility.

Antidiabetics + **Digoxin**

Some but not all studies have found that digoxin plasma levels can be markedly reduced by acarbose.

> Just why there is an inconsistency between these reports is not understood but it would clearly be prudent to consider monitoring digoxin levels for any evidence of a reduced effect.

Antidiabetics + **Disopyramide**

Disopyramide occasionally and unpredictably causes hypoglycaemia, which may be severe. Isolated reports describe severe hypoglycaemia when disopyramide was given to diabetic patients taking gliclazide, or metformin and/or insulin.

> Patients at particular risk of hypoglycaemia are the elderly, the malnourished and diabetics. Impaired renal function or cardiac function may also be predisposing factors. It has been suggested that blood glucose levels should be closely monitored and the disopyramide stopped if problems arise.

Antidiabetics + **Diuretics**

Loop diuretics

The control of diabetes is not usually significantly disturbed by etacrynic acid, furosemide, or torasemide, although there are a few reports showing that etacrynic acid and furosemide can sometimes raise blood glucose levels.

No action needed.

Thiazide diuretics

By raising blood glucose levels, the thiazide and related diuretics can reduce the effects of the antidiabetics and impair the control of diabetes. However, this effect appears to be dose-related, and is less frequent at the low doses now commonly used for hypertension. Hyponatraemia has rarely been reported with chlorpropamide combined with a thiazide and potassium-sparing diuretic.

This interaction is of only moderate practical importance. Guidelines on the treatment of hypertension in diabetes (2009) recommend the use of thiazides. However, if higher doses are used, increased monitoring of diabetic control would seem prudent. The full effects may take many months to develop in some patients.

Antidiabetics + Endothelin receptor antagonists

There appears to be an increased risk of liver toxicity if bosentan is used with glibenclamide (glyburide). Glibenclamide (glyburide) modestly reduces the plasma levels of bosentan, and bosentan reduces the plasma levels of glibenclamide (glyburide).

The manufacturers suggest the combination should be avoided.

Antidiabetics + Fibrates

Sulfonylureas or Insulin

TA number of reports describe hypoglycaemia and/or an enhancement of the effects of insulin and sulfonylureas in patients given fibrates.

There would seem to be no good reason for avoiding concurrent use, but be aware that the dose of the antidiabetic may need adjustment. Patients should be warned that excessive hypoglycaemia occurs occasionally and unpredictably.

Nateglinide

Only a modest pharmacokinetic interaction occurs between gemfibrozil and nateglinide.

The manufacturer of nateglinide recommends particular caution, but this seems a very wary approach. Consider increasing the frequency of blood glucose monitoring until treatment is stabilised.

Pioglitazone or Rosiglitazone

Gemfibrozil causes large increases in the AUCs of pioglitazone and rosiglitazone.

The clinical relevance of this interaction has not been assessed. Until further experience is gained, caution is warranted. Consider an increased frequency of

A

blood glucose monitoring if gemfibrozil is started or stopped, adjusting the pioglitazone or rosiglitazone dose as necessary.

Repaglinide

Gemfibrozil markedly increases the levels and blood glucose-lowering effects of repaglinide and cases of serious hypoglycaemia have been reported.

On the basis of studies and reports of serious hypoglycaemic episodes with gemfibrozil and repaglinide, the European Medicines Agency contraindicate concurrent use.

Antidiabetics + Grapefruit juice ❓

Diltiazem (a moderate inhibitor of CYP3A4) increases saxagliptin levels. Grapefruit juice is predicted to interact similarly.

No initial saxagliptin dose adjustment is recommended; however, consider monitoring blood glucose levels more closely and reduce the dose if clinically indicated.

Antidiabetics + H$_2$-receptor antagonists

Metformin ⚠

Cimetidine appears to reduce the clearance of metformin, and may have contributed to a case of metformin-associated lactic acidosis.

The dose of metformin may need to be reduced if cimetidine is used, bearing in mind the possibility of lactic acidosis if levels become too high.

Miglitol ⚠

Miglitol decreases the AUC of ranitidine by 60%.

The clinical significance of this effect is unknown. It may be prudent to monitor for ranitidine efficacy.

Sulfonylureas ❓

Cimetidine and ranitidine generally cause no clinically important changes in the pharmacokinetics or pharmacodynamics of the sulfonylureas, although isolated cases of raised sulfonylurea levels and hypoglycaemia have been seen.

The evidence suggests that most diabetics do not experience any marked changes in their diabetic control if they are given cimetidine or ranitidine. However, consider the possibility of an interaction if any unexplained loss of diabetic control occurs.

A

Antidiabetics + Herbal medicines or Dietary supplements

Glucosamine +/- Chondroitin

In a controlled study glucosamine with chondroitin had no effect on the glycaemic control of patients taking oral antidiabetics, but one report notes that unexpected increases in blood glucose levels have occurred.

It may be prudent to increase monitoring of blood glucose if glucosamine supplements are taken. Also, if glucose control unexpectedly deteriorates, bear in mind the possibility of self-medication with supplements such as glucosamine.

Karela (Momordica charantia)

The blood glucose-lowering effects of antidiabetics can be increased by karela.

Karela is used to flavour foods such as curries, and also used as a herbal medicine for the treatment of diabetes mellitus. Health professionals should therefore be aware that patients may possibly be using karela as well as more orthodox drugs to control their diabetes. Irregular consumption of karela as part of the diet could possibly contribute to unexplained fluctuations in diabetic control.

St John's wort (Hypericum perforatum)

St John's wort decreased the AUC of rosiglitazone (modest decrease of about 25%). Pioglitazone may be similarly affected.

The clinical relevance of the modest reduction in rosiglitazone levels has not been assessed, but an interaction with rosiglitazone or pioglitazone seems unlikely to be important. However, note that the UK manufacturer of pioglitazone advises caution on concurrent use.

Antidiabetics + HRT

Some women may require small increases or decreases in their dose of antidiabetic while taking HRT, but it is unusual for the control of diabetes to be seriously disturbed.

Routine monitoring should be adequate to detect any interaction as the effects seem to be gradual. However, note that occasionally severe disturbances in control do occur. Menopausal HRT should be used with caution in diabetics because of the increased risk of arterial disease.

Antidiabetics + Lanreotide

Lanreotide may affect glucose levels in diabetic patients.

The manufacturer of lanreotide recommends that blood glucose levels should be checked in diabetic patients to determine whether antidiabetic treatment needs to be adjusted. This seems prudent.

A

Antidiabetics + Leflunomide

The active metabolite of leflunomide (A771726) has been shown by *in vitro* studies to be an inhibitor of CYP2C9, which is concerned with the metabolism of tolbutamide. The manufacturers advise caution if leflunomide is given with tolbutamide as increased tolbutamide levels may result.

It may be prudent to monitor blood glucose levels on concurrent use.

Antidiabetics + Macrolides

Sulfonylureas

Isolated cases of hypoglycaemia have been described in patients taking glibenclamide (glyburide) or glipizide with clarithromycin or erythromycin. Studies in healthy subjects have found that hypoglycaemia may occur if tolbutamide is given with clarithromycin and that glibenclamide levels are modestly increased by clarithromycin.

It may be prudent to consider monitoring blood glucose levels. Adjust the dose of the antidiabetic medications as necessary.

Repaglinide

Clarithromycin and telithromycin appear to increase the AUC of repaglinide and may enhance its blood glucose-lowering effects: a case of hypoglycaemia has been reported with clarithromycin. Erythromycin may interact similarly.

It may be prudent to increase blood glucose monitoring on concurrent use and adjust the dose of repaglinide if necessary.

Saxagliptin

Ketoconazole (a potent inhibitor of CYP3A4) increases saxagliptin levels. Clarithromycin and telithromycin are predicted to interact similarly. Erythromycin may also interact, although to a lesser extent.

The US manufacturer recommends that the dose of saxagliptin should be limited to 2.5 mg daily with clarithromycin or telithromycin. It would seem prudent to increase blood glucose level monitoring and adjust treatment accordingly. No initial saxagliptin dose adjustment is recommended with erythromycin; however, consider monitoring blood glucose levels more closely and reduce the dose if clinically indicated.

Antidiabetics + MAOIs

The blood glucose-lowering effects of insulin and the oral antidiabetics can be increased by MAOIs. This may improve the control of blood glucose levels in most diabetics, but in a few it may cause undesirable hypoglycaemia.

It may be prudent to increase blood glucose monitoring on concurrent use.

Antidiabetics + **Neomycin**

Neomycin alone can reduce postprandial blood glucose levels, and may enhance the reduction in postprandial glucose levels associated with acarbose. Neomycin also appears to increase the unpleasant gastrointestinal adverse effects (flatulence, cramps and diarrhoea) of acarbose.

> The manufacturers suggest that if these adverse effects are severe the dose of acarbose should be reduced.

Antidiabetics + **Nicotinic acid (Niacin)**

Nicotinic acid causes deterioration in glucose tolerance, which may be dose-related, and can result in the need for dose adjustment of a patient's antidiabetic drugs. Nevertheless, its beneficial effects on lipids may outweigh its effects on glucose tolerance in some diabetics.

> Diabetic control should be closely monitored, recognising that some adjustment of the antidiabetic drugs may be needed.

Antidiabetics + **NSAIDs**

Antidiabetics with Azapropazone or Phenylbutazone

Although in general NSAIDs do not appear to interact with antidiabetics (see below) azapropazone and particularly phenylbutazone seem to cause a consistent lowering of blood glucose levels (probably by inhibiting the metabolism of the sulphonylureas), which has resulted in severe hypoglycaemia in a number of cases.

> Concurrent use with phenylbutazone should be well monitored and a reduction in the dosage of the sulphonylurea may be necessary to avoid excessive hypoglycaemia. The manufacturers of azapropazone say that the concurrent use of sulphonylureas is not recommended.

Pioglitazone or Rosiglitazone with NSAIDs

The risk of fluid retention with pioglitazone or rosiglitazone is increased by NSAIDs, and this may exacerbate or precipitate heart failure and/or oedema, particularly in those with limited cardiac reserve.

> Caution is appropriate, and patients should be monitored for signs of fluid retention and heart failure (e.g. shortness of breath or swollen ankles). Patients who develop these symptoms should seek a medical review.

Antidiabetics, general with NSAIDs

No adverse interaction normally occurs between most NSAIDs and antidiabetics, although in some isolated cases hypoglycaemia has occurred.

> No action needed, but be aware that NSAIDs may rarely and unpredictably cause hypoglycaemia.

A

Antidiabetics + Octreotide ⚠️

Octreotide decreases insulin resistance so that the dose of insulin used by patients with type 1 diabetes can be reduced. Octreotide appears to have no benefits in those with intact insulin reserves (type 2 diabetes). In addition, octreotide has been reported to reduce sulfonylurea-induced hypoglycaemia.

> If octreotide is used with insulin, anticipate the need to reduce the insulin dose (studies suggest by up to 50%). Octreotide may affect insulin secretion, and therefore glucose tolerance, and so it would be prudent to monitor the effects of giving octreotide with any of the oral antidiabetics.

Antidiabetics + Orlistat

Acarbose ❌

The manufacturers of orlistat recommend avoiding the concurrent use of acarbose because of a lack of interaction studies.

> Avoid concurrent use.

Other antidiabetics ⚠️

Orlistat improved glycaemic control, which resulted in the need to reduce the dose of glibenclamide (glyburide) or glipizide in almost half of the patients in one study. In other studies, orlistat reduced the dose requirement for metformin and insulin.

> Monitor the outcome of concurrent use on blood sugar levels and adjust the antidiabetic treatment accordingly.

Antidiabetics + Pancreatic enzymes ❌

The manufacturers of acarbose and miglitol reasonably suggest that digestive enzyme preparations (such as amylase, pancreatin) would be expected to reduce the effects of these antidiabetics.

> The manufacturers advise avoiding concurrent use.

Antidiabetics + Phenobarbital

Repaglinide ⚠️

Rifampicin, a potent inducer of CYP2C8 and CYP3A4, reduces the levels of repaglinide, and the manufacturers state that they cannot exclude the possibility that other enzyme inducers, such as phenobarbital (and therefore probably primidone, which is metabolised to phenobarbital), may also interact.

> It would seem prudent to increase blood glucose level monitoring if phenobarbital or primidone is started to ensure that repaglinide is still effective, and adjust the antidiabetic treatment accordingly.

Saxagliptin ❓

Rifampicin (*rifampin*), a potent CYP3A4 and CYP2C8 inducer, markedly reduces the levels of saxagliptin without affecting the levels of its active metabolite (which is about half as potent as saxagliptin). Other potent inducers of CYP3A4, such as phenobarbital and primidone (which is metabolised to phenobarbital), might be expected to interact similarly.

The US manufacturer considers that no dose adjustment of saxagliptin is needed as overall dipeptidylpeptidase-4 inhibitory activity was unaffected. However, as it cannot be ruled out that enzyme inducers might reduce the blood-glucose lowering effect of saxagliptin the UK manufacturer advises caution. Bear this interaction in mind should any reduced saxagliptin effects occur.

Antidiabetics + Phenytoin

Repaglinide ⚠

Rifampicin (*rifampin*) an inducer of CYP2C8 and CYP3A4, reduces repaglinide levels and the manufacturers state that they cannot exclude the possibility that other enzyme inducers, such as phenytoin (and therefore probably its prodrug, fosphenytoin), may interact similarly.

It would seem prudent to increase blood glucose level monitoring if phenytoin or fosphenytoin is started to ensure that repaglinide is still effective, and adjust the antidiabetic treatment accordingly.

Saxagliptin ❓

Rifampicin, a potent CYP3A4 inducer, markedly reduces the levels of saxagliptin without affecting the levels of its active metabolite (which is about half as potent as saxagliptin). Other potent inducers of CYP3A4, such as phenytoin (and therefore probably its prodrug, fosphenytoin), are predicted to interact similarly.

The US manufacturer considers that no dose adjustment of saxagliptin is needed as overall dipeptidylpeptidase-4 inhibitory activity was unaffected. However, as it cannot be ruled out that enzyme inducers might reduce the blood-glucose lowering effect of saxagliptin the UK manufacturer advises caution. Bear this interaction in mind should any reduced saxagliptin effects occur.

Other antidiabetics ❓

Large and toxic doses of phenytoin have been observed to cause hyperglycaemia, but normal therapeutic doses do not usually affect the control of diabetes. Two isolated cases of phenytoin toxicity have been attributed to the use of tolbutamide.

No interaction of clinical importance normally occurs and so no special precautions would seem to be necessary, but bear it in mind in the case of an unexpected response to treatment. Indicators of phenytoin toxicity include blurred vision, nystagmus, ataxia or drowsiness.

Antidiabetics + Probenecid ⚠

The clearance of chlorpropamide is prolonged by probenecid, but the clinical importance of this is uncertain.

Monitor the effect of concurrent use on blood glucose levels and adjust the chlorpropamide dose if necessary. Tolbutamide appears not to interact with probenecid, and so may be a suitable alternative.

Antidiabetics + Protease inhibitors

Ketoconazole (a potent inhibitor of CYP3A4) increases saxagliptin levels, but reduces the levels of its active metabolite. The manufacturer predicts that atazanavir, indinavir, nelfinavir, ritonavir and saquinavir will interact similarly. Amprenavir and fosamprenavir are also predicted to increase saxagliptin levels, but to a lesser extent.

The US manufacturer recommends that the dose of saxagliptin should be limited to 2.5 mg daily with most of these protease inhibitors, although no dose adjustment is necessary with amprenavir and fosamprenavir. It would seem prudent to increase blood glucose level monitoring with any protease inhibitor, and adjust treatment accordingly.

Antidiabetics + Quinolones

A number of reports describe severe hypoglycaemia (and, rarely, hyperglycaemia) in diabetic patients taking gatifloxacin with various antidiabetics including some sulfonylureas, insulin, metformin, pioglitazone, repaglinide, rosiglitazone, and voglibose. Isolated cases describe hypoglycaemia in diabetic patients taking glibenclamide (glyburide) with ciprofloxacin, levofloxacin, or norfloxacin.

Studies have shown that systemic gatifloxacin may cause hypoglycaemia and hyperglycaemia with at least a 10-fold higher incidence than other quinolones. Studies using ciprofloxacin and levofloxacin with glibenclamide (glyburide) suggest plasma glucose levels are not usually affected to a clinically relevant extent. Therefore in general these interactions seem unlikely to be clinically significant with most quinolones; however, the use of systemic gatifloxacin in patients with diabetes has been contraindicated. Gatifloxacin eye drops are not expected to interact.

Antidiabetics + Rifabutin

The manufacturers and the CSM in the UK warn that rifabutin may possibly reduce the effects of oral antidiabetics, although this is likely to be to at lesser extent than rifampicin. For information on the effects *rifampicin* has on antidiabetics, see Antidiabetics + Rifampicin (Rifampin), below.

Monitor the outcome of concurrent use on blood glucose levels and adjust the antidiabetic treatment accordingly. In many cases an increase in the dose of the antidiabetic may possibly be needed. Note that the US manufacturer considers that no dose adjustment of saxagliptin is needed with *rifampicin* (*rifampin*), and therefore an initial dose adjustment seems unlikely to be needed with rifabutin.

Antidiabetics + Rifampicin (Rifampin)

Rifampicin reduces the levels and blood glucose-lowering effects of tolbutamide, gliclazide, chlorpropamide (single case) and glibenclamide (glyburide), and to a lesser extent glimepiride, glipizide and glymidine. Rifampicin also reduces the AUC and effects of repaglinide, and possibly nateglinide. Rifampicin reduces the AUCs of pioglitazone and rosiglitazone by about 50%, which could be clinically relevant. Rifampicin markedly reduces the levels of saxagliptin without affecting the levels of the active metabolite (which is about half as potent as saxagliptin).

> Monitor the outcome of concurrent use on blood glucose levels and adjust the antidiabetic treatment accordingly. In many cases an increase in the dose of the antidiabetic seems likely to be needed. The US manufacturer states that no dose adjustment of saxagliptin is needed as overall efficacy was unaffected. However, as it cannot be ruled out that carbamazepine might reduce the blood-glucose lowering effect of saxagliptin the UK manufacturer advises caution. Bear this interaction in mind should any reduced saxagliptin effects occur.

Antidiabetics + SSRIs

In various clinical studies in patients with diabetes, the SSRIs have generally caused minor improvements in glycaemic control. However, isolated cases of severe hypoglycaemia, hyperglycaemia and hypoglycaemia unawareness have been reported.

> It may be prudent to consider increasing the frequency of blood glucose monitoring if an SSRI is started or stopped, adjusting the antidiabetic therapy as necessary.

Antidiabetics + Statins

Glibenclamide

Fluvastatin may raise glibenclamide levels, but this possibly only occurs with doses above 40 mg daily. Blood glucose levels were not affected by concurrent use.

> The UK manufacturers of fluvastatin suggest that concurrent use should be avoided because of the risk of hypoglycaemia. The US manufacturers advise close monitoring, which should continue if the fluvastatin dose is increased to 40 mg twice daily. This seems prudent.

Other antidiabetics

One study reported an increased incidence of adverse effects when repaglinide was given with simvastatin, and there is a possibility of increased liver and muscle effects when pioglitazone or rosiglitazone are used with atorvastatin.

> As yet there is insufficient evidence to recommend special precautions when the statins are used with any antidiabetic drug. No clinically relevant adverse interactions appear to have been reported between statins and sulfonylureas. The use of statins in patients with diabetes is known to be beneficial for both primary and secondary prevention of cardiovascular events.

Antidiabetics + Sulfinpyrazone

Sulfinpyrazone reduces the clearance of tolbutamide by about 40%.

> There appear to be no reports of a clinically relevant interaction with these or any other sulfonylureas; however what is known suggests that increased blood

A

glucose-lowering effects, and possibly hypoglycaemia, could occur. It would therefore seem prudent to consider monitoring blood-glucose levels, and warn patients that hypoglycaemia may occur.

Antidiabetics + Sulfonamides

The blood glucose-lowering effects of some of the sulfonylureas are increased by some, but not all, sulfonamides. The sulfonamides now available appear less likely to interact. Nevertheless, occasionally and unpredictably acute hypoglycaemia has occurred.

Information is limited and serious adverse effects appear to be rare. Nevertheless, the cautious approach would be to increase the frequency of blood glucose monitoring and warn the patient that increased blood glucose-lowering effects, sometimes excessive, are a possibility.

Antidiabetics + Tibolone

Tibolone may slightly impair glucose tolerance and therefore possibly reduce the effects of antidiabetics. Strictly speaking this is a drug-disease interaction.

The manufacturers of tibolone state that patients with diabetes should be closely supervised. It would therefore seem prudent to increase the frequency of blood glucose monitoring if tibolone is started or stopped.

Antidiabetics + Tricyclics ?

Interactions between antidiabetics and tricyclic antidepressants appear to be rare, but isolated cases of hypoglycaemia have been recorded in patients given insulin or a sulfonylurea with a tricyclic.

These isolated cases seem unlikely to be of general importance.

Antidiabetics + Trimethoprim

Repaglinide

In one study trimethoprim increased the AUC of single-dose repaglinide by about 60% without changing its blood-glucose lowering effects.

The UK manufacturers advise that concurrent use should be avoided as the effect of larger doses of both drugs are unknown. However, the US manufacturers suggest that repaglinide dose adjustments may be necessary. If both drugs are used it would seem prudent to increase the frequency of blood glucose monitoring until the effects are known.

Rosiglitazone ?

Trimethoprim appears to modestly increase the AUC of rosiglitazone and pioglitazone.

This interaction is not expected to be clinically significant, but, until more experience is gained, some caution is warranted.

Sulphonylureas

Trimethoprim does not appear to significantly affect the pharmacokinetics of tolbutamide. Consider also co-trimoxazole, page 74, which may interact.

> No action needed.

Antidiabetics + **Warfarin and other oral anticoagulants**
Exenatide

A controlled study found that exenatide had no effect on the pharmacokinetics and only slightly raised the INR (by 12%). However, the manufacturer states that cases of raised INRs have been reported with concurrent use, and predict that other coumarins will interact similarly.

> A clinically significant interaction seems unlikely. However, the manufacturer advises that the INR should be closely monitored when exenatide is started, stopped, or the dose altered.

Other antidiabetics

Although isolated cases of interactions (raised prothrombin times, bleeding or hypoglycaemia) have been seen in patients taking anticoagulants and acarbose, metformin or sulfonylureas, in general no important interaction appears to occur. A decrease in prothrombin time has also been seen with acarbose or metformin.

> The isolated cases of bleeding are not expected to represent a general interaction.

Antihistamines

No specific interaction studies have been performed with antihistamine eye drops. However, interactions are not anticipated since very little drug is expected to reach the systemic circulation. Note also that the sedative antihistamines may cause additive sedation with any other CNS depressant drug.

Antihistamines + **Azoles**
Mizolastine

Ketoconazole raises mizolastine levels, which caused a small increase in the QT interval in one study.

> The manufacturer of mizolastine contraindicates the concurrent use of azoles.

Ebastine

Ketoconazole very markedly raised ebastine levels. Itraconazole is expected to interact similarly.

> Although the risk of an interaction seems small, because of the potential for

life-threatening torsade de pointes arrhythmia, the manufacturer of ebastine advises against the use of itraconazole or ketoconazole.

Other antihistamines

Ketoconazole markedly raised loratadine levels. In one study, this was associated with a small increase in the QT interval for both antihistamines, but there was no obvious alteration in the adverse event profile. Ketoconazole and itraconazole markedly raised the plasma levels of fexofenadine and rupatadine, and modestly raised those of desloratadine and emedastine.

Because there are no data on acrivastine with ketoconazole, the manufacturer advises caution. As no change in QT interval or in adverse events occurred, the combination of ketoconazole or itraconazole with fexofenadine, desloratadine or emedastine is assumed to be safe in terms of cardiac effects. The manufacturer cautions the use of rupatadine with ketoconazole. No special precautions appear to have been recommended for the use of loratadine with azoles. Azelastine, cetirizine (and therefore probably its isomer levocetirizine)and levocabastine do not appear to interact with the azole antifungals and may therefore be suitable alternatives.

Antihistamines + Benzodiazepines

An enhanced sedative effect would be expected if known sedative antihistamines are given with benzodiazepines.

Warn all patients taking sedating antihistamines of the potential effects, and counsel against driving or undertaking other skilled tasks. The degree of impairment will depend on the individual patient.

Antihistamines + Betahistine

A single report describes the re-emergence of labyrinthine symptoms in a patient taking betahistine with terfenadine. This interaction had been predicted on theoretical grounds because betahistine is an analogue of histamine. Betahistine may therefore oppose the effects of all antihistamines.

Although the general relevance of this isolated case report is unclear, the use of antihistamines should be carefully considered in patients taking betahistine.

Antihistamines + Grapefruit juice

Rupatadine

Grapefruit juice increases the exposure to rupatadine 3.5-fold.

The manufacturer advises that grapefruit juice should not be taken at the same time as rupatadine.

A

Other antihistamines

Grapefruit juice has been found to reduce the AUC of fexofenadine by up to 67%, which may reduce its efficacy.

> The general importance of reduction in fexofenadine levels is unclear, but bear it in mind in case of a lack of response to treatment. Note that the manufacturer of acrivastine advises caution with grapefruit juice but notes that there are no data to demonstrate an interaction.

Antihistamines + H$_2$-receptor antagonists

Cimetidine moderately raises hydroxyzine levels and considerably raises loratadine levels, but this is not thought to be of clinical significance. The manufacturer of mizolastine predicts that cimetidine may raise mizolastine levels.

> No action is generally needed. Note that the manufacturer of mizolastine recommends caution because raised mizolastine levels may prolong the QT interval.

Antihistamines + Herbal medicines or Dietary supplements

Some studies have found that St John's wort increased the clearance of fexofenadine up to 2-fold, whereas another study found no clinically relevant effect.

> If fexofenadine is less effective in a patient taking regular St John's wort, consider this interaction as a possible cause.

Antihistamines + Macrolides

Ebastine or Mizolastine ❌

Erythromycin markedly raises ebastine levels, which caused a modest prolongation of the QT interval in one study. Erythromycin also raises mizolastine levels, although this has no effect on the QT interval.

> The manufacturer of ebastine advises against the concurrent use of erythromycin, clarithromycin and josamycin. The manufacturer of mizolastine contraindicates the concurrent use of the macrolides.

Other antihistamines

Erythromycin raises fexofenadine and rupatadine levels, although this has no effect on the QT interval. Azithromycin has also been reported to raise fexofenadine levels, but this also had no effect on the QT interval, or on adverse events. One study found that the combination of erythromycin and loratadine caused a very slight increase in the QT interval.

> The manufacturer of rupatadine advises caution with concurrent use. The situation with erythromycin and loratadine is unclear; however, no special precautions appear to have been recommended. Because there are no data on acrivastine with erythromycin, the manufacturer advises caution. Azelastine,

A

cetirizine (and probably levocetirizine), desloratadine, levocabastine may be suitable non-interacting alternatives. As the use of fexofenadine with erythromycin did not result in significant adverse cardiac effects, concurrent use with erythromycin is considered safe. Note that the macrolides differ in the likely extent of their interaction, see macrolides, page 361.

Antihistamines + MAOIs

Antihistamines, general ⊗

The alleged interaction between MAOIs and most antihistamines appears to be based on a single animal study, and is probably more theoretical than real. The exception seems to be cyproheptadine and promethazine (see below).

In general, there would appear to be no good reason to avoid the concurrent use of sedating or non-sedating antihistamines with an MAOI. However, the UK manufacturers of some of the sedating antihistamines (chlorphenamine, diphenhydramine) state that MAOIs may intensify the antimuscarinic effect of antihistamines, and many contraindicate or advise caution on concurrent use, both with and for 14 days after stopping an MAOI. The US manufacturers of isocarboxazid and tranylcypromine contraindicate all antihistamines.

Cyproheptadine ⊗

Isolated reports describe delayed hallucinations in a patient taking phenelzine and cyproheptadine, and the rapid re-emergence of depression when cyproheptadine was given to two other patients taking brofaromine or phenelzine.

It would be prudent to monitor for a reduction in efficacy or an adverse response if cyproheptadine is given with any MAOI or RIMA. The manufacturer of cyproheptadine contraindicates concurrent use with MAOIs, however, there appears to be no reason why cyproheptadine cannot be used to treat serotonin syndrome occurring in a patient taking an MAOI.

Promethazine ⊗

Promethazine is a phenothiazine antihistamine. Rarely, cases of neuroleptic malignant syndrome or extrapyramidal symptoms have been seen when phenothiazines have been given with MAOIs.

The UK manufacturer contraindicates the use of promethazine, both with and for 14 days after stopping treatment with an MAOI.

Antihistamines + Protease inhibitors

Mizolastine ⚠

The manufacturers of mizolastine predict that the protease inhibitors will raise mizolastine levels.

The manufacturer advises caution on concurrent use. However, note that they contraindicate the use of the azoles, page 85, which would not be expected to interact to the same extent as the protease inhibitors.

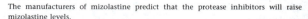

Other antihistamines

Ritonavir modestly increases cetirizine levels. Ritonavir and ritonavir-boosted lopinavir raise the levels of fexofenadine.

> These interactions are not expected to be clinically significant. No action needed.

Antihistamines + **Rifampicin (Rifampin)**

Rifampicin increases the oral clearance of fexofenadine, more than 5-fold in some cases, but the clinical significance of this is unclear.

> Until more is known it would seem prudent to monitor the efficacy of fexofenadine if it is given with rifampicin.

Antihypertensives

The hypotensive effect of antihypertensives can be enhanced by other antihypertensives, as would be expected. Although first-dose hypotension' (dizziness, light-headedness, fainting) can occur with some combinations (e.g. see ACE inhibitors, page 1 and alpha blockers, page 35), the additive effects are usually clinically useful. Perhaps of more concern is the use of antihypertensives with drugs that have hypotension as an adverse effect, where the effects may not be anticipated or deliberately sought. The situation with alcohol is slightly more complex. Chronic moderate to heavy drinking raises blood pressure and reduces, to some extent, the effectiveness of antihypertensive drugs. A few patients taking antihypertensives may experience postural hypotension, dizziness and fainting shortly after having an alcoholic drink. See also alpha blockers, page 14, beta blockers, page 17 and calcium-channel blockers, page 17, for more specific information on these individual groups. Patients with hypertension who are moderate to heavy drinkers should be encouraged to reduce their intake of alcohol. It may then become possible to reduce the dose of the antihypertensive. It should be noted that epidemiological studies show that regular light to moderate alcohol consumption is associated with a *lower* risk of cardiovascular disease. Drugs where hypotension is the main effect include:

- ACE inhibitors
- Aliskiren
- Alpha blockers
- Angiotensin II receptor antagonists
- Beta blockers
- Calcium-channel blockers
- Clonidine
- Diazoxide
- Diuretics
- Guanethidine
- Hydralazine
- Methyldopa
- Minoxidil
- Moxonidine
- Nitrates
- Nitroprusside

Drugs where hypotension is a significant adverse effect include:

- Alcohol
- Aldesleukin
- Alprostadil
- Antipsychotics
- Dopamine agonists (e.g. apomorphine, bromocriptine, pergolide)
- Levodopa
- MAOIs
- Moxisylyte
- Nicorandil
- Tizanidine

Antimuscarinics

Remember that other drugs, (e.g. clozapine, nefopam, tricyclic antidepressants) have antimuscarinic adverse effects, and therefore may interact similarly.

Antimuscarinics + **Antimuscarinics**

Additive antimuscarinic effects can develop if two or more drugs with antimuscarinic effects are used together. The easily recognised and common peripheral antimuscarinic effects are blurred vision, dry mouth, constipation, difficulty in urination, reduced sweating and tachycardia. Central effects include confusion, disorientation, visual hallucinations, agitation, irritability, delirium, memory problems, belligerence and even aggressiveness. Problems are most likely to arise in patients with particular physical conditions such as glaucoma, prostatic hypertrophy or constipation, in whom antimuscarinic drugs should be used with caution, if at all. It has been pointed out that the antimuscarinic adverse effects can mimic the effects of normal ageing. Consider also antipsychotics, below.

> Concurrent use need not be avoided but some caution is warranted, especially in the disease states mentioned.

Antimuscarinics + **Antipsychotics**

Antipsychotics and antimuscarinics are often given together advantageously and uneventfully, but occasionally serious and even life-threatening interactions occur. These include heat stroke in hot and humid conditions, severe constipation and adynamic ileus, and atropine-like psychoses. Antimuscarinics used to counteract the extrapyramidal adverse effects of antipsychotics may also reduce or abolish their therapeutic effects. See also antimuscarinics, above, as many antipsychotics also have antimuscarinic adverse effects.

> These drugs have been widely used together with apparent advantage and often without problems. However, be aware that low-grade antimuscarinic toxicity can easily go undetected, particularly in the elderly. Also note that serious problems

can sometimes develop, particularly if high doses are used. Consider:

- warning patients (particularly those on high doses) to minimise outdoor exposure and/or exercise in hot and humid climates.
- being alert for severe constipation and for the development of complete gut stasis, which can be fatal.
- that the symptoms of central antimuscarinic psychosis can be confused with the basic psychotic symptoms of the patient.
- withdrawal of one or more of the drugs, or a dose reduction and/or appropriate symptomatic treatment if any of these interactions occur.
- that the concurrent use of antimuscarinics to control the extrapyramidal adverse effects of neuroleptics is necessary, and be aware that the therapeutic effects may possibly be reduced as a result.

Some antipsychotics and antimuscarinics prolong the QT interval. For interactions resulting from additive effects on the QT interval see drugs that prolong the QT interval, page 277. Remember that many drugs have antimuscarinic adverse effects (e.g. tricyclics, page 105).

Antimuscarinics + Donepezil

The effects of donepezil are expected to oppose the actions of drugs with antimuscarinic effects, and in turn to be opposed by antimuscarinics. However, two cases describe confusional states resulting from the concurrent use of anticholinesterases and drugs with antimuscarinic effects, which is the opposite effect to that expected.

> Whether this interaction is of real practical importance awaits confirmation, but it would seem prudent to monitor concurrent use for an increase in adverse effects.

Antimuscarinics + Galantamine

The effects of galantamine are expected to oppose the actions of drugs with antimuscarinic effects, and in turn to be opposed by antimuscarinics. However, two cases describe confusional states resulting from the concurrent use of other anticholinesterases and drugs with antimuscarinic effects, which is the opposite effect to that expected.

> Whether this interaction is of real practical importance awaits confirmation, but it may be prudent to monitor concurrent use for an increase in adverse effects.

Antimuscarinics + Levodopa

Antimuscarinics may modestly reduce the rate and possibly the extent of levodopa absorption. One case describes levodopa toxicity, which occurred after the withdrawal of an antimuscarinic.

> Concurrent use is of established benefit. The presence of a dopa-decarboxylase inhibitor would be expected to minimise the effects of any interaction, however reduced levodopa absorption has still been reported with this combination. There is certainly no need to avoid concurrent use, but it would be prudent to be alert for any evidence of a reduced levodopa response if antimuscarinics are added, or for levodopa toxicity if they are withdrawn.

A

Antimuscarinics + MAOIs

No adverse interactions between the MAOIs and antimuscarinics appear to have been reported. However, some manufacturers of non-selective MAOIs and antimuscarinics advise caution because of the theoretical possibility that concurrent use may lead to increased antimuscarinic effects.

Bear this possible interaction in mind on concurrent use.

Antimuscarinics + Nitrates

Drugs with antimuscarinic effects, such as the tricyclic antidepressants and disopyramide, depress salivation and many patients complain of having a dry mouth. In theory sublingual glyceryl trinitrate (nitroglycerin) tablets will dissolve less readily under the tongue in these patients, thereby reducing their absorption and effects.

A possible alternative is to use a glyceryl trinitrate (nitroglycerin) spray in patients who suffer from dry mouth.

Antimuscarinics + Rivastigmine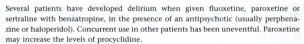

The effects of rivastigmine are expected to oppose the actions of drugs with antimuscarinic effects, and in turn to be opposed by antimuscarinics. However, in practice two cases describe confusional states resulting from the concurrent use of anticholinesterases and drugs with antimuscarinic effects, which is the opposite effect to that expected.

Whether this interaction is of real practical importance awaits confirmation, but it may be prudent to monitor concurrent use for an increase in adverse effects.

Antimuscarinics + SSRIs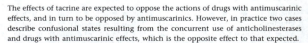

Several patients have developed delirium when given fluoxetine, paroxetine or sertraline with benzatropine, in the presence of an antipsychotic (usually perphenazine or haloperidol). Concurrent use in other patients has been uneventful. Paroxetine may increase the levels of procyclidine.

The general clinical importance of this interaction is uncertain, but be alert for evidence of confusion and possible delirium in patients given SSRIs with benzatropine, particularly if they are also taking other drugs with antimuscarinic actions. If antimuscarinic effects are seen in patients taking paroxetine and procyclidine, the dose of procyclidine should be reduced.

Antimuscarinics + Tacrine

The effects of tacrine are expected to oppose the actions of drugs with antimuscarinic effects, and in turn to be opposed by antimuscarinics. However, in practice two cases describe confusional states resulting from the concurrent use of anticholinesterases and drugs with antimuscarinic effects, which is the opposite effect to that expected.

Whether this interaction is of real practical importance awaits confirmation, but it may be prudent to monitor concurrent use for an increase in adverse effects.

Antipsychotics

Antipsychotics + **Antipsychotics**

Quetiapine

Thioridazine moderately reduces quetiapine levels and a case report describes a seizure in a patient taking olanzapine and quetiapine.

Concurrent use need not be avoided. Monitor concurrent use of thioridazine with quetiapine for efficacy, being alert for the need to raise the quetiapine dose. The case highlights the importance of considering seizure potential when prescribing multiple antipsychotic medications.

Other antipsychotics

Additive QT-prolonging effects are likely with some antipsychotic combinations.

For more information on the effects of using multiple drugs with QT-prolonging effects, see drugs that prolong the QT interval, page 277.

Antipsychotics + **Apomorphine**

Centrally-acting dopamine antagonists (such as the antipsychotics, including prochlorperazine used at an antiemetic dose) may antagonise the effects of apomorphine. However, note that clozapine may be used to reduce the symptoms of neuropsychiatric complications of Parkinson's disease. Additive hypotensive effects are also possible, see antihypertensives, page 89.

Concurrent use should be avoided, or monitored closely to ensure apomorphine remains effective. Note that prochlorperazine has been used safely in patients taking apomorphine for erectile dysfunction.

Antipsychotics + **Aprepitant**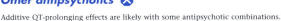

Aprepitant inhibits the enzymes involved in the metabolism of pimozide, and is therefore expected to raise pimozide levels, which may result in potentially fatal torsade de pointes, (see Drugs that prolong the QT interval, page 277). Fosaprepitant, a prodrug of aprepitant, would be expected to interact similarly.

Concurrent use is contraindicated. Caution is needed in the 2 weeks after aprepitant is stopped because it is also a mild *inducer* of CYP3A4 and the induction is transient. Therefore, it may *induce* the metabolism of pimozide leading to *reduced* pimozide levels.

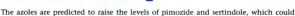

A

Antipsychotics + **Azoles**

Pimozide and Sertindole

The azoles are predicted to raise the levels of pimozide and sertindole, which could lead to potentially fatal torsade de pointes.

> The concurrent use of azoles with pimozide or sertindole is contraindicated. Note that miconazole oral gel may be swallowed in sufficient amounts to cause a systemic effect, and the manufacturer also contraindicates its use with sertindole.

Quetiapine ✕

Quetiapine levels are increased 3.4-fold by ketoconazole. Other azoles are predicted to interact similarly.

> The UK manufacturer contraindicates concurrent use. The US manufacturer advises that lower quetiapine doses may be needed. If both drugs are given monitor for quetiapine adverse effects (such as somnolence, dry mouth, tachycardia) and adjust the quetiapine dose accordingly.

Other antipsychotics ⚠

The levels of some antipsychotics may be raised by azole antifungals:

- Aripiprazole levels are increased by itraconazole and ketoconazole by about 20 to 40%.
- Haloperidol levels are raised by 30% or more by itraconazole, but there was wide variation between subjects. Adverse neurological effects were seen in some subjects.
- Risperidone levels were raised by about 80% by itraconazole in one study. Ketoconazole would be expected to interact similarly.

> Monitor for signs of adverse antipsychotic effects (such as sedation, agitation, movement disorders) if these azoles are given, and consider reducing the antipsychotic dose, in particular quetiapine. The manufacturers of aripiprazole suggest halving its dose if itraconazole or ketoconazole are given.

Antipsychotics + **Benzodiazepines**

Antipsychotics, general ⚠

Additive sedative effects would be expected when antipsychotics are given with benzodiazepines or related drugs (such as zopiclone or zolpidem). Concurrent use has resulted in severe hypotension, respiratory depression and, in rare cases, the neuroleptic malignant syndrome. Rarely, fatal hypotension and respiratory arrest have been reported when clozapine was given with benzodiazepines. Note that the parenteral use of these drugs is frequent in the more severe cases.

> Be aware of these potential adverse effects, but note that concurrent use is common and most often uneventful.

Olanzapine ⚠

Excessive sedation and hypotension may occur if parenteral benzodiazepines are given with intramuscular olanzapine: fatalities have been reported.

> Parenteral benzodiazepines should not be given until at least one hour after intramuscular olanzapine. If a parenteral benzodiazepine has already been given, intramuscular olanzapine should be given with care and the patient should be closely monitored for sedation and cardiorespiratory depression.

Antipsychotics + **Beta blockers**

Sotalol ❌

Additive QT-prolonging effects likely, see drugs that prolong the QT interval, page 277.

> Concurrent use should generally be avoided.

Beta blockers, general ⚠

The concurrent use of chlorpromazine and propranolol can result in a marked rise in the levels of both drugs. Propranolol also markedly increases thioridazine levels. Additive hypotensive effects are also possible, see antihypertensives, page 89.

> Monitor the outcome of concurrent use, adjusting the doses of both drugs as necessary.

Antipsychotics + **Bupropion**

Bupropion is predicted to inhibit the metabolism of haloperidol, risperidone, and thioridazine.

> The manufacturers recommend that if any of these drugs are added to treatment with bupropion, they should be given in doses at the lower end of the range. If bupropion is added to existing treatment, decreased doses of the antipsychotics should be considered. However, there appear to be no reports of problems with the concurrent use of any of these drugs. Note that both bupropion and antipsychotics can lower the seizure threshold, and a maximum dose of 150 mg of bupropion should be considered for patients prescribed other drugs that may lower the convulsive threshold.

Antipsychotics + **Buspirone**

Two studies found that buspirone can cause a rise in haloperidol levels, while another found that no interaction occurred.

> There would seem to be no reason for avoiding concurrent use. However, be aware that some patients seem to experience large rises in haloperidol levels, so consider this interaction if the adverse effects of haloperidol (e.g. sedation, agitation, movement disorders) become troublesome.

A

Antipsychotics + Calcium-channel blockers

Aripiprazole or Droperidol ⚠

Diltiazem is predicted to increase aripiprazole and droperidol levels. Verapamil would be expected to interact similarly.

Patients should be closely monitored for signs of aripiprazole or droperidol toxicity (such as sedation, hypotension, dizziness). An initial dose reduction of aripiprazole is probably not required, but if adverse effects develop, consider adjusting the dose.

Sertindole ✖

Diltiazem and verapamil reduce the clearance of sertindole by about 20%.

The concurrent use of these calcium-channel blockers is contraindicated as raised sertindole levels may prolong the QT interval, see Drugs that prolong the QT interval, page 277.

Antipsychotics, general ❓

In general, the hypotensive adverse effects of phenothiazines would be expected to be additive with the blood pressure-lowering effects of the calcium-channel blockers, see antihypertensives, page 89.

Bear the possibility of hypotension in mind on concurrent use. Warn patients to take time in getting up to minimise orthostatic hypotension.

Antipsychotics + Carbamazepine ❓

Clozapine, haloperidol and risperidone plasma levels can be roughly halved by carbamazepine. Aripiprazole, bromperidol, fluphenazine, olanzapine, paliperidone, quetiapine, sertindole, tiotixene, and possibly chlorpromazine, levels are also reduced by carbamazepine. An increase in the levels of carbamazepine or its epoxide metabolite (which is thought to cause some of the adverse effects of carbamazepine) has been reported in patients given loxapine, haloperidol, quetiapine, risperidone, or chlorpromazine with amoxapine. Toxicity has occurred. Isolated cases of neuroleptic malignant syndrome have occurred in patients taking antipsychotics with carbamazepine. The combination of clozapine and carbamazepine is predicted to increase agranulocytosis and one case of fatal pancytopenia has been reported.

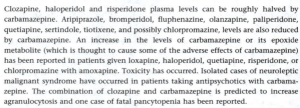

Monitor carbamazepine levels if loxapine, haloperidol, quetiapine, risperidone, or chlorpromazine are given. Also monitor concurrent use to ensure that the antipsychotics remain effective, (especially risperidone, clozapine, olanzapine and haloperidol) and consider a dose increase if needed. The manufacturers recommend using double the dose of aripiprazole in patients taking carbamazepine. The manufacturers advise that clozapine should not be given with carbamazepine; if both drugs are necessary, full blood counts should be closely monitored, as should clozapine efficacy (increase the clozapine dose as required). The general significance of the raised levels of the carbamazepine epoxide metabolite is unclear but the possibility of an interaction should be considered in patients who develop neurotoxic adverse effects. It is also important to consider the seizure potential when prescribing antipsychotic medications.

Antipsychotics + **Darifenacin**

Darifenacin increases the levels of CYP2D6 substrates such as the *tricyclics* (imipramine AUC increased by 70%). The manufacturers therefore advise caution with other CYP2D6 substrates, and specifically name thioridazine.

If the combination is used it would be prudent to closely monitor for thioridazine adverse effects, and consider the possibility of ventricular arrhythmias.

Antipsychotics + **Dopamine agonists**

Centrally-acting dopamine antagonists (such as the antipsychotics, including prochlorperazine used at an antiemetic dose) are expected to oppose the effects of the dopamine agonists.

Concurrent use should be avoided, or monitored closely to ensure that the dopamine agonist remains effective. Additive hypotensive effects are possible, see antihypertensives, page 89.

Antipsychotics + **Duloxetine**

Duloxetine is predicted to inhibit the metabolism of thioridazine and risperidone.

In the US concurrent use of duloxetine and thioridazine is contraindicated. If the combination is used it would be prudent to closely monitor for thioridazine or risperidone adverse effects (such as sedation, hypotension, dizziness). With thioridazine, consider the possibility of ventricular arrhythmias.

Antipsychotics + **Grapefruit juice**

The manufacturers predict that grapefruit juice will, like other CYP3A4 inhibitors, raise pimozide levels. This may lead to potentially life-threatening torsade de pointes. Grapefruit juice is also predicted to increase quetiapine levels.

The concurrent intake of grapefruit juice is contraindicated with pimozide and is not recommended with quetiapine.

Antipsychotics + **Guanethidine**

Large doses of chlorpromazine may reduce or even abolish the antihypertensive effects of guanethidine. However, in some patients the hypotensive effect of chlorpromazine may predominate. The antihypertensive effects of guanethidine can also be reduced by haloperidol and thiothixene. Note also, that the antipsychotics can cause postural hypotension, therefore additive hypotensive effects are possible with combined use, see antihypertensives, page 89.

Increases or decreases in blood pressure may occur as a result of concurrent use. Monitor blood pressure adjusting the guanethidine dose as necessary.

A

Antipsychotics + H₂-receptor antagonists

Chlorpromazine, Clozapine or Droperidol ⚠

One study found that chlorpromazine levels are reduced by cimetidine, while another study suggested that chlorpromazine levels can be increased. A single case report describes clozapine toxicity when cimetidine was also taken. The manufacturers predict that cimetidine will inhibit the metabolism of droperidol.

> The general significance of these interactions is unclear, but it would seem prudent to monitor concurrent use for both excessive antipsychotic adverse effects (such as drowsiness, hypotension) and/or loss of efficacy. Consider monitoring clozapine levels

Sertindole ✖

Cimetidine is predicted to increase sertindole levels (by inhibiting CYP3A4), which may result in potentially fatal torsade de pointes, see Drugs that prolong the QT interval, page 277.

> The manufacturers contraindicate concurrent use.

Antipsychotics + Herbal medicines or Dietary supplements

Evening primrose oil ❓

Although seizures have occurred in a few patients with schizophrenia taking phenothiazines with evening primrose oil, no adverse effects were seen in others, and there appears to be no firm evidence that evening primrose oil should be avoided by epileptic patients.

> No action needed; it seems likely that the phenothiazine rather than the evening primrose oil caused this adverse reaction.

St John's wort (Hypericum perforatum) ⚠

The manufacturers of aripiprazole and paliperidone say that St John's wort may be expected to reduce the level of these drugs.

> The manufacturers recommend using double the dose of aripiprazole, then titrating to effect, in patients taking potent inducers of aripiprazole metabolism. The manufacturer of paliperidone advise monitoring paliperidone effects and adjusting the dose of paliperidone if necessary.

Antipsychotics + Levodopa ✖

Centrally-acting dopamine antagonists (such as the antipsychotics, including prochlorperazine used at an antiemetic dose) may antagonise the effects of levodopa. The antipsychotic effects and extrapyramidal adverse effects of these drugs can be opposed by levodopa. Of the atypical antipsychotics, risperidone, and olanzapine cause deterioration in motor function in Parkinson's disease. Ziprasidone and paliperidone may act similarly, and there have been reports of mild motor deterioration with quetiapine. However, note that clozapine does not appear to have this effect and may be used to reduce the symptoms of neuropsychiatric complications of Parkinson's disease. Additive hypotensive effects possible, see antihypertensives, page 89.

> Concurrent use should be avoided, or monitored closely, to ensure levodopa remains effective.

Antipsychotics + Lithium

Chlorpromazine levels can be reduced to subtherapeutic concentrations by lithium, and one study suggested that lithium may reduce olanzapine levels. Lithium may increase amisulpride levels. The development of severe extrapyramidal adverse effects or severe neurotoxicity has been seen in one or more patients given lithium with chlorpromazine, chlorprothixene, clopenthixol, clozapine, flupentixol, fluphenazine, haloperidol, levomepromazine, loxapine, mesoridazine, molindone, olanzapine, perphenazine, prochlorperazine, risperidone, sulpiride, thioridazine, tiotixene, trifluoperazine or zuclopenthixol. Sleep-walking has been described in some patients taking chlorpromazine-like drugs and lithium. Additive QT-prolonging effects are also possible, see drugs that prolong the QT interval, page 277.

> Monitor the outcome of concurrent use being aware that on occasion dose adjustments may be needed to manage adverse effects. Withdraw one or both drugs if severe neurotoxicity occurs.

##

Clozapine

A study in healthy subjects found no evidence of an interaction between clozapine and erythromycin, but three case reports describe clozapine toxicity (seizures in one patient, drowsiness, incoordination and incontinence in another, and neutropenia in the third) when the patients also took erythromycin. Clarithromycin and telithromycin may interact similarly. Note that not all macrolides would be expected to interact, see macrolides, page 361.

> An interaction seems rare; however, bear the possibility in mind should an increase in clozapine adverse effects (e.g. agitation, dizziness, orthostatic hypotension, neutropenia) occur in patients given any of these macrolides.

Quetiapine ✖

Quetiapine levels are increased by erythromycin. Clarithromycin and telithromycin may interact similarly. Note that not all macrolides would be expected to interact, see macrolides, page 361.

> The UK manufacturer contraindicates concurrent use, whereas the US manufacturer advises that lower quetiapine doses may be needed. If quetiapine is given with any of these drugs, monitor closely for quetiapine adverse effects (e.g. dizziness, anxiety, orthostatic hypotension) and monitor closely for cardiac adverse effects.

Pimozide or Sertindole ❌

Clarithromycin can increase the levels of pimozide. Erythromycin slightly raises the levels of sertindole, and concurrent use increases the incidence of adverse effects (diarrhoea, abdominal pain, dizziness) but no ECG changes appear to occur. Raised pimozide and sertindole levels may increase the risk of QT interval prolongation, see drugs that prolong the QT interval, page 277.

> The UK manufacturer of pimozide contraindicates the concurrent use of all macrolides, whereas the US manufacturer specifically contraindicates azithromycin, clarithromycin, dirithromycin, and erythromycin. The manufacturers of sertindole specifically contraindicate clarithromycin and erythromycin, and an interaction with other macrolides should be considered. Note that not all macrolides inhibit CYP3A4 to the same extent, and therefore the severity of the interaction will vary; macrolides such as azithromycin would not be expected to interact, see macrolides, page 361.

Antipsychotics + Melatonin

The concurrent use of melatonin and thioridazine does not appear to affect the pharmacokinetics of either drugs, but it may lead to additive CNS effects.

> The degree of sedation will depend on the individual patient. However, warn all patients of the potential effects, and counsel against driving or undertaking other skilled tasks.

Antipsychotics + NNRTIs

Efavirenz and nevirapine are potent inducers of CYP3A4 and are predicted increase the metabolism of aripiprazole.

> The manufacturers recommend using double the dose of aripiprazole when it is taken with potent inducers of CYP3A4, then titrating to effect.

Antipsychotics + NSAIDs

Profound drowsiness and confusion have been described in patients given haloperidol and indometacin. Celecoxib is predicted to increase the metabolism of a number of antipsychotics (haloperidol, clozapine, risperidone) by inhibiting CYP2D6.

> Evidence of an interaction with haloperidol appears to be very limited, but the incidence (6 out of 20) is high. If concurrent use is thought appropriate, consider warning patients to be alert for this effect. Monitor the concurrent use of celecoxib and these antipsychotics for adverse effects, and consider reducing the dose of the antipsychotic if they become troublesome.

Antipsychotics + Opioids

Pethidine (meperidine) and chlorpromazine can be used together to enhance analgesia and for premedication before anaesthesia, but increased respiratory depression, sedation, CNS toxicity and hypotension can also occur. Similar effects would be expected with other phenothiazines and opioids.

The combination need not be avoided, but care obviously needs to be taken. Patients should be monitored carefully and dosage reductions made if necessary. The US manufacturer suggests that the dose of pethidine (meperidine) should be proportionally reduced (usually by 25 to 50%) when it is given with phenothiazines. Note that the manufacturers of methadone generally advise caution with other CNS depressants; however, one advises against concurrent use. Note that additive QT-prolonging effects are possible with methadone, see drugs that prolong the QT interval, page 277.

Antipsychotics + Phenobarbital

Haloperidol levels, and possibly clozapine levels, are roughly halved by phenobarbital. Aripiprazole, chlorpromazine, sertindole, and possibly thioridazine, levels are also reduced by phenobarbital. The levels of quetiapine are predicted to be reduced by barbiturates. Chlorpromazine, mesoridazine, and thioridazine appear to reduce barbiturate levels, and other phenothiazines may possibly have a similar effect.

Monitor concurrent use to ensure that the antipsychotics remain effective, adjusting the dose if necessary. The manufacturers of aripiprazole suggest doubling its dose. The manufacturer of sertindole states that the dose may need to be increased towards the upper end of the maximum dose range. It is also important to consider the seizure potential when prescribing antipsychotic medications, but be alert for evidence of reductions in response to both drugs if a phenothiazine and a barbiturate are given, and to increased responses if one of the drugs is withdrawn. Primidone is metabolised in the body to phenobarbital. It would therefore be expected to interact similarly.

Antipsychotics + Phenytoin

Haloperidol levels, and possibly clozapine levels, are more than halved by phenytoin. Sertindole levels are also significantly reduced, and the levels of aripiprazole and risperidone are predicted to be reduced, by phenytoin. The clearance of quetiapine is increased by phenytoin. The levels of the active metabolite of thioridazine may be reduced by phenytoin, however it is unclear if other phenothiazines interact similarly. The levels of phenytoin can be raised or lowered by the use of chlorpromazine, prochlorperazine or thioridazine. Fosphenytoin, a prodrug of phenytoin, may interact similarly with any of these antipsychotics.

Monitor phenytoin levels if chlorpromazine, prochlorperazine or thioridazine are given. Also monitor concurrent use to ensure that the antipsychotics remain effective; consider a dose increase of the antipsychotic where necessary, remembering to reduce the dose if phenytoin is withdrawn. The manufacturers of aripiprazole suggest doubling its dose. The manufacturer of sertindole states that the dose may need to be increased towards the upper end of the maximum dose range. It is also important to consider the seizure potential when prescribing antipsychotic medications.

A

Antipsychotics + Protease inhibitors

Antipsychotics with Saquinavir ⊗

Saquinavir is associated with a high risk of prolonging the QT interval. The manufacturer predicts that a serious QT prolongation is possible if it is given with antipsychotics, and they name haloperidol, pimozide, the phenothiazines, and ziprasidone. QT prolongation may lead to the potentially fatal torsade de pointes, see Drugs that prolong the QT interval, page 277.

> The UK manufacturers of saquinavir contraindicate concurrent use.

Aripiprazole ⚠

Aripiprazole is metabolised by CYP3A4, which is strongly inhibited by the protease inhibitors. Increased aripiprazole levels are therefore expected.

> Caution and monitoring are recommended. The manufacturers suggest that the dose of aripiprazole should be halved.

Clozapine ⊗

Clozapine levels are predicted to be raised by ritonavir, resulting in serious haematological toxicity.

> Concurrent use is therefore contraindicated. Note that concurrent use with saquinavir is predicted to increase the risk of QT prolongation.

Haloperidol ⚠

The manufacturer predicts that ritonavir will increase haloperidol levels.

> Monitor for haloperidol adverse effects (e.g. sedation, agitation, movement disorders)and consider a haloperidol dose reduction, if necessary. Note that concurrent use with saquinavir is predicted to increase the risk of QT prolongation, see under Antipsychotics with Saquinavir, above.

Olanzapine ⚠

Olanzapine levels are roughly halved by ritonavir.

> If concurrent use is necessary monitor olanzapine efficacy and increase the dose if necessary.

Pimozide or Sertindole ⊗

Pimozide and sertindole are metabolised by CYP3A4, which is inhibited by the protease inhibitors. Raised pimozide or sertindole levels, which increase the risk of potentially fatal arrhythmias, would be expected.

> Concurrent use is contraindicated. Note that concurrent use with saquinavir is predicted to increase the risk of QT prolongation.

Quetiapine ⊗

Quetiapine levels are increased 6-fold by *ketoconazole*, a potent inhibitor of CYP3A4.

Protease inhibitors are also inhibitors of CYP3A4 and are therefore predicted to interact similarly.

> Monitor for signs of quetiapine adverse effects (e.g. dizziness, anxiety, orthostatic hypotension) if a protease inhibitor is also given, and expect the need to reduce the quetiapine dose.

Risperidone

Neuroleptic malignant syndrome, ataxia and severe lethargy leading to coma, and extrapyramidal adverse effects have been seen in patients given risperidone with indinavir and ritonavir.

> If risperidone is given to any patient taking ritonavir (including ritonavir given as a pharmacokinetic enhancer) be alert for risperidone adverse effects (e.g. agitation, insomnia, headache, extrapyramidal effects). If these become troublesome consider decreasing the risperidone dose.

Thioridazine

Antiretroviral doses of ritonavir (300 mg twice daily or more) may increase thioridazine levels.

> The manufacturer of ritonavir recommends monitoring for thioridazine adverse effects during concurrent use. Note that concurrent use with saquinavir is predicted to increase the risk of QT prolongation, see under Antipsychotics with Saquinavir, above.

Antipsychotics + Quinidine

Quinidine appears to double aripiprazole and haloperidol levels. Additive QT-prolonging effects may also occur.

> Concurrent use need not be avoided, but consider this interaction if haloperidol or aripiprazole adverse effects (e.g. sedation, agitation, movement disorders) become troublesome. Of more concern is the potential for additive effects on the QT interval, see drugs that prolong the QT interval, page 277. The manufacturers of aripiprazole suggest halving its dose.

Antipsychotics + Quinolones

A small number of case reports suggest that ciprofloxacin may increase clozapine levels leading to toxicity, and a study supports this observation. Increased olanzapine levels and QT prolongation have been reported in two patients taking olanzapine and given ciprofloxacin. Additive QT-prolonging effects are possible with gatifloxacin, levofloxacin, moxifloxacin, and particularly sparfloxacin, and with several of the antipsychotics, see drugs that prolong the QT interval, page 277.

> Monitor the outcome of concurrent use closely for clozapine adverse effects (e.g. agitation, dizziness, sedation, hypersalivation). The manufacturers of olanzapine recommend a lower starting dose. Other quinolones may also interact to varying degrees, see quinolones, page 444.

A

Antipsychotics + **Rifabutin**

Rifabutin is predicted to reduce aripiprazole levels.

The manufacturers recommend using double the dose of aripiprazole then titrating to effect. Remember to re-adjust the dose if rifabutin is stopped.

Antipsychotics + **Rifampicin (Rifampin)**

Rifampicin decreases risperidone and sertindole levels and is also predicted to decrease aripiprazole, paliperidone and quetiapine levels. Case reports suggest that rifampicin reduces clozapine levels. Haloperidol levels appear to be decreased by rifampicin.

Clozapine levels should be well monitored if rifampicin is added. Be alert for the need to increase the dose of any of these antipsychotics in the presence of rifampicin. The manufacturers recommend that the dose of aripiprazole should be doubled. Note that increasing the dose of clozapine may not be successful in managing this interaction; it may be prudent to consider the use of other drugs.

Antipsychotics + **SSRIs**

Pimozide

Pimozide levels are expected to be increased by inhibition of CYP2D6 by fluoxetine, fluvoxamine, paroxetine, or sertraline. The use of SSRIs and pimozide has also led to extrapyramidal adverse effects, oculogyric crises and sedation in rare cases. QT prolongation may occur with the concurrent use of pimozide and citalopram.

Raised pimozide levels can cause torsade de pointes arrhythmias, which can be fatal. The manufacturers of pimozide contraindicate its use with most SSRIs. They do not specifically mention fluoxetine but as this has a greater effect than other SSRIs on CYP2D6, it would be prudent to avoid concurrent use.

Thioridazine

Thioridazine levels are expected to be increased by fluvoxamine (225% rise seen), and are predicted to be increased by fluoxetine or paroxetine.

The US manufacturers of fluoxetine, fluvoxamine, and paroxetine contraindicate the concurrent use of as raised levels increase the risk of QT prolongation, see drugs that prolong the QT interval, page 277. The use of thioridazine is also contraindicated for 5 weeks after fluoxetine has been stopped. It has been suggested that the dose of thioridazine may need to be reduced when it is given with escitalopram. Note that caution is advised when thioridazine is taken with other drugs that may lower the seizure threshold such as the SSRIs.

Other antipsychotics

On the whole no significant adverse interactions appear to occur between most antipsychotics and the SSRIs. However, a number of case reports describe extrapyramidal adverse effects and serotonin syndrome following the use of fluoxetine or paroxetine with an antipsychotic. The levels of some antipsychotics are raised by SSRIs:

- Aripiprazole levels are predicted to be raised by fluoxetine and paroxetine.
- Clozapine levels are raised by fluoxetine, paroxetine, sertraline and possibly citalopram: particularly large increases can occur with fluvoxamine. Toxicity has been seen in some patients.
- Haloperidol levels raised up to twofold by fluoxetine and by 20 to 60% by fluvoxamine. Sertraline may also possibly interact and escitalopram is predicted to interact with haloperidol.
- Olanzapine levels are significantly raised by fluvoxamine, increasing olanzapine adverse effects. Other SSRIs have modest or no significant effect.
- Perphenazine levels possibly raised by fluoxetine and paroxetine, which increased extrapyramidal adverse effects in a few cases.
- Risperidone levels are significantly raised by fluoxetine and paroxetine, and modestly by fluvoxamine and sertraline.
- Sertindole levels are raised 2- to 3-fold by fluoxetine and paroxetine.
- Zotepine levels are slightly raised by fluoxetine by 10%; however, the levels of norzotepine are doubled.

Where antipsychotic levels are raised monitor the outcome of concurrent use and adjust the doses as necessary. Some have suggested that the antipsychotic dose should be re-evaluated before the SSRI is started. The manufacturers of sertindole suggest that low maintenance doses of sertindole are used and that ECG monitoring is necessary as sertindole can prolong the QT interval. A risperidone dose reduction by one-third has been suggested with fluoxetine use. The manufacturers recommend halving the dose of aripiprazole with fluoxetine or paroxetine. A dose adjustment of olanzapine with SSRIs other than fluvoxamine is not expected to be necessary. A dose adjustment of risperidone with SSRIs other than fluoxetine or paroxetine is not expected to be necessary. Note that both groups of drugs lower the seizure threshold. Caution is advised when paliperidone or phenothiazines are taken with other drugs that may lower the seizure threshold, such as the SSRIs.

Antipsychotics + Sucralfate

Sucralfate can reduce the absorption of sulpiride by about 40%.

Separating dosing by 1 to 2 hours appears to minimise this interaction.

Antipsychotics + Tricyclics

Studies and case reports have described increased tricyclic antidepressant levels with phenothiazines. There is currently evidence for this interaction between:

- chlorpromazine and imipramine
- flupentixol and imipramine or desipramine
- fluphenazine and imipramine
- haloperidol and desipramine
- levomepromazine and nortriptyline
- perphenazine and amitriptyline, imipramine, desipramine or nortriptyline
- thioridazine and desipramine, imipramine or nortriptyline

Further, antipsychotic levels may be raised or their clearance reduced by the tricyclics, and this has been seen with:

- amitriptyline, imipramine or nortriptyline and chlorpromazine

The concurrent use of antipsychotics and tricyclics has also resulted in extrapyramidal reactions and seizures (both groups of drugs lower the seizure threshold). Despite these reactions these drugs are widely used in combination, and a number of fixed-dose combinations have been marketed. Also note that additive QT-prolonging effects are possible with certain combinations, see drugs that prolong the QT interval, page 277.

> Concurrent use is common. No action is generally needed but bear the interaction in mind in case of problems. Additive antimuscarinic adverse effects are also possible, see antimuscarinics, page 90.

Antipsychotics + Valproate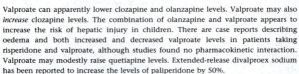

Valproate can apparently lower clozapine and olanzapine levels. Valproate may also *increase* clozapine levels. The combination of olanzapine and valproate appears to increase the risk of hepatic injury in children. There are case reports describing oedema and both increased and decreased valproate levels in patients taking risperidone and valproate, although studies found no pharmacokinetic interaction. Valproate may modestly raise quetiapine levels. Extended-release divalproex sodium has been reported to increase the levels of paliperidone by 50%.

> Bear in mind the potential for a change in the levels of clozapine and/or an increase in its adverse effects, and adjust the dose as necessary. With olanzapine, it has been suggested that liver enzymes should be monitored every 3 to 4 months for the first year of treatment, thereafter monitoring every 6 months if no adverse effects are detected. Bear the cases of an interaction with risperidone in mind in if unexpected changes in valproate levels or oedema occurs. Consider a dose reduction of paliperidone if it is given with divalproex sodium. Consider the possibility of an interaction with valproate if quetiapine adverse effects increase.

Antipsychotics + Venlafaxine

Venlafaxine can almost double haloperidol levels. Adverse effects resulting from this interaction have been seen in practice.

> Be aware that increased haloperidol adverse effects (e.g. sedation, agitation, movement disorders) may occur. It may be necessary to reduce the haloperidol dose.

Apomorphine

Apomorphine + 5-HT$_3$-receptor antagonists

Extrapyramidal adverse effects, profound hypotension and loss of consciousness have been reported with the concurrent use of ondansetron and subcutaneous apomorphine (for Parkinsoñs disease). Other 5-HT₃-receptor antagonists may interact similarly.

> The US manufacturer of subcutaneous apomorphine for Parkinson's disease contraindicates concurrent use of all 5-HT₃-receptor antagonists. However, the manufacturers of sublingual apomorphine used for erectile dysfunction state that it may be used safely with ondansetron.

Apomorphine + Metoclopramide

Metoclopramide is a centrally-acting dopamine antagonist and can oppose the effects of apomorphine, and also worsen Parkinson's disease.

> Concurrent use should generally be avoided. Domperidone is the antiemetic of choice in Parkinson's disease, and may also be used safely in patients taking sublingual apomorphine for erectile dysfunction.

Aprepitant

Fosaprepitant is a prodrug of aprepitant, and therefore has the potential to interact similarly.

Aprepitant + Azoles

Ketoconazole increases the AUC of aprepitant 5-fold. The manufacturer predicts that itraconazole, posaconazole and voriconazole may interact similarly. Fosaprepitant, a prodrug of aprepitant, would be expected to interact similarly.

> The manufacturers recommend caution when aprepitant is given with these azoles. The lowest dose of aprepitant may be appropriate. Counsel patients about aprepitant adverse effects (e.g. hiccups, fatigue, constipation, headache).

Aprepitant + Benzodiazepines ⚠️

Aprepitant inhibits the metabolism of midazolam and doubles the levels of oral midazolam after 5 days of concurrent use. A few days after aprepitant treatment is stopped a transient slight reduction in midazolam plasma levels may occur. Other benzodiazepines metabolised by CYP3A4 (alprazolam, triazolam) would be expected to interact similarly. Aprepitant appears to have less effect on *intravenous* midazolam. Fosaprepitant, a prodrug of aprepitant, would be expected to interact similarly.

> Aprepitant may be expected to increase the drowsiness and length of sedation and amnesia in patients given midazolam (and possibly alprazolam or triazolam). Consider reducing the midazolam dose and monitor the outcome of concurrent use carefully.

A

Aprepitant + **Calcium-channel blockers**

The concurrent use of aprepitant and diltiazem increases the levels of both drugs by almost 2-fold, although this did not result in any significant cardiovascular effects. Fosaprepitant moderately raises diltiazem levels, and a small decrease in blood pressure was reported. It seems likely that verapamil will interact with both drugs in the same way as diltiazem.

Consider giving the lowest dose of aprepitant and be alert for aprepitant adverse effects such as hiccups, fatigue, constipation and headache. Also be aware of a potential decrease in blood pressure if either of these antiemetics is given to a patient taking diltiazem or verapamil.

Aprepitant + **Carbamazepine**

Rifampicin, a potent inducer of CYP3A4, reduces the AUC of aprepitant by 91%; reduced efficacy would be expected. Carbamazepine, another potent inducer of CYP3A4, is predicted to interact similarly, both with aprepitant, and its prodrug, fosaprepitant.

The UK manufacturer recommends that concurrent use should be avoided.

Aprepitant + **Contraceptives**

Aprepitant reduces the levels of ethinylestradiol and norethisterone (given as a combined hormonal contraceptive). Greater effects were seen in another study when dexamethasone was also given with aprepitant. Contraceptive efficacy would be expected to be reduced. Fosaprepitant, a prodrug of aprepitant, would be expected to interact similarly. The contraceptive efficacy of oral progestogen-only contraceptives, the etonogestrel implant and emergency hormonal contraceptives (both progestogen-only and combined hormonal preparations) are also expected to be reduced.

The manufacturer recommends that alternative or additional contraceptive methods should be used during aprepitant therapy and for 2 months (UK advice) or one month (US advice) after the last dose of aprepitant. The same advice is given for fosaprepitant. For general advice on the use of enzyme inducers and contraceptives, see contraceptives, page 233.

Aprepitant + **Corticosteroids**

In the short-term, aprepitant increases the AUC of dexamethasone (by about 2.2-fold) and methylprednisolone (by up to 2.5-fold). Fosaprepitant, a prodrug of aprepitant, would be expected to interact similarly.

The manufacturers recommend that the usual dose of dexamethasone should be reduced by about 50% when given with aprepitant. In clinical studies a dexamethasone regimen of 12 mg on day one and 8 mg on days 2 to 4 was used, and this is the recommended regimen. They also recommend that the usual dose of intravenous methylprednisolone is reduced by 25%, and the usual oral dose by 50%, in the presence of aprepitant. However, the manufacturer also notes that during continuous treatment with methylprednisolone, levels would be expected to *decrease* over the following 2 weeks. The effect is expected to be greater if methylprednisolone is given orally rather than intravenously.

Aprepitant + **Ergot derivatives** ✖

Aprepitant is predicted to increase the levels of the ergot derivatives in the short-term, then reduce them within 2 weeks. Ergotism could occur. Fosaprepitant, a prodrug of aprepitant, would be expected to interact similarly.

> The effect may persist for 2 weeks after aprepitant is stopped. Avoid the combination where possible. Concurrent use needs close monitoring (e.g. for cold extremities and other signs of ergot adverse effects).

Aprepitant + **Herbal medicines or Dietary supplements** ✖

Rifampicin, a potent inducer of CYP3A4, reduces the AUC of aprepitant by 91%; reduced efficacy would be expected. St John's wort, another inducer of CYP3A4, is predicted to interact similarly, both with aprepitant, and its prodrug, fosaprepitant.

> The UK manufacturer recommends that concurrent use should be avoided.

Aprepitant + **HRT**

Aprepitant reduces the levels of ethinylestradiol and norethisterone (given as a combined hormonal contraceptive). Greater effects were seen in another study when dexamethasone was also given with aprepitant. The hormones in HRT are similar to those used in hormonal contraceptives, and so may be affected by enzyme-inducing drugs in the same way. Note that fosaprepitant, a prodrug of aprepitant, would also be expected to reduce HRT levels.

> Consider the possibility of reduced HRT efficacy. This effect would be most likely noticed where HRT is prescribed for menopausal vasomotor symptoms, but might be difficult to detect where the indication is osteoporosis. The interaction is not relevant to HRT applied locally for menopausal vaginitis.

Aprepitant + **Macrolides** ⚠

Ketoconazole, a potent CYP3A4 inhibitor, increases the AUC of aprepitant 5-fold. The manufacturer predicts that clarithromycin and telithromycin will interact similarly. Fosaprepitant, a prodrug of aprepitant, would also be expected to interact with these macrolides in this way.

> The manufacturer recommends caution when aprepitant is used with any potent inhibitor of CYP3A4 (they name clarithromycin and telithromycin). The lowest dose of aprepitant may be appropriate. Counsel patients about adverse effects (e.g. hiccups, fatigue, constipation, headache). Other macrolides may also interact, although it seems unlikely that they all will, see macrolides, page 361.

Aprepitant + **Phenobarbital** ✖

Rifampicin, a potent inducer of CYP3A4, reduces the AUC of aprepitant (and probably its prodrug, fosaprepitant) by 91%; reduced efficacy would be expected. Phenobarbital

A

(and therefore probably primidone), another potent inducer of CYP3A4, is predicted to interact similarly.

> The UK manufacturer recommends that concurrent use should be avoided.

Aprepitant + **Phenytoin**

The manufacturers predict that phenytoin (and therefore probably its prodrug, fosphenytoin) may reduce the levels of aprepitant and therefore reduce its efficacy. Phenytoin levels may also be reduced by aprepitant. Fosaprepitant, a prodrug of aprepitant, would be expected to interact similarly.

> Avoid concurrent use. If both drugs are given monitor aprepitant (and fosaprepitant) and phenytoin (and fosphenytoin) efficacy carefully.

Aprepitant + **Protease inhibitors**

Ketoconazole increases the AUC of aprepitant 5-fold. The manufacturer suggests that potent inhibitors of CYP3A4 may interact similarly; they specifically name ritonavir and nelfinavir although other protease inhibitors could also interact in this way. Fosaprepitant, a prodrug of aprepitant, would be expected to interact with the protease inhibitors in the same way as aprepitant.

> The lowest dose of aprepitant may be appropriate. Counsel patients about adverse effects (e.g. hiccups, fatigue, constipation, headache).

Aprepitant + **Rifampicin (Rifampin)**

Rifampicin reduced the AUC of aprepitant by 91%, and reduced efficacy would be expected. Fosaprepitant, a prodrug of aprepitant, would be expected to interact similarly.

> The UK manufacturer recommends that concurrent use should be avoided.

Aprepitant + **Warfarin and other oral anticoagulants**

Aprepitant modestly reduces warfarin levels and slightly decreases the INR in healthy subjects. Fosaprepitant, a prodrug of aprepitant, would be expected to interact similarly.

> The manufacturer recommends that the INR should be monitored closely for 2 weeks, particularly 7 to 10 days after each 3-day course of aprepitant. They also recommend similar caution with acenocoumarol.

Artemether

Co-artemether is a combination product containing artemether and lumefantrine, and its interactions are discussed under the individual constituents.

Artemether + Azoles

Ketoconazole doubled the AUC of artemether in one study. However, this is within the range of inter-individual variability and no changes in ECG parameters or increases in adverse events were reported. Itraconazole is likely to interact similarly, as are posaconazole and voriconazole.

> This increase is unlikely to be clinically relevant, and no dose adjustment is necessary when artemether with lumefantrine is used with ketoconazole.

Artemether + Food

Food, especially high-fat food, moderately increases the absorption of artemether.

> As soon as patients can tolerate food, artemether should be taken with food to increase absorption. Patients who are unable to eat during treatment should be closely monitored as they may be at greater risk of treatment failure.

Artemether + Grapefruit juice

Grapefruit juice doubles the AUC of artemether.

> Based on the evidence with ketoconazole, above, this increase is not expected to be clinically significant and no dose adjustment of artemether is required.

Aspirin

Aspirin + Contraceptives

Hormonal contraceptives lower aspirin levels. A few early reports suggest that the very occasional failure of copper IUDs to prevent pregnancy may have been due to an interaction with aspirin.

> The evidence is insufficient to justify general precautions. No action is needed.

Aspirin + Corticosteroids

Salicylate levels are reduced by corticosteroids, and therefore salicylate levels may rise, possibly to toxic concentrations, if the corticosteroid is withdrawn without salicylate dose adjustment. Concurrent use increases the risk of gastrointestinal bleeding and ulceration.

Patients taking high-dose salicylates should be monitored to ensure that the levels remain adequate when corticosteroids are added and do not become excessive if they are withdrawn.

Aspirin + Diuretics

Loop diuretics

Aspirin may reduce the diuretic effect of bumetanide, furosemide, and piretanide, and the combination of aspirin and furosemide may increase the risk of acute renal failure and salicylate toxicity. The risk of ototoxicity with high doses of salicylates may theoretically be increased by loop diuretics.

The clinical significance of this interaction is unclear. However, aspirin should be avoided in patients with recurrent hospital admissions for worsening heart failure. Salicylate toxicity may occur if furosemide is given concurrently in patients receiving high doses of salicylates. Be aware that renal impairment and ototoxicity are a possibility in patients receiving high dose of salicylates, and consider increasing monitoring for these effects.

Spironolactone

Although studies in healthy subjects have found that the spironolactone-induced loss of sodium in the urine is reduced, a study in hypertensive patients showed that the blood pressure-lowering effects of spironolactone were not affected by analgesic dose aspirin.

Concurrent use need not be avoided, but if the diuretic response to spironolactone is less than expected, consider this interaction as a cause.

Aspirin + Food

Food delays the absorption of aspirin but does not affect the overall amount absorbed.

Avoid food if rapid analgesia is needed. Otherwise aspirin is better taken with or after food to minimise gastric irritation.

Aspirin + Gold

A study in patients given analgesic doses of aspirin suggested that the concurrent use of gold can increase aspirin-induced hepatotoxicity.

Other analgesics, such as fenoprofen, appear safer than aspirin (in analgesic doses) so it is probably wise to consider an alternative analgesic.

Aspirin + Heparin

Although the concurrent use of aspirin and heparin is indicated in specific situations (such as acute coronary syndromes), combined use slightly increases the risk of haemorrhage, and may contribute to the development of epidural or spinal haematoma after epidural anaesthesia.

> Unless specifically indicated, it may be prudent to avoid the combined use of aspirin with heparin because of the likely increased risk of bleeding. Patients should be monitored closely for signs of bleeding. Extreme caution is needed if combined use is considered appropriate in patients undergoing epidural anaesthesia.

Aspirin + Herbal medicines or Dietary supplements

Ginkgo biloba

Ginkgo biloba alone has been associated with platelet, bleeding, and clotting disorders, and there are isolated reports of clinically significant bleeding after its concurrent use with antiplatelet drugs such as aspirin. However, several studies have found no evidence of an increased risk of bleeding with concurrent use.

> The evidence is too slim to advise patients against taking aspirin with *Ginkgo biloba*, but some do recommend caution. This seems prudent as caution is generally recommended with concurrent use of more than one conventional antiplatelet drugs. Patients should be told to seek professional advice if any bleeding problems arise.

Tamarindus indica

Tamarindus indica (tamarind) fruit extract markedly increased the absorption of aspirin and caused a 3-fold increase in its levels.

> The clinical relevance of this interaction is unknown, but large rises in the levels of analgesic dose aspirin may result in toxicity. Bear this in mind if analgesic doses of aspirin are taken with this fruit extract.

Aspirin + Kaolin

Kaolin-pectin causes a small reduction in the absorption of aspirin, which is not clinically relevant.

> No action needed.

Aspirin + Low-molecular-weight heparins

Although the concurrent use of aspirin and a low-molecular-weight-heparin is indicated in specific situations (such as acute coronary syndromes), combined use slightly increases the risk of haemorrhage. Cases of retroperitoneal and spinal haematoma have been reported with concurrent use of low-molecular-weight heparins (e.g. enoxaparin) and aspirin.

> Unless specifically indicated, it may be prudent to avoid the combined use of aspirin with a low-molecular-weight-heparin because of the likely increased risk of bleeding. Patients should be monitored closely for signs of bleeding. Extreme

A

caution is needed if combined use is considered appropriate in patients undergoing epidural anaesthesia.

Aspirin + Methotrexate ⚠

Analgesic-dose aspirin slightly reduces the clearance of methotrexate. Concurrent use may increase the incidence of methotrexate toxicity (pancytopenia, pneumonitis).

Regular antiplatelet-dose aspirin in patients stabilised on methotrexate seems unlikely to cause a significant problem. With analgesic-dose aspirin the risks are likely to be lowest in those taking low-dose methotrexate for psoriasis or rheumatoid arthritis. Patients should be counselled regarding non-prescription aspirin use. Patients should be told to report any sign or symptom suggestive of infection, particularly sore throat (which might possibly indicate that white cell counts have fallen) or dyspnoea or cough (suggestive of pulmonary toxicity).

Aspirin + Metoclopramide ✓

Although some studies have found that metoclopramide increases the rate of aspirin absorption, others have found no change, and the clinical efficacy of aspirin seems unaltered.

No action needed. This may be a beneficial interaction if a faster onset of analgesia is needed.

Aspirin + Mifepristone ❓

Theoretically NSAIDs (including aspirin) might reduce the efficacy of mifepristone, and combined use is often not recommended. However, evidence from two studies with naproxen and diclofenac suggests no reduction in mifepristone efficacy.

Because of theoretical concerns of antagonistic effects, NSAID analgesics have been avoided in protocols for medical abortion. However, the limited available evidence suggests that this might not be necessary.

Aspirin + NSAIDs ❓

Non-selective NSAIDs may antagonise the antiplatelet effects of aspirin and reduce its cardioprotective effects. Some NSAIDs (particularly coxibs) are also associated with an increased thrombotic/cardiovascular risk. Combined use of NSAIDs (including coxibs) and aspirin, even in low-dose, increases the risk of gastrointestinal bleeds.

The CHM in the UK considers that there may be a small increased risk of thrombotic events with the non-selective NSAIDs, particularly when used at high doses and for long-term treatment. They advise that the combination of a non-aspirin NSAID and low-dose aspirin should only be used if absolutely necessary, and patients taking long-term aspirin should be reminded to avoid NSAIDs, including non-prescription NSAIDs. In addition, the European Society of Cardiology guidelines recommend that patients resistant to antiplatelet treatment should not be given either coxibs or non-selective NSAIDs with aspirin, and recommend that coxibs and NSAIDs should not be used after myocardial infarction. If antiplatelet dose aspirin is used with NSAIDs, gastroprotection (e.g. a proton pump inhibitor) should be considered, especially when other risk factors (e.g. corticosteroids) are present. There is no clinical rationale for the combined use of anti-inflammatory/analgesic doses of aspirin and NSAIDs, and such use should be avoided.

Aspirin + Phenytoin

Although it has been suggested that aspirin enhances the effects of phenytoin, there appears to be no good evidence to show that a clinically significant interaction occurs.

No action needed.

Aspirin + Probenecid

The uricosuric effects of high doses of aspirin or other salicylates and probenecid are mutually antagonistic. Low dose, enteric-coated aspirin appears not to interact.

Regular dosing with substantial amounts of salicylates should be avoided, but small very occasional analgesic doses probably do not matter. Salicylate levels of 50 to 100 mg/L are necessary before this interaction occurs.

Aspirin + Quinidine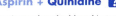

A patient and two healthy subjects given quinidine with aspirin (325 mg twice daily or more) showed a 2- to 3-fold increase in bleeding times. The patient developed petechiae and gastrointestinal bleeding.

This interaction appears to result from the additive effects of the two drugs. Be aware of the potential for this interaction if the combination is used. However, significant interactions seem rare.

Aspirin + SSRIs

The SSRIs may increase the risk of upper gastrointestinal bleeding and the risk appears to be further increased by the concurrent use of antiplatelet drugs including aspirin. The overall evidence for an increased risk of bleeding when giving an SSRI with antiplatelet-dose aspirin is conflicting, with some studies demonstrating an increased risk and others suggesting no additional antiplatelet effect occurs.

The manufacturers of the SSRIs warn that patients should be cautioned about the concurrent use of aspirin. For analgesic dose aspirin, alternatives such as paracetamol (acetaminophen), or less gastrotoxic NSAIDs, such as ibuprofen, may be considered. If the combination of an SSRI and aspirin cannot be avoided, consider giving a gastroprotective drug (such as a proton pump inhibitors), especially in elderly patients or those with a history of gastrointestinal bleeding.

Aspirin + **Sulfinpyrazone** ⚠

The uricosuric effects of the salicylates, including analgesic-dose aspirin, and sulfinpyrazone are mutually antagonistic.

Concurrent use for uricosuria should be avoided. Analgesic doses of aspirin as low as 700 mg can cause an appreciable fall in uric acid excretion. Regular dosing with substantial amounts of salicylates should be avoided, but small very occasional analgesic doses probably do not matter. Salicylate levels of 50 to 100 mg/L are necessary before this interaction occurs. Note that sulfinpyrazone can cause gastric bleeding and inhibit platelet aggregation which may be additive with aspirin.

Aspirin + **Valproate** ❓

Sodium valproate toxicity developed in several patients given large and repeated doses of aspirin and one elderly patient given regular low-dose aspirin.

Any interaction seems rare. Bear the potential for an interaction in mind should any unexpected valproate adverse effects occur in patients taking aspirin, particularly in high doses, and consider advising patients to monitor for indicators of valproate toxicity (such as nausea, vomiting, dizziness, rash, ataxia).

Aspirin + **Vitamin C** ✅

Aspirin appears to reduce the absorption of vitamin C by about one-third.

The clinical importance of this interaction is unclear, however it has been suggested that normal physiological requirements of vitamin C (30 to 60 mg ascorbic acid daily) may need to be increased to 100 to 200 mg daily.

Aspirin + **Warfarin and other oral anticoagulants** ⚠

High doses of aspirin (4 g daily or more) can increase prothrombin times. It also damages the stomach wall, which increases the risks of bleeding. Low-dose aspirin (75 to 325 mg daily) increases the risk of bleeding when given with warfarin by about 1.5- to 2.5-fold, although, in most studies the absolute risks have been small. Increased warfarin effects have been seen when the salicylates methyl salicylate or trolamine salicylate, were used on the skin.

It is usual to avoid normal analgesic and anti-inflammatory doses of aspirin while taking any anticoagulant. Patients should be told that many non-prescription analgesic, antipyretic, cold and influenza preparations may contain substantial amounts of aspirin. Warn them that it may be listed as acetylsalicylic acid. Paracetamol (acetaminophen) is a safer analgesic substitute (but not entirely without problems). Low-dose aspirin is also associated with an increased risk of bleeding. However, in certain patient groups (for example, those with prosthetic heart valves at high risk of thromboembolism) the benefits may outweigh the risks. Consider adding a gastroprotective drug in those who are at risk of gastrointestinal bleeding. In addition, in the long-term, aspirin doses should be limited to no more than 81 mg daily in those taking oral anticoagulants. Any interaction with topical salicylates seems likely to be rare.

Aspirin + Zafirlukast

Aspirin 650 mg four times daily increases zafirlukast levels by 45%.

The clinical importance of this interaction awaits assessment, although it is likely to be limited. The manufacturers do not suggest any alteration in the zafirlukast dose.

Atomoxetine

Atomoxetine + MAOIs

The manufacturer notes that other drugs that affect brain monoamine levels (like atomoxetine) have caused serious reactions (including symptoms of serotonin syndrome, page 454 and symptoms similar to neuroleptic malignant syndrome) when taken with MAOIs.

The manufacturer contraindicates the use of atomoxetine during and for 2 weeks after stopping an MAOI.

Atomoxetine + Mirtazapine

Atomoxetine is a sympathomimetic that acts as a noradrenaline (norepinephrine) reuptake inhibitor. The manufacturers therefore predict that it may have additive or synergistic pharmacological effects with other drugs that affect noradrenaline, such as mirtazapine.

The manufacturer recommends caution. Be aware that additive effects are possible and monitor e.g. somnolence or agitation, as appropriate.

Atomoxetine + Nasal decongestants

Atomoxetine is a sympathomimetic that acts as a noradrenaline (norepinephrine) reuptake inhibitor. The manufacturers therefore predict that it may have additive or synergistic pharmacological effects with other drugs that affect noradrenaline, such as pseudoephedrine.

The manufacturer recommends caution. Be aware that additive effects are possible and monitor e.g. somnolence or agitation, as appropriate.

Atomoxetine + Quinidine

Paroxetine increases the AUC and levels of atomoxetine by 6.5-fold and 3.5-fold, respectively by inhibiting its metabolism by CYP2D6. Quinidine, also a CYP2D6 inhibitor, is expected to interact similarly.

It would seem prudent to monitor for an increase in atomoxetine adverse effects (somnolence, agitation). The atomoxetine dose should be titrated slowly with the

A

dose increased only if symptoms fail to improve and if the initial dose is well tolerated. The UK manufacturers say that the initial dose should be maintained for a minimum of 7 days before considering an increase.

Atomoxetine + Salbutamol (Albuterol) and related bronchodilators

Atomoxetine potentiated the increase in heart rate and blood pressure caused by salbutamol infusions in one study, but another study found no adverse interaction.

The manufacturers recommend caution when atomoxetine is given to patients receiving intravenous, oral, or high-dose nebulised salbutamol or other beta$_2$ agonists. Monitor heart rate and blood pressure carefully in the initial stages of concurrent use.

Atomoxetine + SSRIs

Paroxetine increases the AUC and levels of atomoxetine by 6.5-fold and 3.5-fold, respectively, which may increase the incidence of adverse effects. Fluoxetine interacts similarly.

It would seem prudent to monitor for an increase in adverse effects (somnolence, agitation). The atomoxetine dose should be started low and titrated slowly. The UK manufacturers say that the initial dose should be maintained for a minimum of 7 days before considering an increase.

Atomoxetine + Terbinafine

Paroxetine increases the AUC and levels of atomoxetine by 6.5-fold and 3.5-fold, respectively, by inhibiting its metabolism by CYP2D6. Terbinafine, also a CYP2D6 inhibitor, is expected to interact similarly.

It would seem prudent to monitor for an increase in adverse effects (somnolence, agitation). The atomoxetine dose should be started low and titrated slowly, with the dose increased only if symptoms fail to improve and if the initial dose is well tolerated. The UK manufacturers say that the initial dose should be maintained for a minimum of 7 days before considering an increase.

Atomoxetine + Tricyclics

Atomoxetine is a sympathomimetic that acts as a noradrenaline (norepinephrine) reuptake inhibitor. The manufacturers therefore predict that it may have additive or synergistic pharmacological effects with other drugs that affect noradrenaline, such as imipramine, and other tricyclics.

The manufacturer recommends caution. Be aware that additive effects are possible and monitor e.g. somnolence or agitation, as appropriate.

Atomoxetine + **Venlafaxine**

Atomoxetine is a sympathomimetic that acts as a noradrenaline (norepinephrine) reuptake inhibitor. The manufacturers therefore predict that it may have additive or synergistic pharmacological effects with other drugs that affect noradrenaline, such as venlafaxine.

The manufacturer recommends caution. Be aware that additive effects are possible and monitor e.g. somnolence or agitation, as appropriate.

Atovaquone

Atovaquone + **Food**

Fatty foods markedly increase the AUC of atovaquone tablets and suspension 2- to 3-fold.

Atovaquone (with proguanil) tablets should be taken with food, a milky drink or an enteral supplement, and atovaquone suspension should be taken with food. Monitor patients who are unable to tolerate taking atovaquone with food for treatment failure; consider intravenous treatment in the case of pneumocystis pneumonia.

Atovaquone + **Metoclopramide**

Metoclopramide appears to halve the levels of atovaquone.

The manufacturers advise caution on concurrent use. It has been suggested that metoclopramide should be given only if other antiemetics are unavailable, and, if it is used, that parasitaemia should be closely monitored.

Atovaquone + **NRTIs**

Moderate increases in the AUC of zidovudine have been seen with atovaquone in one study, whereas another study found no significant pharmacokinetic changes.

The increased zidovudine levels are unlikely to increase its adverse effects during a short-course of atovaquone and no dose adjustments are required. Nevertheless, the manufacturers recommend regular monitoring for zidovudine-associated adverse effects, particularly if atovaquone suspension is used, as this achieves higher atovaquone levels.

Atovaquone + **Protease inhibitors**

Atovaquone decreases the minimum levels of indinavir by almost 25%. The manufacturer of ritonavir predicts that it will decrease atovaquone levels; however, there appears to be no published data of an interaction with any other protease inhibitors.

The manufacturers recommend caution because of the potential risk of indinavir treatment failure, although the effect on indinavir alone was small. However, indinavir is usually used with ritonavir as a pharmacological booster and with other antiretrovirals, which might modify the interaction. The manufacturers recommend careful monitoring of atovaquone levels and/or therapeutic effects when it is used with ritonavir-boosted protease inhibitors.

Atovaquone + Rifabutin

In one study the concurrent use of atovaquone and rifabutin resulted in a 34% decrease in the AUC of atovaquone and a small 19% decrease in rifabutin levels.

It has been suggested that no atovaquone dose adjustment is needed. However, in the UK, the manufacturer of atovaquone still considers that rifabutin use could result in subtherapeutic atovaquone levels and so they advise against the use of this combination.

Atovaquone + Rifampicin (Rifampin)

Rifampicin reduces atovaquone levels by about 50% whereas atovaquone modestly raises rifampicin levels.

Concurrent use should be avoided because of the likelihood of sub-therapeutic atovaquone levels.

Atovaquone + Tetracyclines

Tetracycline reduces atovaquone levels by about 40%.

The manufacturers suggest that parasitaemia should be closely monitored in patients taking atovaquone (with proguanil) and tetracycline. In the UK, they also say that tetracycline should be given with caution to patients taking atovaquone for pneumocystis pneumonia.

Azathioprine

Azathioprine is rapidly and extensively metabolised to mercaptopurine. Mercaptopurine is therefore expected to share the interactions of azathioprine.

Azathioprine + Balsalazide

The haematological toxicity of azathioprine and mercaptopurine may be increased by 5-aminosalicylates. Balsalazide may be less likely to interact although this requires confirmation.

Full blood counts should be monitored routinely if azathioprine or mercaptopurine is used; however, it may be prudent to increase the frequency of monitoring when starting this combination. If any abnormalities arise, consider this interaction as a possible cause.

Azathioprine + **Co-trimoxazole**

There is some evidence that the risk of haematological toxicity may be increased in renal transplant patients taking azathioprine if they are also given co-trimoxazole (which contains sulfamethoxazole with trimethoprim) or trimethoprim, particularly if both drugs are taken for extended periods. However, other evidence suggests that the drugs may be used together safely, and the combination is commonly used in practice. Azathioprine is rapidly and extensively metabolised to mercaptopurine. Mercaptopurine is therefore expected to interact similarly.

Full blood count should be monitored if azathioprine or mercaptopurine is used. If any abnormalities arise, consider this interaction as a possible cause.

Azathioprine + **Leflunomide**

The manufacturers state that the concurrent use of leflunomide and azathioprine has not yet been studied but it would be expected to increase the risk of serious adverse reactions (haematological toxicity or hepatotoxicity). Azathioprine is rapidly and extensively metabolised to mercaptopurine. Mercaptopurine is therefore expected to interact similarly.

The manufacturers advise avoiding concurrent use. As the active metabolite of leflunomide has a long half-life of 1 to 4 weeks, a washout with colestyramine or activated charcoal should be given if patients are to be switched to other DMARDs.

Azathioprine + **Mesalazine (Mesalamine)**

The haematological toxicity of azathioprine and mercaptopurine may be increased by mesalazine.

Full blood counts should be monitored if azathioprine or mercaptopurine is used; however it may be prudent to increase the frequency of monitoring when starting this combination. If any abnormalities arise, consider this interaction as a possible cause.

Azathioprine + **Mycophenolate**

The manufacturers have recommended that mycophenolate should not be given with azathioprine because concurrent use has not been studied and both drugs have the potential to cause bone marrow suppression. Azathioprine is rapidly and extensively metabolised to mercaptopurine. Mercaptopurine is therefore expected to interact similarly.

Avoid concurrent use.

Azathioprine + **Olsalazine**

The haematological toxicity of azathioprine and mercaptopurine may be increased by olsalazine.

Full blood counts should be monitored if azathioprine or mercaptopurine is used; however, it may be prudent to increase the frequency of monitoring when starting this combination. If any abnormalities arise, consider this interaction as a possible cause.

Azathioprine + Sulfasalazine

The haematological toxicity of azathioprine and mercaptopurine may be increased by sulfasalazine.

Full blood counts should be monitored if azathioprine or mercaptopurine is used; however, it may be prudent to increase the frequency of monitoring when starting this combination. If any abnormalities arise, consider this interaction as a possible cause.

Azathioprine + Sulfonamides

There is some evidence that the risk of haematological toxicity may be increased in renal transplant patients taking azathioprine if they are also given co-trimoxazole (which contains the sulfonamide, sulfamethoxazole, and trimethoprim), particularly if both drugs are taken for extended periods. However, other evidence suggests that the drugs may be used together safely, and the combination is commonly used in practice. Azathioprine is rapidly and extensively metabolised to mercaptopurine. Mercaptopurine is therefore expected to interact similarly.

Full blood count should be monitored if azathioprine or mercaptopurine is used. If any abnormalities arise, consider this interaction as a possible cause.

Azathioprine + Trimethoprim

There is some evidence that the risk of haematological toxicity may be increased in renal transplant patients taking azathioprine if they are also given trimethoprim, particularly if both drugs are taken for extended periods. However, other evidence suggests that the drugs may be used together safely, and the combination of azathioprine or mercaptopurine and trimethoprim with sulfamethoxazole is commonly used in practice. Azathioprine is rapidly and extensively metabolised to mercaptopurine. Mercaptopurine is therefore expected to interact similarly.

Full blood count should be monitored if azathioprine or mercaptopurine is used. If any abnormalities arise, consider this interaction as a possible cause.

Azathioprine + Vaccines

The immune response of the body is suppressed by cytotoxic antineoplastics. The effectiveness of vaccines may be poor and generalised infection may occur in patients immunised with live vaccines. In one study the antibody response to pneumococcal vaccination was reduced by 60% in patients receiving antineoplastics, and suboptimal responses to influenza and measles vaccines have been reported.

Live vaccines should not be given to patients who are receiving cytotoxics or other immunosuppressant antineoplastics. In the UK, it is recommended that live vaccines should not be given during or within at least 6 months of such treatment.

Monitor the immune response to other types of vaccine. Consider whether vaccination can be carried out before or after azathioprine or mercaptopurine use.

Azathioprine + **Warfarin and other oral anticoagulants**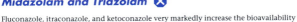

Azathioprine appears to increase warfarin requirements, and cases of bleeding have occurred when azathioprine is stopped. Dose increases of up to 4-fold have been needed. Mercaptopurine appears to interact similarly with acenocoumarol.

Monitor the anticoagulant effect closely if azathioprine or mercaptopurine is added or withdrawn and adjust the warfarin dose as necessary. Similar precautions would seem necessary with any coumarin.

Azoles

The azole antifungals are potent enzyme inhibitors, but they do not all affect the same isoenzymes. This explains their differing interaction profiles.

- Fluconazole is a potent inhibitor of CYP2C9 and CYP2C19, and generally only inhibits CYP3A4 at high doses (greater than 200 mg daily). Interactions are less likely with single doses used for genital candidiasis than with longer term use.
- Itraconazole and its major metabolite, hydroxy-itraconazole, are potent inhibitors of CYP3A4.
- Ketoconazole is a potent inhibitor of CYP3A4.
- Miconazole is a potent inhibitor of CYP2C9.
- Posaconazole is an inhibitor of CYP3A4.
- Voriconazole is an inhibitor of CYP2C9, CYP2C19 and CYP3A4.

A number of other azoles are only used topically in the form of skin creams or intravaginal preparations, and are not usually been associated with drug interactions, presumably because their systemic absorption is so low. Fluconazole, ketoconazole and voriconazole have been associated with prolongation of the QT interval, although generally not to a clinically relevant extent. However, they may also raise the levels of other drugs that prolong the QT interval, and these combinations are often contraindicated

Azoles + **Benzodiazepines**

Midazolam and Triazolam ✖

Fluconazole, itraconazole, and ketoconazole very markedly increase the bioavailability of oral midazolam and triazolam (AUCs increased by 3.5-fold to about 15-fold), thereby increasing and prolonging their sedative and amnesic effects. Voriconazole and posaconazole also markedly increase midazolam levels.

Most manufacturers contraindicate concurrent use of oral midazolam or triazolam with itraconazole or ketoconazole. Similarly, the manufacturer of miconazole oral gel also contraindicates triazolam and oral midazolam. Expect increased and prolonged sedation. If concurrent use is necessary, it may be prudent to reduce the dose of midazolam or triazolam by about 75% with itraconazole or ketoconazole. Other azoles are likely to interact similarly. Patients should be warned about increased sedation and counselled against driving or undertaking other skilled tasks.

Other benzodiazepines ▲

The effects of the benzodiazepines may be increased and prolonged by azole antifungals. Moderate interactions have been seen between alprazolam and itraconazole or ketoconazole, brotizolam and itraconazole. Fluconazole and voriconazole increase the levels of diazepam. Ketoconazole or itraconazole cause modest increases in the levels of the non-benzodiazepine hypnotics, zolpidem, eszopiclone, and zopiclone. Alprazolam and brotizolam should also be used with caution with oral miconazole.

The deepness of sleep and its duration may be increased. Monitor the outcome of concurrent use and consider decreasing the benzodiazepine or zopiclone, eszopiclone or zolpidem dose. Patients should be warned about increased sedation and counselled against driving or undertaking other skilled tasks.

Azoles + Bexarotene ❓

The manufacturers say that, in theory, itraconazole and ketoconazole may possibly raise oral bexarotene levels. An interaction is not expected to occur with a low to moderate intensity topical regimen of bexarotene as systemic exposure is low.

This interaction does not appear to have been studied in patients, so the clinical importance of these predictions are unknown. However, bear it in mind should any unexpected increase in bexarotene adverse effects (such as headache, pruritus, hyperlipidaemia, leucopenia) occur.

Azoles + Buspirone ▲

Buspirone levels are markedly increased by itraconazole (13-fold). Ketoconazole and miconazole oral gel (which at high doses, may be sufficiently absorbed to potentially have systemic effects) are predicted to interact similarly.

The manufacturers recommend reducing the buspirone dose to 2.5 mg either daily or twice daily if ketoconazole or itraconazole are used. The manufacturer of miconazole oral gel also advises caution and suggests that buspirone dose reductions may be needed on concurrent use.

Azoles + Busulfan ▲

Itraconazole reduces the clearance of busulfan by a modest 20%. There is some limited evidence that ketoconazole may increase the risk of hepatic veno-occlusive disease in those given high-dose busulfan. The manufacturer of miconazole oral gel (which may be sufficiently absorbed to potentially have systemic effects) predicts that it will also inhibit the metabolism of busulfan.

Although the rise in levels is only moderate, it would be prudent to monitor for busulfan toxicity. The manufacturer of miconazole oral gel suggests that dose reductions of busulfan may be necessary. Fluconazole appears not to interact, and so may be a useful alternative.

Azoles + Calcium-channel blockers
Lercanidipine

Ketoconazole markedly increases lercanidipine levels up to about 8-fold. Itraconazole, posaconazole and voriconazole are expected to interact similarly. Fluconazole is only likely to interact in doses of greater than 200 mg daily. At the maximum doses miconazole oral gel is sufficiently absorbed to potentially have systemic effects, and may also interact.

> The concurrent use of lercanidipine with itraconazole or ketoconazole is contraindicated. If other azoles are given with lercanidipine, be alert for the need to lower the lercanidipine dose and monitor for adverse effects, such as hypotension, headache, flushing, and oedema.

Other calcium-channel blockers

Itraconazole can raise felodipine levels up to 8-fold, which increases its adverse effects, in particular ankle and leg oedema. Ketoconazole can have a similar effect on nisoldipine levels. A few case reports suggest that isradipine and nifedipine can interact similarly with itraconazole, and that fluconazole can also interact with nifedipine. It is likely that all calcium-channel blockers will be affected in the same way, although probably to a greater or lesser extent. Posaconazole and voriconazole are expected to increase calcium-channel blocker levels. Fluconazole is only likely to interact in doses of greater than 200 mg daily. At the maximum doses miconazole oral gel is sufficiently absorbed to potentially have systemic effects, and may also interact.

> Monitor the outcome of concurrent use, being prepared to reduce the dose of calcium-channel blocker as necessary. Monitor for calcium-channel blocker adverse effects, such as hypotension, headache, flushing, and oedema.

Azoles + Carbamazepine
Fluconazole or Miconazole ⚠

Carbamazepine toxicity has been caused by fluconazole and miconazole.

> Evidence is limited. Nevertheless, monitor for signs of carbamazepine toxicity, which may present as nausea, vomiting, ataxia or drowsiness. It has been suggested that azoles may increase carbamazepine levels; consider monitoring and adjust the dose if necessary. Carbamazepine adverse effects include nausea, vomiting, ataxia and drowsiness).

Other azoles ⚠

Carbamazepine, either alone or when given with phenobarbital or phenytoin, has been shown to markedly decrease itraconazole levels resulting in treatment failure. Carbamazepine is predicted to decrease posaconazole and voriconazole levels. Carbamazepine levels may be raised by 30% by ketoconazole; other azoles may interact similarly.

> Concurrent use should be avoided unless the benefits are expected to outweigh the

risks, although note that the use of voriconazole is specifically contraindicated. If concurrent use is necessary it seems likely that the antifungal dose will need to be increased. It would seem prudent to use other alternatives wherever possible or monitor efficacy very closely. Be alert for any evidence of increased carbamazepine adverse effects (e.g. nausea, vomiting, ataxia and drowsiness).

Azoles + Ciclosporin (Cyclosporine)

Posaconazole

Three heart transplant patients required ciclosporin dose reductions of about 15 to 30% when posaconazole was added. The manufacturers also report cases of ciclosporin toxicity which resulted in significant adverse effects, including nephrotoxicity and one case of fatal leukoencephalopathy.

The manufacturers suggest that the dose of ciclosporin should be reduced by about 25% when posaconazole is started, with careful monitoring of ciclosporin levels and further dose adjustment as needed.

Voriconazole

Voriconazole increases the AUC of ciclosporin in stable renal transplant patients by between about 1.7- and 2.5-fold.

The dose of ciclosporin should be halved when initiating voriconazole, and ciclosporin levels should be carefully monitored during treatment. The ciclosporin dose should be increased again when voriconazole is withdrawn.

Other azoles

Ciclosporin levels may be increased by the azoles to a greater or lesser extent. Ketoconazole may cause 5- to 10-fold rises, while itraconazole and fluconazole may cause 2- to 3-fold rises. A case report suggests that intravenous miconazole interacts similarly and, in theory, miconazole oral gel may also interact (in high doses it may be sufficiently absorbed to interact systemically). However, many patients may not be affected. Rhabdomyolysis has been reported with the combination of ciclosporin and itraconazole, but four of these cases were complicated by the presence of statins.

Ciclosporin levels and/or effects (e.g. on renal function) should be monitored as a matter of routine, but the frequency of monitoring should be increased and the dose of ciclosporin adjusted accordingly if these azoles are stopped, started, or if the doses are altered. Dose reductions of up to 80% have been reported to be needed with itraconazole and ketoconazole.

Azoles + Cilostazol

Ketoconazole increases the AUC of cilostazol more than 2-fold, and increased cilostazol adverse effects (such as headache and diarrhoea) may occur. Itraconazole is predicted to interact similarly. Fluconazole and miconazole may also interact, but probably to a lesser extent.

The manufacturers recommend reducing the dose of cilostazol to 50 mg twice daily in the presence of itraconazole, ketoconazole, fluconazole or miconazole.

Azoles + Cinacalcet

Ketoconazole raises cinacalcet levels 2-fold and increased the incidence of cinacalcet adverse effects. Itraconazole and voriconazole are predicted to interact similarly.

It may be prudent to monitor parathyroid hormone and serum calcium more frequently if any of these azoles is started or stopped.

Azoles + Colchicine

Several case reports describe acute life-threatening colchicine toxicity caused by the concurrent use of macrolides that are known to inhibit CYP3A4. The manufacturers predict that itraconazole and ketoconazole will interact similarly.

If any patient is given colchicine and itraconazole or ketoconazole be alert for colchicine adverse effects such as nausea, vomiting, and diarrhoea, especially in patients with pre-existing renal impairment. Note that one UK manufacturer of colchicine contraindicates the concurrent use of colchicine with itraconazole or ketoconazole in patients with renal or hepatic impairment.

Azoles + Contraceptives

There are isolated reports of breakthrough bleeding and failure of oral combined hormonal contraceptives with fluconazole, itraconazole and ketoconazole. However, fluconazole, itraconazole, ketoconazole and voriconazole have been shown to modestly *increase* the levels of contraceptive steroids. In the case of voriconazole, the increase was considered roughly equivalent to increasing the ethinylestradiol dose from 35 micrograms to 50 micrograms. Intravaginal miconazole slightly increases the levels of ethinylestradiol and etonogestrel during the use of an intravaginal contraceptive ring. Oral combined hormonal contraceptives modestly increase the AUC of voriconazole.

Although anecdotal reports suggest that these antifungals can rarely make hormonal contraception less reliable, the pharmacokinetic data suggest that, if anything, an *enhanced* effect of the combined hormonal contraceptives is likely. Note that, of all the drugs proven to decrease the efficacy of combined hormonal contraceptives, all have also been shown to decrease contraceptive steroid levels. Furthermore, the manufacturers do not advise any additional precautions when taking oral contraceptives and azoles. However, some consider that the data warrant consideration being given to the use of additional contraceptive measures. The theoretical teratogenic risk from these azoles may have a bearing on this. The clinical relevance of the increase in voriconazole levels is unclear; however, bear the possibility of increased voriconazole adverse effects in mind on concurrent use.

Azoles + Corticosteroids

There is some evidence that itraconazole can increase the levels and/or effects of the active metabolite of ciclesonide, oral deflazacort, dexamethasone, methylprednisolone, and to a lesser extent, prednisolone and prednisone, as well as inhaled budesonide and fluticasone. Cases of Cushing's syndrome have been reported. One manufacturer predicts that inhaled beclometasone may be similarly affected.

Similarly, ketoconazole reduces the metabolism and clearance of methylprednisolone, increases the levels of the active metabolite of ciclesonide, modestly increases the systemic effect of inhaled budesonide and possibly inhaled fluticasone, and markedly increases the AUC of oral budesonide. One manufacturer predicts that inhaled beclometasone may be similarly affected.

Monitor the outcome of concurrent use of these azoles with the corticosteroids, and adjust the steroid dose according to the patients' response. Be alert for evidence of adrenal suppression (e.g. moonface, flushing, increased bruising and acne). Dose reductions of up to 50% have been recommended if ketoconazole is given with methylprednisolone. The manufacturer advises against the concurrent use of inhaled budesonide with itraconazole. However, if the concurrent use of inhaled budesonide and itraconazole or ketoconazole cannot be avoided, the interaction may be reduced by about half by separating the doses by 12 hours; consider reducing the budesonide dose if adverse effects occur. The manufacturers of ciclesonide suggest that the concurrent use of ketoconazole or itraconazole should be avoided unless the benefits outweigh the risks. Similarly, the manufacturer of fluticasone recommends caution, and, if possible, the avoidance of long-term treatment with itraconazole. Voriconazole appears to have less of an effect on prednisolone than itraconazole and may therefore be a suitable alternative. Note that increased corticosteroid immunosuppression may be undesirable in those with a fungal infection.

Azoles + Cyclophosphamide

Fluconazole and itraconazole inhibit the metabolism of cyclophosphamide. There is some evidence that, compared with fluconazole, itraconazole might increase cyclophosphamide toxicity.

Until more is known caution is advised when azoles are used in patients taking cyclophosphamide (other than therapies established in randomised clinical studies) being alert for unexpected toxicity or reduced efficacy.

Azoles + Darifenacin

Fluconazole

Fluconazole almost doubles darifenacin levels.

The UK manufacturers recommend an initial dose of darifenacin of 7.5 mg daily, increasing to 15 mg daily if the initial dose is well tolerated. The US manufacturers suggest that no dose adjustment is needed. Bear in mind the possibility of an interaction if antimuscarinic adverse effects (dry mouth, constipation, drowsiness) are increased.

Itraconazole, Ketoconazole and Voriconazole

Ketoconazole markedly increases the AUC of darifenacin by up to 10-fold. Itraconazole and possibly voriconazole would be expected to interact similarly.

The UK manufacturers contraindicate concurrent use whereas the US manufacturers recommend that the daily dose of darifenacin is limited to 7.5 mg daily. It may be prudent to assess adverse effects (such as dry mouth, constipation, and drowsiness) in these patients, and withdraw the drug if it is not tolerated.

Azoles + Digoxin

Itraconazole can cause a marked increase in digoxin levels (usually doubled, but a 6-fold increase was seen in one case). Toxicity may occur unless the digoxin dose is suitably reduced. Ketoconazole and posaconazole are predicted to interact similarly. Itraconazole may have significant negative inotropic effects, and this may oppose the pharmacological effects of digoxin.

> Monitor concurrent use for digoxin toxicity (e.g. bradycardia or nausea), taking digoxin levels as necessary. Adjust the dose accordingly. Note that, based on the interaction with itraconazole, the manufacturer of posaconazole advises monitoring digoxin levels.

Azoles + Disopyramide

Itraconazole and ketoconazole are predicted to increase disopyramide levels, which increases the risk of arrhythmias. Other azoles are likely to interact similarly, although probably to a greater or lesser extent.

> It would seem prudent to monitor the outcome of concurrent use carefully. It has been suggested that the use of azoles and disopyramide should be avoided. The UK manufacturers of ketoconazole and itraconazole contraindicate concurrent use, whereas the US manufacturer of itraconazole advises caution. If the concurrent use of disopyramide and any azole is essential, monitor the patient for an increase in disopyramide adverse effects (such as dry mouth, blurred vision, urinary retention and nausea).

Azoles + Diuretics

Eplerenone with Fluconazole

Fluconazole increases the AUC of eplerenone 2.2-fold.

> The dose of eplerenone should not exceed 25 mg daily. Monitor for an increase in dose-related adverse effects such as hyperkalaemia.

Eplerenone with Itraconazole or Ketoconazole

Ketoconazole increases the AUC of eplerenone 5.4-fold. Itraconazole is predicted to interact similarly.

> Concurrent use of either itraconazole or ketoconazole is contraindicated.

Hydrochlorothiazide with Fluconazole

A very brief report describes a 40% increase in fluconazole serum levels in a small group of healthy subjects also given hydrochlorothiazide.

> It has been suggested that the fluconazole dose need not be altered, but bear this interaction in mind in case of an unexpected response to treatment.

A

Azoles + **Domperidone**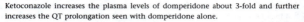

Ketoconazole increases the plasma levels of domperidone about 3-fold and further increases the QT prolongation seen with domperidone alone.

The manufacturers state that the concurrent use of domperidone with ketoconazole should be avoided. This seems to be a very cautious approach, but may be prudent because alternatives to this combination would usually be available.

Azoles + **Donepezil**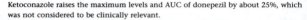

Ketoconazole raises the maximum levels and AUC of donepezil by about 25%, which was not considered to be clinically relevant.

Despite this finding the manufacturer recommends that donepezil should be used with ketoconazole or itraconazole with care.

Azoles + **Dopamine agonists** ⚠

Two patients taking cabergoline had improvements in their Parkinson's disease symptoms while taking itraconazole. In one case a 300% increase in cabergoline levels occurred, and the other patient reduced the dose of her medications without adversely affecting disease control. Bromocriptine is predicted to interact in the same way as cabergoline.

It would be prudent to monitor toxicity and efficacy in any patient taking cabergoline with itraconazole, or similar potent inhibitors of CYP3A4 such as ketoconazole. Similar caution would seem prudent with bromocriptine.

Azoles + **Dutasteride** ⚠

Potent CYP3A4 inhibitors (itraconazole, ketoconazole) may cause a clinically significant rise in dutasteride levels.

The manufacturers suggest reducing the dosing frequency if increased dutasteride adverse effects occur.

Azoles + **Endothelin receptor antagonists**

Fluconazole or Voriconazole ❌

Fluconazole is predicted to dramatically raise bosentan levels. Voriconazole may interact similarly. This may be expected to increase bosentan adverse effects, such as hepatotoxicity.

The manufacturers do not recommend the concurrent use of bosentan and fluconazole or voriconazole in the presence of other inhibitors of CYP3A4. If either drug is given with bosentan it would seem prudent to monitor the outcome, particularly for any effect on liver function tests.

Itraconazole or Ketoconazole

Ketoconazole increases bosentan levels 2-fold. Itraconazole is expected to interact similarly.

The clinical significance of the raised bosentan levels is unclear. The manufacturer suggests that no adjustment of the bosentan dose is likely to be required when it is used with ketoconazole (and therefore probably itraconazole).

Azoles + **Ergot derivatives**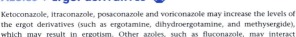

Ketoconazole, itraconazole, posaconazole and voriconazole may increase the levels of the ergot derivatives (such as ergotamine, dihydroergotamine, and methysergide), which may result in ergotism. Other azoles, such as fluconazole, may interact similarly, although to a lesser extent.

The UK manufacturers of various ergot derivatives contraindicate the concurrent use of all azoles. The US manufacturers of ergotamine and dihydroergotamine advise caution with fluconazole and clotrimazole, which are moderate CYP3A4 inhibitors. Any patient taking an ergot derivative with an azole should be closely monitored for signs of ergotism.

Azoles + **Fesoterodine**

Itraconazole, Ketoconazole, or Voriconazole 🔺

Ketoconazole increases fesoterodine levels by up to about 2.5-fold. Itraconazole and probably voriconazole would be expected to interact similarly.

The manufacturers state that the dose of fesoterodine should be restricted to 4 mg daily. Concurrent use is contraindicated in those with moderate to severe hepatic impairment.

Fluconazole ❓

Fluconazole is predicted to increase fesoterodine levels, although this is expected to be to a lesser extent than ketoconazole.

If fluconazole is added monitor for an increase in fesoterodine adverse effects (e.g. dry mouth, dizziness, insomnia), and consider reducing the fesoterodine dose if these become troublesome.

Azoles + **Food** ❓

Some foods increase the absorption of itraconazole capsules or tablets, but appear to decrease the bioavailability of itraconazole solution. Studies with ketoconazole have shown little effect of food on absorption although one found a decrease. Food increases the bioavailability of posaconazole suspension. The bioavailability of voriconazole is modestly reduced by food.

Itraconazole capsules are best taken with or after food, whereas the acidic solution should be taken at least 1 hour before food. Similarly, posaconazole should be taken with food. A confusing and conflicting picture is presented by the studies with ketoconazole; however, one manufacturer of ketoconazole says that it should always be taken with meals. The manufacturers of voriconazole recommend that it should be taken at least one hour before or at least one to two hours after a meal. Food does not appear to affect fluconazole capsules. Cola drinks may increase itraconazole and ketoconazole bioavailability, see H_2-receptor antagonists, below, and proton pump inhibitors, page 141.

Azoles + Galantamine

Ketoconazole increases the bioavailability of galantamine by 30%, which is predicted to increase galantamine adverse effects (e.g. nausea and vomiting).

A clinically significant interaction is not expected, however a decrease in the galantamine maintenance dose should be considered in patients who develop galantamine adverse effects. Note that, all azoles, to a greater or lesser extent, inhibit this isoenzyme, and therefore, until more is known, similar caution would seem prudent.

Azoles + H_2-receptor antagonists

H_2-receptor antagonists reduce the absorption of itraconazole (AUC reduced by about 50%), ketoconazole (AUC reduced by 60% and even 95% in some reports) and posaconazole (AUC reduced by about 40%).

The manufacturers recommend that if H_2-receptor antagonists are used, itraconazole and ketoconazole should be given with an acidic drink (such as cola), which increase their bioavailability. Itraconazole *solution* would not be expected to be affected. The US manufacturer advises caution on concurrent use. Posaconazole may also be given with an acidic drink to improve its bioavailability with H_2-receptor antagonists. However, the manufacturers currently recommend avoiding concurrent use, unless the benefits outweigh the risk. Fluconazole and voriconazole do not appear to interact and may therefore be suitable alternatives in some cases.

Azoles + Herbal medicines or Dietary supplements

Two weeks of treatment with St John's wort (*Hypericum perforatum*) halved the AUC of a single dose of voriconazole.

Patients requiring voriconazole should be asked about current or recent use of St John's wort, because they may be at risk of treatment failure. The manufacturers contraindicate concurrent use.

Azoles + Imatinib

Ketoconazole increases the AUC of imatinib by 40%. Voriconazole increased imatinib levels 2-fold in one patient, leading to adverse effects. The manufacturers of imatinib predict that itraconazole will interact similarly.

Caution is warranted on concurrent use, being alert for increased imatinib adverse effects (such as bone marrow suppression and diarrhoea).

Azoles + Isoniazid

Ketoconazole levels can be reduced by 50 to 80% by *rifampicin* (*rifampin*), and there seems to be a modest additional effect when isoniazid is also given.

Monitor efficacy closely and consider increasing the dose of ketoconazole if required. It may be prudent to consider an alternative antifungal.

Azoles + Lumefantrine

Ketoconazole doubled the AUC of lumefantrine in one study. However, this is within the range of inter-individual variability and no changes in ECG parameters or increases in adverse events were reported. Itraconazole and voriconazole are likely to interact similarly.

This increase is not expected to be clinically relevant, and the manufacturer advises that no dose adjustment is necessary when artemether with lumefantrine is used with these azoles.

Azoles + Macrolides

Although some moderate pharmacokinetic interactions occur between the azoles and macrolides, most do not appear to be of clinical significance. However, clarithromycin appears to almost double itraconazole levels, whereas erythromycin modestly increases itraconazole levels by about 44%. The manufacturer predicts that posaconazole levels will be increased by clarithromycin and erythromycin. Ketoconazole and itraconazole may increase telithromycin levels by about 52% and 22%, respectively, but no increase in adverse effects occurred.

Monitor the effects of concurrent use of these azoles with clarithromycin or telithromycin. Consider either reducing the dose of the affected drug if adverse effects occur or using a different combination. No dose adjustment is considered necessary when itraconazole is taken with erythromycin.

Azoles + Mefloquine

Ketoconazole increases the AUC of mefloquine by 79%. Itraconazole and voriconazole may interact similarly.

The clinical relevance of this is uncertain, but it may be prudent to exercise caution on the concurrent use of mefloquine and these azoles in case of an increase in adverse events. As mefloquine has a long half-life, the manufacturers also advise caution with the use of ketoconazole for up to 15 weeks after a course of mefloquine.

Azoles + Mirtazapine

Ketoconazole is reported to increase the peak plasma levels and AUC of mirtazapine by about 30% and 45%, respectively.

The manufacturers of mirtazapine advise caution on concurrent use with potent inhibitors of CYP3A4 such as the azoles. However note that the azoles differ in their effects on CYP3A4, see under Azoles, page 123 for further information. Monitor for adverse effects (e.g. oedema, sedation).

Azoles + NNRTIs

Delavirdine with Ketoconazole

Ketoconazole appears to raise delavirdine levels by 50%.

The clinical significance of this interaction is unclear. Monitor concurrent use for delavirdine adverse effects.

Delavirdine with Voriconazole

Voriconazole is predicted to increase delavirdine levels, and delavirdine is predicted to increase voriconazole levels.

The manufacturers suggest that patients be carefully monitored for evidence of drug toxicity and/or loss of efficacy during concurrent use.

Efavirenz with Itraconazole

Efavirenz appears to modestly decrease the levels and the AUC of itraconazole; however, cases of antifungal treatment failure and subtherapeutic itraconazole levels have been reported. The pharmacokinetics of efavirenz are not affected by itraconazole.

The manufacturers of efavirenz say that alternatives to itraconazole should be considered. If there are no appropriate alternatives, it might be prudent to increase the dose of itraconazole, with increased monitoring for efficacy and toxicity of the combination.

Efavirenz with Ketoconazole

Efavirenz appears to halve the levels of ketoconazole, although there appears to be no information on the clinical outcome of this interaction. Efavirenz levels may be raised by ketoconazole, which might increase adverse effects.

The risk of antifungal treatment failure should be considered with concurrent use. Cautious monitoring of the efficacy of ketoconazole and of an increase in the adverse effects of efavirenz would be prudent if concurrent use is deemed necessary.

Efavirenz with Posaconazole

Efavirenz appears to reduce the levels of posaconazole by about 50%. Posaconazole is predicted to increase efavirenz levels but no effect was seen in one study.

The manufacturer of posaconazole advises avoiding concurrent use of efavirenz unless the benefits outweigh the risks. If concurrent use is necessary, monitor for signs of posaconazole treatment failure and/or efavirenz toxicity, and adjust the dose accordingly.

Efavirenz with Voriconazole

Efavirenz markedly decreases voriconazole levels, and voriconazole modestly increases efavirenz levels.

> The dose of voriconazole should be doubled to 400 mg twice daily, and the efavirenz dose should be halved to 300 mg once daily. The dose of efavirenz should be increased back to 600 mg daily when the voriconazole course is finished.

Etravirine with Fluconazole

The manufacturer of etravirine predicts that fluconazole will increase the levels of etravirine, although this has not been specifically studied. Etravirine is not expected to affect the metabolism of fluconazole.

> Despite these predictions, the manufacturer advises that no dose adjustment of etravirine is needed when it is taken with fluconazole.

Etravirine with Ketoconazole

The manufacturers of etravirine predict that ketoconazole will increase the levels of etravirine, whereas etravirine is expected to reduce the levels of ketoconazole.

> The US manufacturer advises that dose adjustments of ketoconazole may be required. However, the UK manufacturer advises that no dose adjustment of either ketoconazole or etravirine is required with concurrent use.

Etravirine with Itraconazole

The manufacturers of etravirine predict that itraconazole will increase the levels of etravirine, whereas etravirine is expected to reduce the levels of itraconazole.

> The US manufacturer advises that dose adjustments of itraconazole may be required. However, the UK manufacturer advises that no dose adjustment of either itraconazole or etravirine is required with concurrent use.

Etravirine with Voriconazole

The manufacturers of etravirine predict the levels of both etravirine and voriconazole are likely to be raised on concurrent use.

> The US manufacturer advises that dose adjustments of voriconazole may be required. However, the UK manufacturer advises that no dose adjustment of either voriconazole or etravirine is required with concurrent use.

Nevirapine with Fluconazole

Fluconazole appears to double the exposure to nevirapine. However, studies have found no increase in adverse effects such as hepatitis, skin rashes or raised LFTs.

> Caution is warranted. Monitor the effects of nevirapine carefully, although an increase in adverse effects appears to be rare.

Nevirapine with Itraconazole

Nevirapine decreases the AUC and levels of itraconazole by 61% and 38%, respectively. Itraconazole does not appear to affect the pharmacokinetics of nevirapine.

> Monitor itraconazole efficacy carefully and anticipate the need to increase the dose.

A

Nevirapine with Ketoconazole

Ketoconazole slightly raises nevirapine levels, and nevirapine markedly lowers the AUC of ketoconazole.

The manufacturers of nevirapine state that ketoconazole should be avoided because of the risk of antifungal treatment failure.

Nevirapine with Voriconazole

Voriconazole is predicted to increase levels of nevirapine whereas nevirapine is predicted to decrease voriconazole levels.

The manufacturers suggest that patients be carefully monitored for evidence of drug toxicity and/or loss of efficacy during concurrent use.

Azoles + NRTIs

Didanosine

Itraconazole levels may become undetectable if buffered didanosine is taken at the same time. In one case this resulted in treatment failure. A similar interaction would be expected with ketoconazole.

Itraconazole and ketoconazole should be taken at least 2 hours before buffered didanosine. Consider changing to enteric-coated didanosine as it does not appear to affect absorption of these azoles. Itraconazole *solution* is not expected to be affected by buffered didanosine.

Zidovudine

In one study fluconazole increased the AUC of zidovudine by 74% but other studies have found that fluconazole causes only slight changes in zidovudine pharmacokinetics. Increased zidovudine levels, thought to be caused by itraconazole, have been seen in two cases.

Be aware that concurrent use may rarely result in zidovudine toxicity, however the minor interaction between zidovudine and fluconazole is not expected to be clinically significant.

Azoles + NSAIDs **A**

Fluconazole increases the AUC of celecoxib by 130% and increases the AUC of the active metabolite of parecoxib (valdecoxib) by 62%. Fluconazole almost doubles flurbiprofen and ibuprofen exposure. Voriconazole increases the levels of and/or exposure to diclofenac and ibuprofen 2-fold.

The manufacturers recommend that half the dose of celecoxib should be used in patients taking fluconazole whereas the US manufacturer suggests starting with the lowest recommended dose. A dose reduction of parecoxib is recommended in patients taking fluconazole. The clinical relevance of the interaction between voriconazole and diclofenac or ibuprofen and fluconazole with ibuprofen or flurbiprofen is unknown but lower doses of these NSAIDs may be adequate to accommodate it.

Azoles + Opioids

Alfentanil or Fentanyl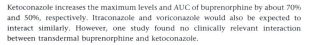

Some patients experience prolonged and increased alfentanil effects if they are also given fluconazole or voriconazole. Itraconazole and ketoconazole are expected to interact similarly. Fluconazole and voriconazole inhibit the metabolism of fentanyl. Posaconazole is predicted to interact similarly. There is a case report of a fatality possibly due to the interaction with fluconazole and transdermal fentanyl. Opioid toxicity has been reported when itraconazole was given to a patient with a fentanyl patch, however no interaction was seen in healthy subjects. Note that, at high doses, miconazole oral gel may be absorbed in sufficient quantities to have systemic effects, and the manufacturer predicts it will inhibit the metabolism of alfentanil.

A small, single dose of alfentanil is not expected to need adjustment, however, multiple doses or continuous infusions of alfentanil should be given with care. Be alert for evidence of prolonged alfentanil or fentanyl effects and respiratory depression. Consider using smaller doses of these opioids.

Buprenorphine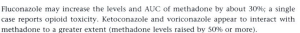

Ketoconazole increases the maximum levels and AUC of buprenorphine by about 70% and 50%, respectively. Itraconazole and voriconazole would also be expected to interact similarly. However, one study found no clinically relevant interaction between transdermal buprenorphine and ketoconazole.

Monitor for an increase in buprenorphine adverse effects (such as drowsiness, nausea and vomiting) with sublingual or intravenous and consider a buprenorphine dose reduction as necessary. One manufacturer advises that the dose of sublingual buprenorphine for opioid addiction should be halved when starting ketoconazole, although some manufacturers of sublingual and intravenous buprenorphine recommend avoiding concurrent use. One manufacturer states that no precaution is necessary with ketoconazole in patients using *transdermal* buprenorphine.

Methadone

Fluconazole may increase the levels and AUC of methadone by about 30%; a single case reports opioid toxicity. Ketoconazole and voriconazole appear to interact with methadone to a greater extent (methadone levels raised by 50% or more).

Patients given these azoles with methadone should be monitored for signs of opioid toxicity and a methadone dose alteration should be considered. However, note that the interaction with fluconazole is considered unlikely to be of general clinical significance.

Azoles + Phenobarbital

Itraconazole, Posaconazole, or Voriconazole ⊗

Limited evidence suggests phenobarbital causes a marked decrease in itraconazole levels, and might decrease ketoconazole levels. Phenobarbital is predicted to decrease posaconazole and voriconazole levels. Note that primidone is metabolised to phenobarbital and therefore may interact similarly with these azoles.

Concurrent use should be avoided unless the benefits are expected to outweigh the

A

risks, although note that the manufacturers contraindicate the use of voriconazole. If concurrent use is necessary it seems likely that the antifungal dose will need to be increased. It would seem prudent to use other alternatives wherever possible or monitor concurrent use very closely.

Ketoconazole

Phenobarbital (with phenytoin) has been reported to reduce the levels of ketoconazole and its antifungal effects. Note that primidone is metabolised to phenobarbital and therefore may interact similarly.

Be alert for any signs of a reduced antifungal response. Consider adjusting the dose of ketoconazole.

Azoles + Phenytoin

Fluconazole or Miconazole

Phenytoin levels are raised by fluconazole or miconazole, and toxicity has been reported. Fluconazole levels are not usually affected by phenytoin, although there is one report of reduced efficacy. Fosphenytoin, a prodrug of phenytoin, may interact similarly.

Toxicity can develop within 2 to 7 days unless the phenytoin dose is reduced. Monitor phenytoin levels closely and reduce the dose appropriately. Also be alert for any evidence of reduced antifungal effects and consider increasing the dose. Note that, at high doses, miconazole oral gel has the potential to interact.

Itraconazole or Ketoconazole

Phenytoin reduces itraconazole levels (by about 90%). Ketoconazole may interact similarly with phenytoin, and fosphenytoin, a prodrug of phenytoin, may interact similarly with these azoles.

Concurrent use of phenytoin and itraconazole (and probably ketoconazole) should be avoided unless the benefits are expected to outweigh the risks. It seems highly likely that these azoles will be ineffective.

Posaconazole or Voriconazole

Phenytoin decreases the levels of voriconazole and posaconazole by about 50%. Also, voriconazole increases the maximum levels and AUC of phenytoin by 67% and 81%, respectively. Potentially clinically significant increases in phenytoin levels have been reported in some patients taking posaconazole. Fosphenytoin, a prodrug of phenytoin, may interact similarly.

Concurrent use should be avoided unless the benefits outweigh the risks. If both drugs are used be alert for evidence of phenytoin toxicity (blurred vision, nystagmus, ataxia or drowsiness) and, if necessary, adjust the dose based on phenytoin levels. The dose of oral voriconazole should be increased from 200 to 400 mg twice daily, or from 100 mg to 200 mg twice daily in patients who weigh less than 40 kg, and intravenous voriconazole should be increased from 4 to 5 mg/kg twice daily. Similarly, consideration should be given to increasing the posaconazole dose.

Azoles + **Phosphodiesterase type-5 inhibitors**

Ketoconazole markedly raises the levels of tadalafil and very markedly raises the levels of vardenafil. There is some evidence that ketoconazole also reduces sildenafil clearance. Itraconazole, posaconazole and voriconazole are predicted to interact similarly. Note that at the maximum doses, miconazole oral gel is sufficiently absorbed to potentially have systemic effects and the manufacturers predict it will interact with sildenafil.

The manufacturers of sildenafil recommend that a low starting dose (25 mg) of sildenafil should be used for erectile dysfunction. The manufacturers say that for pulmonary hypertension the use of sildenafil with ketoconazole or itraconazole is contraindicated (UK) or not recommended (US). If itraconazole or ketoconazole is given with tadalafil, decrease the dose of tadalafil if adverse effects become troublesome. The US manufacturer advises that the dose of tadalafil should not exceed 10 mg in a 72-hour period, or 2.5 mg daily for patients taking ketoconazole (and therefore probably itraconazole). The UK manufacturer of vardenafil advises avoiding the concurrent use of ketoconazole or itraconazole in all patients, but specifically contraindicates concurrent use in those over 75-years-old. In contrast, the US manufacturer recommends that the dose of vardenafil should not exceed 5 mg in 24 hours when used with itraconazole or ketoconazole 200 mg daily, or 2.5 mg in 24 hours with itraconazole or ketoconazole 400 mg daily. Similar advice should be used in patients taking these phosphodiesterase type-5 inhibitors with posaconazole or voriconazole, and possibly miconazole.

Azoles + **Praziquantel**

Ketoconazole almost doubles the AUC of praziquantel, which appears to increase the incidence of mild adverse effects (headache and gastrointestinal adverse effects, including nausea and vomiting).

Information is limited, but all azoles have the potential to interact, to a greater or lesser extent (see azoles, page 123). It may be prudent to be alert for an increase in the adverse effects of praziquantel, although an increase in efficacy is also possible.

Azoles + **Protease inhibitors**

Ritonavir-boosted tipranavir with Fluconazole

Fluconazole increases tipranavir bioavailability and levels by about 50%.

The manufacturer of tipranavir states that fluconazole, in doses of greater than 200 mg daily, is not recommended. No dose adjustments are recommended for lower doses of fluconazole.

Protease inhibitors with Itraconazole

Itraconazole increases the levels of fosamprenavir, indinavir, ritonavir-boosted lopinavir, and saquinavir, and may theoretically increase the levels of other protease inhibitors. Some protease inhibitors, especially ritonavir and possibly indinavir, may increase itraconazole levels and cases of raised itraconazole levels and adverse effects have been reported. No significant interaction is predicted to occur between itraconazole and nelfinavir.

The manufacturers of indinavir advise modestly reducing the indinavir dose to

600 mg every 8 hours if it is to be given with itraconazole. The UK manufacturer of saquinavir recommends monitoring for saquinavir toxicity if itraconazole is used but states that no data are available for ritonavir-boosted saquinavir. Most manufacturers say that doses of itraconazole greater than 200 mg a day are not recommended with ritonavir-boosted protease inhibitors. Be alert for itraconazole adverse effects (e.g. abdominal pain, dyspepsia).

Protease inhibitors with Ketoconazole

Most protease inhibitors increase the levels of ketoconazole (up to about 3.5-fold with ritonavir). Ketoconazole may increase the levels of protease inhibitors, but this is usually not clinically significant. The exception may be indinavir, see below.

Ritonavir alone, ritonavir combined with darunavir, fosamprenavir, lopinavir, saquinavir and theoretically tipranavir may increase the adverse effects of ketoconazole. Most protease inhibitor manufacturers (although, see amprenavir or fosamprenavir, below) say that doses greater than 200 mg a day of ketoconazole are not recommended. Dose changes of the protease inhibitors are generally not needed (but see indinavir, below).

Amprenavir or Fosamprenavir with Ketoconazole

Amprenavir (the active metabolite of fosamprenavir) increases the levels of ketoconazole by about 50%. Ketoconazole only modestly increases the AUC of amprenavir. Ritonavir-boosted fosamprenavir increased the levels of ketoconazole 2.7-fold, but had no clinically significant effect on the pharmacokinetics of amprenavir or ritonavir.

The US manufacturer states that the ketoconazole dose may need to be reduced if unboosted fosamprenavir is given with a dose of ketoconazole greater than 400 mg daily. The US and UK manufacturers advise against the use of ketoconazole doses greater than 200 mg daily with ritonavir-boosted fosamprenavir. Increased monitoring for ketoconazole adverse effects is advised.

Indinavir with Ketoconazole

Ketoconazole raises the AUC of indinavir by 62%.

The US manufacturer of indinavir recommends that the dose of indinavir be reduced to 600 mg every 8 hours when used with ketoconazole.

Protease inhibitors with Posaconazole

Posaconazole appears to increase the AUC of atazanavir and ritonavir-boosted atazanavir. Other protease inhibitors are predicted to be similarly affected.

Patients should be monitored for atazanavir adverse effects and toxicity during concurrent use. Other protease inhibitors are predicted to interact similarly, and the same precautions are advisable.

Protease inhibitors with Voriconazole

In vitro studies suggest that the concurrent use of protease inhibitors with voriconazole may inhibit the metabolism of both drugs, although no interaction appears to occur with indinavir. Most protease inhibitors are combined with ritonavir as a pharmacological booster, see also ritonavir with voriconazole, below.

The manufacturers suggest that patients be carefully monitored for evidence of drug toxicity and/or loss of efficacy during concurrent use with ritonavir-boosted protease inhibitors.

Ritonavir with Voriconazole

Ritonavir decreases the AUC of voriconazole by 82%.

> Ritonavir, in doses of 400 mg twice daily or more, is contraindicated with voriconazole. Low doses of ritonavir (pharmacokinetic booster doses) should only be given if the benefits outweigh the risks.

Azoles + Proton pump inhibitors

The bioavailability of ketoconazole is reduced by omeprazole (AUC reduced by about 80%) and rabeprazole (bioavailability reduced by 30%). Other proton pump inhibitors are expected to behave similarly. Omeprazole also markedly reduces the absorption of itraconazole capsules (AUC decreased by 65%), but not the oral solution. Posaconazole absorption is predicted to be reduced by proton pump inhibitors. Omeprazole levels may be increased by ketoconazole (and therefore possibly itraconazole), and markedly increased by fluconazole and voriconazole. Voriconazole may more than double the levels of esomeprazole.

> An increase in the antifungal dose has been suggested to overcome the reduction in the bioavailability of the affected azoles by the proton pump inhibitors, as has giving ketoconazole or itraconazole with an acidic drink such as cola, which increases its bioavailability. The manufacturers of posaconazole advise avoiding concurrent use. Fluconazole and oral itraconazole solution appear to be unaffected, and they may therefore be alternatives. However, as fluconazole increases omeprazole levels, and an omeprazole dose adjustment may be required with long-term treatment. Voriconazole does not require a dose adjustment when given with omeprazole. However, the manufacturers of voriconazole recommend halving the dose of omeprazole, but this is probably only necessary with higher doses. The dose of esomeprazole will only need adjusting in those taking voriconazole if the esomeprazole dose is very high (e.g. 240 mg).

Azoles + Quinidine

Itraconazole increases quinidine levels by 60%, and ketoconazole caused a marked increase in quinidine levels in one patient. Fluconazole, posaconazole and voriconazole are predicted to increase quinidine levels, although the effect of fluconazole may be more modest. Note that, a large proportion of miconazole oral gel may be swallowed, and therefore adequate systemic absorption may occur to produce an interaction.

> The manufacturers of ketoconazole, itraconazole, miconazole, posaconazole and voriconazole contraindicate the concurrent use of quinidine. Therefore, it may be prudent to avoid using fluconazole with quinidine. However if concurrent use is essential, the patient should be very closely monitored and the dose of quinidine reduced accordingly.

A

Azoles + Ranolazine

Ketoconazole increases the AUC, peak and trough levels, and half-life of ranolazine 2.5- to 4.5-fold. The dose-related adverse effects of ranolazine such as nausea and dizziness were increased by ketoconazole. Further, increases in plasma levels of ranolazine may cause significant QT prolongation and increase the risk of arrhythmias.

> The manufacturers of ranolazine contraindicate its use with ketoconazole and other potent CYP3A4 inhibitors. They specifically name itraconazole, posaconazole, and voriconazole.

Azoles + Reboxetine

Ketoconazole decreases the clearance of single-dose reboxetine, without apparently altering its adverse effect profile. Other azoles are predicted to interact similarly.

> It has been suggested that caution should be used, and a reduction in reboxetine dose considered, if it is given with ketoconazole. The manufacturers recommend that azoles should not be given with reboxetine as it has a narrow therapeutic index, but this seems overly cautious.

Azoles + Rifabutin

Fluconazole or Miconazole

The AUC of rifabutin is increased by about 80% by fluconazole. This carries an increased risk of uveitis. Miconazole oral gel may be absorbed in sufficient quantities to have systemic effects, and it is therefore predicted to interact similarly.

> The concurrent use of rifabutin with fluconazole can be advantageous but because of the increased risk of uveitis, the CSM in the UK says that the dose of rifabutin should be reduced to 300 mg daily. The manufacturer of miconazole oral gel advises caution and suggest that rifabutin dose reductions may be necessary.

Itraconazole or Ketoconazole

Itraconazole may increase rifabutin levels and increase the risk of toxicity. Rifabutin reduces the levels of itraconazole and reduces efficacy leading to treatment failure. Uveitis was attributed to the concurrent use of rifabutin and itraconazole in one report. Ketoconazole is predicted to interact similarly.

> Information is sparse, but based on what is known monitor for reduced antifungal activity, raising the azole dose as necessary, and watch for increased rifabutin levels and toxicity (in particular uveitis). The manufacturers of itraconazole and ketoconazole do not recommend concurrent use.

Posaconazole

Rifabutin reduces posaconazole levels by about 50% and posaconazole increases the AUC of rifabutin. Uveitis has been attributed to the concurrent use of these drugs.

> Concurrent use should be avoided unless the benefits are expected to outweigh the

risks. If used together, the efficacy of posaconazole and toxicity of rifabutin should both be closely monitored, particularly full blood counts and uveitis.

Voriconazole

Rifabutin decreases voriconazole levels, while voriconazole dramatically increases rifabutin levels.

Concurrent use should be avoided unless the benefits are expected to outweigh the risks. The UK manufacturers recommend that the dose of voriconazole should be increased from 200 mg twice daily to 350 mg twice daily (and from 100 to 200 mg twice daily in patients under 40 kg). The intravenous dose should also be increased from 4 to 5 mg/kg twice daily. Patients should be closely monitored for rifabutin adverse effects (e.g. check full blood counts, monitor for uveitis). In the US concurrent use is contraindicated.

Azoles + **Rifampicin (Rifampin)**

Fluconazole

Although rifampicin causes only a modest increase in fluconazole clearance, the reduction in its effects may possibly be clinically important. Fluconazole does not appear to affect rifampicin pharmacokinetics.

Monitor concurrent use and increase the fluconazole dose if necessary.

Itraconazole, Ketoconazole, Posaconazole, or Voriconazole

Rifampicin causes a marked reduction in itraconazole, ketoconazole and voriconazole serum levels (almost undetectable in some instances) and had similar effects on posaconazole levels in one case. Rifampicin levels can be halved by ketoconazole, but are possibly unaffected if the drugs are given 12 hours apart.

The manufacturers do not recommend the concurrent use of itraconazole and rifampicin, and the manufacturers of ketoconazole and posaconazole advise against concurrent use unless the benefit to the patient outweighs the risk. If concurrent use is necessary, monitor closely, being alert for the need to increase the dose of these azoles. With ketoconazole, a rifampicin dose increase may also be needed. Note that the concurrent use of rifampicin with voriconazole is contraindicated.

Azoles + **Salbutamol (Albuterol) and related bronchodilators**

Ketoconazole increases the AUC of inhaled salmeterol 16-fold, which may result in systemic adverse effects adverse effects of salmeterol. Although, clinically significant effects were not seen on blood pressure, heart rate, blood glucose and blood potassium levels, this increase in the exposure to salmeterol increases the risk of QT prolongation. Itraconazole and voriconazole are expected to interact in the same way as ketoconazole.

Avoid unless the benefits outweigh the risks. If ketoconazole and salmeterol are given be alert for salmeterol adverse effects such as hypokalaemia and tachycardia.

Azoles + Sibutramine

Ketoconazole can cause moderate increases in sibutramine levels and its two metabolites. Itraconazole and voriconazole may interact similarly. Small increases in heart rates have also been reported seen although there were no associated ECG changes.

A clinically relevant interaction between sibutramine and any of these azoles seems unlikely; however, unless more is known it may be prudent to be alert for an increase in sibutramine adverse effects (e.g. dry mouth, headache, insomnia, and constipation) and adjust treatment accordingly.

Azoles + Sirolimus

Fluconazole and Miconazole ⚠

Two cases of raised sirolimus levels and toxicity, one of which was fatal, have been reported with fluconazole. Note that miconazole oral gel may be swallowed in large enough quantities to have a systemic interaction with sirolimus.

Close monitoring of sirolimus levels is recommended with a dose reduction of sirolimus as required.

Itraconazole, Ketoconazole or Posaconazole

Itraconazole, ketoconazole and posaconazole markedly increase the maximum levels of sirolimus and sirolimus dose reductions of up to 90% have been required in some patients in order to manage this interaction.

Concurrent use is not recommended by the manufacturers. However, if these azoles are required in a patient taking sirolimus, a pre-emptive sirolimus dose reduction would appear to be prudent, and trough sirolimus levels should be very closely monitored both during use and after the azoles are stopped.

Voriconazole ⊗

Voriconazole raised the maximum levels and AUC of a single 2 mg dose of sirolimus by about 5.5-fold and 10-fold, respectively.

These rises are probably too large to be easily accommodated by reducing the dose of the sirolimus. Concurrent use is contraindicated.

Azoles + Solifenacin

Ketoconazole increases solifenacin levels 2- to 3-fold by inhibiting CYP3A4. Other CYP3A4 inhibitors (e.g. itraconazole and voriconazole) would be expected to have the same effect.

It is recommended that the daily dose of solifenacin is limited to 5 mg in patients taking these azoles. The concurrent use of solifenacin and these azoles is contraindicated in patients with severe renal impairment or moderate hepatic impairment.

Azoles + **Statins**

Atorvastatin with Posaconazole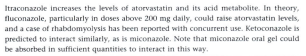

Itraconazole causes a marked increase in atorvastatin levels, which increases the risk of myopathy and rhabdomyolysis. Posaconazole is predicted to interact similarly.

> The UK manufacturer contraindicates concurrent use, whereas the US manufacturer suggests reducing the dose of the statin during concurrent use. All patients should be warned to report promptly any unexplained muscle aches, tenderness, cramps, stiffness or weakness.

Atorvastatin with other Azoles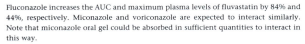

Itraconazole increases the levels of atorvastatin and its acid metabolite. In theory, fluconazole, particularly in doses above 200 mg daily, could raise atorvastatin levels, and a case of rhabdomyolysis has been reported with concurrent use. Ketoconazole is predicted to interact similarly, as is miconazole. Note that miconazole oral gel could be absorbed in sufficient quantities to interact in this way.

> Because of the potentially serious reactions that can result, any patient given atorvastatin with an azole should be told to report any unexplained muscle pain, tenderness or weakness. Because large increases in atorvastatin levels can occur (most likely with itraconazole or ketoconazole), consider using lower atorvastatin doses or, for short courses of the azole, temporarily withdrawing the statin. The UK manufacturer of atorvastatin advises a maximum atorvastatin dose of 40 mg daily with itraconazole and a similar dose reduction would seem prudent with ketoconazole. The manufacturers of voriconazole recommend considering a dose reduction of atorvastatin during concurrent use.

Fluvastatin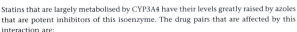

Fluconazole increases the AUC and maximum plasma levels of fluvastatin by 84% and 44%, respectively. Miconazole and voriconazole are expected to interact similarly. Note that miconazole oral gel could be absorbed in sufficient quantities to interact in this way.

> The clinical relevance of the modest changes in fluvastatin levels with fluconazole is unclear. However, because of the potentially serious reactions that can result, any patient given fluvastatin with these azoles should be told to report any unexplained muscle pain, tenderness or weakness.

Simvastatin or Lovastatin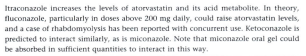

Statins that are largely metabolised by CYP3A4 have their levels greatly raised by azoles that are potent inhibitors of this isoenzyme. The drug pairs that are affected by this interaction are:

- lovastatin with itraconazole (20-fold rises seen)
- lovastatin with ketoconazole
- simvastatin with itraconazole (17-fold rises seen)
- simvastatin with ketoconazole

This interaction has resulted in severe muscle toxicity, including rhabdomyolysis, in a number of cases. Voriconazole may also interact similarly. Fluconazole (particularly in high dose i.e. greater than 200 mg daily), and miconazole (including the oral gel, which can be absorbed sufficiently to have enzyme-inhibitory effects) are also predicted to interact, but probably to a lesser extent.

Concurrent use of itraconazole, ketoconazole and miconazole oral gel with simvastatin or lovastatin is contraindicated. The UK manufacturer of posaconazole also contraindicate simvastatin and lovastatin, whereas the US manufacturer suggests reducing the dose of the statin during concurrent use. If a short course of these azoles is essential, the statin should be temporarily withdrawn. The manufacturers of voriconazole recommend considering a dose reduction of lovastatin or simvastatin during concurrent use. Patients should be warned to report promptly any unexplained muscle aches, tenderness, cramps, stiffness or weakness.

Azoles + Sucralfate

Sucralfate reduces ketoconazole absorption by about 25%, but no significant changes appear to occur if ketoconazole is given 2 hours after sucralfate.

Separate administration by 2 to 3 hours to ensure maximal absorption.

Azoles + Tacrolimus

When tacrolimus is given orally, its serum levels are considerably increased (within 3 days) by oral fluconazole. Itraconazole, ketoconazole, posaconazole, voriconazole, and possibly miconazole oral gel, also raise tacrolimus levels. There is some evidence that the levels of *intravenous* tacrolimus are less affected by the azoles.

Monitor tacrolimus levels closely if any azole is given and adjust the tacrolimus dose as required. One study specifically examining dose adjustments suggests that fluconazole can be safely used if 60% of the original tacrolimus dose is given. Nearly all patients are expected to need tacrolimus dose reductions if azoles are given: the manufacturers of posaconazole and voriconazole suggest a reduction of two-thirds. No interaction would be expected if miconazole is applied to the skin or used intravaginally.

Azoles + Theophylline

No clinically significant interaction is expected between theophylline and the azoles, although a fall in theophylline levels has been seen in rare cases with ketoconazole and a rise in theophylline levels has been seen in rare cases with fluconazole.

A significant interaction is unlikely but bear these reports in mind in case of an unexpected response to treatment.

Azoles + Tolterodine

The AUC of tolterodine is raised more than 2-fold by ketoconazole, a potent inhibitor of CYP3A4. Itraconazole and voriconazole would be expected to interact similarly. The US manufacturer predicts that miconazole will interact similarly.

> The UK manufacturers advise avoiding concurrent use. The US manufacturers suggest reducing the tolterodine dose to 1 mg twice daily, which seems practical. If both drugs are given monitor carefully for tolterodine adverse effects, and further reduce the dose or withdraw the drug if necessary.

Azoles + Toremifene

The manufacturer predicts that inhibitors of CYP3A4, such as ketoconazole, may decrease toremifene metabolism, which may lead to toxicity. Itraconazole and voriconazole would be expected to interact similarly.

> These warnings are based on indirect evidence and therefore their clinical importance awaits confirmation. However, until further information is available, it would seem prudent to monitor for toremifene adverse effects (e.g. hot flushes, uterine bleeding, fatigue, nausea, dizziness).

Azoles + Trazodone

Ketoconazole or itraconazole may inhibit the metabolism of trazodone.

> A lower dose of trazodone should be considered if it is given with these azoles, although in the UK it has been suggested that the combination should be avoided where possible. Monitor for increased trazodone adverse effects such as sedation, if concurrent use is required.

Azoles + Tricyclics

Isolated case reports describe increased amitriptyline or nortriptyline levels in patients also taking fluconazole (tricyclic antidepressant levels at least doubled). There is also a report of a patient who developed a prolonged QT interval and torsades de pointes, which were associated with the concurrent use of amitriptyline and fluconazole. Consider also drugs that prolong the QT interval, page 277.

> The general importance of this interaction is unclear, but bear it in mind in case of an unexpected response to treatment or if tricyclic adverse effects become troublesome. The evidence suggests that other factors (such as renal impairment and other potentially interacting medications) may be necessary before an interaction occurs.

Azoles + Triptans

Fluconazole

Fluconazole modestly increases the plasma levels of eletriptan by 40%.

> Be aware that the effects of eletriptan may be increased in those taking fluconazole. Other triptans would be expected to have little or no interaction with the azoles and may be suitable alternatives.

Itraconazole or Ketoconazole

Ketoconazole raises the plasma levels of eletriptan 2.7-fold. Itraconazole is expected to interact similarly.

> The manufacturer states that the concurrent use of ketoconazole and itraconazole with eletriptan should be avoided. The US manufacturers further recommend that eletriptan should not be given within 72 hours of these azoles. Other triptans would be expected to have little or no interaction with the azoles and may be suitable alternatives.

Azoles + Warfarin and other oral anticoagulants

Fluconazole causes a dose-related inhibition of the metabolism of warfarin, and increases its anticoagulant effect. Voriconazole interacts similarly. Case reports describe raised INRs and bleeding when fluconazole, ketoconazole, or itraconazole were given with warfarin, acenocoumarol or phenprocoumon. The anticoagulant effects of acenocoumarol, phenindione, phenprocoumon, and warfarin can be markedly increased if miconazole is given orally, and bleeding can occur. The interaction can occur with buccal gel, intravaginal miconazole, and possibly with miconazole cream applied to the skin.

> Monitor the INR if an azole is given with an indanedione or coumarin and adjust the dose accordingly. Oral miconazole, fluconazole and voriconazole interfere with the main metabolic pathway of warfarin (and acenocoumarol) and are therefore likely to interact more frequently than the other azoles. Concurrent use of prescription doses of miconazole oral gel should be avoided. The warfarin dose may need to be reduced by about 20% when using fluconazole 50 mg daily ranging to a reduction of about 70% when using fluconazole 600 mg daily. These larger reductions should be gradual over 5 days or more, although individual variations between patients can be considerable. In general, an interaction with topical azoles seems rare, but it would be prudent to consider monitoring any patient receiving a coumarin if they need to use large amounts of a topical azole, particularly on broken or damaged skin.

Aztreonam

Aztreonam + Warfarin and other oral anticoagulants ?

Aztreonam occasionally causes a prolongation in prothrombin times, which in theory might possibly be additive with the effects of conventional anticoagulants.

> The clinical importance of this interaction is unknown, but bear it in mind in case of an increased response to anticoagulant treatment.

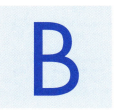

Baclofen

Baclofen + Levodopa

Unpleasant adverse effects (hallucinations, confusion, headache, nausea) and worsening of the symptoms of parkinsonism have occurred in patients taking levodopa who were also given baclofen.

> Information is limited, but what is known suggests that baclofen should be used cautiously in patients taking levodopa.

Baclofen + Lithium

Two patients with Huntington's chorea showed an aggravation of their hyperkinetic symptoms within a few days of starting lithium and baclofen. One patient took lithium first, the other baclofen.

> The clinical significance of this interaction is unclear. Bear it in mind in case of an unexpected response to treatment and consider stopping one of the drugs if hyperkinesis develops.

Baclofen + NSAIDs

An isolated report describes baclofen toxicity (confusion, disorientation, bradycardia, blurred vision, hypotension and hypothermia) in a patient who took ibuprofen. It appeared that the toxicity was caused by ibuprofen-induced acute renal impairment leading to baclofen accumulation.

> The general importance of this interaction is likely to be very small. There appears to be no information about baclofen and other NSAIDs, and little reason for avoiding concurrent use.

B

Baclofen + Tricyclics

An isolated report describes a patient with multiple sclerosis taking baclofen, who was unable to stand within a few days of starting to take nortriptyline, and later imipramine.

The UK manufacturer of baclofen warns that the effect of baclofen may be potentiated by tricyclic antidepressants, resulting in pronounced muscular hypotonia; however, this case report appears to be the only documentation to suggest that a clinically relevant interaction occurs.

Balsalazide

Balsalazide + Digoxin

Because digoxin levels can be reduced by up to 50% by *sulfasalazine* the manufacturers cautiously suggest that an interaction may occur with balsalazide. However, no interactions appear to have been reported.

The manufacturer of balsalazide recommends that plasma levels of digoxin should be monitored in patients starting balsalazide.

Benzodiazepines

Benzodiazepines + Beta blockers

Only small and clinically unimportant pharmacokinetic interactions occur between most benzodiazepines and beta blockers, but there is limited evidence that some psychomotor tests may possibly be impaired in patients taking some benzodiazepines combined with beta blockers, in particular diazepam with metoprolol.

The current evidence does not seem to justify any particular caution, but bear this interaction in mind in case of an unexpected response to treatment.

Benzodiazepines + Calcium-channel blockers

The serum levels and effects of midazolam are markedly increased by diltiazem or verapamil. The effects are likely to be greater with oral than intravenous midazolam. This also occurs with triazolam and diltiazem, and is predicted to occur with triazolam and verapamil. Alprazolam is expected to interact similarly.

Monitor the outcome of concurrent use. Benzodiazepine effects such as sedation may persist for several hours. Consider using a lower initial dose of midazolam or triazolam. It has been suggested that the usual dose of midazolam should be reduced at least 50%. Other benzodiazepines seem generally unlikely to be affected to a clinically relevant extent (although not all combinations have been studied) and may therefore provide suitable alternatives.

Benzodiazepines + Carbamazepine

Alprazolam, Midazolam or Triazolam

Carbamazepine reduces the AUC and peak serum levels of midazolam by about 90%, when compared with control subjects not taking antiepileptics. The effects of midazolam were also reduced. Carbamazepine also increases the oral clearance and reduces the elimination half-life of alprazolam. A patient had a reduction of more than 50% in plasma alprazolam levels when given carbamazepine, and this led to a deterioration in his clinical condition. Triazolam is expected to interact similarly.

Expect to need to use a much larger dose of midazolam in the presence of carbamazepine. An alternative hypno-sedative may be needed. The dose of alprazolam and possibly triazolam may also have to be adjusted.

Other benzodiazepines

The use of benzodiazepines with carbamazepine is common, although some evidence suggests that the effects of the benzodiazepines are sometimes reduced (clobazam, clonazepam, diazepam, etizolam, nitrazepam and zopiclone).

No action is generally needed, but be aware that sometimes the effects of the benzodiazepines may be reduced.

Benzodiazepines + Digoxin

Digoxin toxicity occurred in two elderly patients, and rises in serum digoxin levels have been seen in others, when they were given alprazolam. This interaction seems to occur particularly in patients over 65 years of age.

Given the range of benzodiazepines available it would seem sensible to avoid alprazolam in patients on digoxin. If concurrent use is necessary, monitor heart rate and digoxin levels, and reduce the digoxin dose as necessary. There is no evidence to suggest a clinically significant interaction with other benzodiazepines.

Benzodiazepines + Disulfiram

An isolated and unconfirmed report describes temazepam toxicity, possibly due to disulfiram. The serum levels of chlordiazepoxide and diazepam are increased by the use of disulfiram and some patients may possibly experience increased drowsiness.

If sedation occurs reduce the dose of the benzodiazepine if necessary. Other benzodiazepines that are metabolised similarly may possibly interact in the same way but this needs confirmation. Alprazolam, lorazepam and oxazepam appear to be non-interacting alternatives.

Benzodiazepines + Felbamate

A retrospective study found that felbamate increases the levels of the clobazam metabolite, norclobazam.

> The clinical significance of this interaction is unknown. Both drugs have CNS effects and therefore it would seem prudent to be aware that additive sedative or other adverse effects may occur.

B

Benzodiazepines + H₂-receptor antagonists

The levels of many of the benzodiazepines and related drugs are raised by cimetidine, but normally this appears to be of little or no clinical importance and only the occasional patient may experience an increase in effects (sedation). The interactions with midazolam, and possibly zaleplon may be more significant, but this is not established.

> In general no clinically significant interaction occurs, but note that individual patients may rarely experience increased sedation. If a patient develops increased benzodiazepine effects, consider changing to a non-interacting benzodiazepine (such as lorazepam or temazepam), or to a non-interacting H₂-receptor antagonist (such as ranitidine).

Benzodiazepines + Herbal medicines or Dietary supplements

Kava

A man taking alprazolam became semicomatose a few days after starting to take kava.

> The clinical importance of this isolated case report is uncertain, but bear it in mind in case of an unexpected response to treatment.

St John's wort (Hypericum perforatum)

Long-term use of St John's wort decreases the plasma levels of alprazolam and oral midazolam. Triazolam and zopiclone are expected to interact similarly. St John's wort preparations taken as a single dose, or containing low-hyperforin levels, appear to have less of an effect. Single doses of intravenous midazolam do not appear to be significantly affected.

> Until more is known about the interacting constituents of St John's wort and the amount necessary to provoke an interaction, monitor patients receiving alprazolam and oral midazolam concurrently for any signs of reduced efficacy.

Benzodiazepines + Isoniazid

Isoniazid reduces the clearance of both diazepam and triazolam. Some increase in their effects would be expected.

> The degree of sedation will depend on the individual patient. However, warn all patients of the potential effects, and counsel against driving or undertaking other

skilled tasks. Reduce the benzodiazepine dose as necessary. Clotiazepam and oxazepam appear to be non-interacting alternatives.

B

Benzodiazepines + **Lamotrigine**

Lamotrigine appears to lower clonazepam levels by about 40% in some patients.

The general significance of this interaction is unclear. Both drugs have CNS effects and therefore it would seem prudent to be aware that additive sedative or other adverse effects may occur.

Benzodiazepines + **Levodopa**

On rare occasions it seems that the therapeutic effects of levodopa can be reduced by chlordiazepoxide, diazepam or nitrazepam, but this is not an established interaction.

There is no need to avoid concurrent use, but bear these reports in mind in case of an unexpected response to treatment.

Benzodiazepines + **Lithium** ❓

Neurotoxicity and increased serum lithium levels were reported in 5 patients when they took clonazepam with lithium. Increased serum-lithium levels have been described in one patient taking bromazepam and lithium and an isolated case of hypothermia has been reported during the concurrent use of lithium and diazepam.

It has been recommended that lithium levels should be measured more frequently if clonazepam is added, and the effects of concurrent use should be well monitored. This general significance of the isolated cases is unclear and concurrent use need not be avoided, but bear these cases in mind should any unexpected adverse effects occur.

Benzodiazepines + **Macrolides**

Alprazolam, Brotizolam, Midazolam, Triazolam or Zopiclone ⚠

The plasma levels and effects of midazolam, and triazolam are dramatically increased and prolonged by clarithromycin, probably telithromycin and erythromycin (but to a slightly lesser extent in some cases). Not all macrolides will interact, see macrolides, page 361. Other benzodiazepines and related hypnotics that may interact similarly, although to a lesser extent, include alprazolam, brotizolam and zopiclone.

High doses of intravenous midazolam given long term will need to be carefully titrated: one manufacturer suggests an initial 50% reduction in dose in the presence of the interacting macrolides. Similar precautions are warranted for triazolam, but smaller dose reductions or monitoring should be adequate with the other interacting hypnotics. Single bolus doses of the benzodiazepines probably do not need adjusting. When given orally, the dose of midazolam should be reduced by about 50 to 75% in the presence of the interacting macrolides if excessive effects (marked drowsiness, memory loss) are to be avoided. Note that the hypnotic effects may also be prolonged and patients should be warned about potential hangover effects the following day. Similar precautions are warranted for triazolam but smaller dose reductions or monitoring should be adequate with the other interacting hypnotics.

Other benzodiazepines

Erythromycin has a weak effect on the metabolism of diazepam, flunitrazepam, nitrazepam and zaleplon.

A clinically significant interaction is unlikely and no action is generally needed.

Benzodiazepines + MAOIs

Isolated case reports describe adverse reactions (chorea, severe headache, facial flushing, massive oedema, and prolonged coma), which have been attributed to interactions between phenelzine and chlordiazepoxide, clonazepam or nitrazepam, and between isocarboxazid and chlordiazepoxide.

The case reports of adverse interactions appear to be isolated, and it is by no means certain that all the responses were in fact due to drug interactions. They seem unlikely to be of general significance.

Benzodiazepines + Melatonin

The CNS effects of benzodiazepines and related hypnotics may be additive with those of melatonin.

It would be wise to be aware that increased drowsiness is a possibility if melatonin is given with a benzodiazepine, especially those that are longer-acting.

Benzodiazepines + Mirtazapine

The sedative effects of mirtazapine are increased by the benzodiazepines.

Patients should be warned that the sedative effects of benzodiazepines in general may be potentiated by concurrent use with mirtazapine. Note that the US manufacturer actually recommends that patients taking mirtazapine avoid the use of diazepam and similar drugs, but this is probably overly cautious.

Benzodiazepines + Modafinil

Modafinil reduced the maximum plasma concentration of triazolam by 42% and reduced its elimination half-life by about one hour. Alprazolam and midazolam may be similarly affected. In contrast, diazepam levels are predicted to be increased by modafinil.

Dose adjustments may be necessary on concurrent use. Monitor to ensure that the benzodiazepine effects are adequate, and, in the case of diazepam, not excessive.

Benzodiazepines + **Moxonidine**

Moxonidine increases the cognitive impairment caused by lorazepam. Sedation and dizziness may occur with moxonidine alone, which the manufacturers suggest may be additive with the effects of benzodiazepines.

> The degree of impairment will depend on the individual patient. However, warn all patients of the potential effects, and counsel against driving or undertaking other skilled tasks.

B

Benzodiazepines + **NNRTIs**

Delavirdine

Delavirdine may increase the plasma levels of alprazolam, midazolam and triazolam by inhibiting CYP3A4.

> The concurrent use of delavirdine with alprazolam, midazolam or triazolam is contraindicated.

Efavirenz

Efavirenz appears to increase the metabolism of midazolam. Triazolam would be expected to interact similarly. In contrast, the manufacturers of efavirenz suggest that competition with midazolam for metabolism by CYP3A4 could inhibit midazolam metabolism resulting in prolonged sedation and respiratory depression.

> The study suggests that patients should be monitored for midazolam and probably triazolam efficacy: increase the dose as necessary. However, based on their prediction, the manufacturers of efavirenz contraindicate concurrent use, but note that competition for metabolism rarely results in clinically relevant increases in the levels of either of the two drugs involved.

Etravirine

Etravirine is predicted to increase diazepam levels by inhibiting CYP2C19.

> The UK manufacturers of etravirine suggest that an alternative anxiolytic or sedative drug to diazepam is used but no particular drug is named. The US manufacturer suggests reducing the diazepam dose as necessary.

Nevirapine

Nevirapine may decrease the levels of midazolam (and probably triazolam) by induction of CYP3A4.

> Monitor for benzodiazepine efficacy and increase the dose as necessary.

Benzodiazepines + **NRTIs**

Oxazepam causes a modest increase in the bioavailability of zidovudine and can increase the incidence of headaches. Lorazepam is expected to interact similarly.

> It has been suggested that if headaches occur during concurrent use, the benzodiazepine should be stopped.

B

Benzodiazepines + Opioids ❓

As would be expected, increased sedative and respiratory depressant effects may occur in patients given opioids with benzodiazepines; rarely, hypotension has occurred in patients given intravenous opioids and benzodiazepines. Minor pharmacokinetic interactions may occur, but there is insufficient evidence to suggest that any of these are of general significance.

> Concurrent use is common and is usually beneficial. However, additive adverse effects can occur and the degree of impairment will depend on the individual patient. However, warn all patients of the potential effects, and counsel against driving or undertaking other skilled tasks. Be aware that hypotension may occur if intravenous opioids are given with benzodiazepines.

Benzodiazepines + Phenobarbital ❓

Clobazam has been reported to reduce the clearance of primidone. Clonazepam appears to markedly raise the levels of primidone in children, and toxicity has been seen, however other studies found no change in levels. The use of other benzodiazepines with phenobarbital or primidone may possibly be accompanied by some changes in plasma levels, which are normally of limited clinical importance. However, caution might be necessary with benzodiazepines, such as midazolam, triazolam and alprazolam, which are primarily metabolised by CYP3A4. Similarly, the manufacturer of zopiclone notes that the concurrent use of phenobarbital may decrease the plasma levels of zopiclone. Additive adverse effects such as sedation may occur during the initial use of a benzodiazepine and phenobarbital. More serious effects (hallucinations, violent behaviour) have been reported, but appear rare.

> Adverse effects such as sedation may be more evident when benzodiazepines are given with barbiturates, particularly in the initial stages of treatment, and careful dose adjustment may be required. The general significance of the changes in primidone levels is unclear: it may be prudent to monitor for adverse effects. Indicators of phenobarbital and primidone toxicity include drowsiness, ataxia, and dysarthria.

Benzodiazepines + Phenytoin

Midazolam ⚠

Phenytoin reduced the AUC of midazolam by about 95%, and the peak serum levels by about 90% when compared with control subjects not taking antiepileptics. The effects of midazolam were also reduced.

> Expect to need to use a much larger dose of midazolam in the presence of phenytoin. An alternative hypnotic may be needed.

Other benzodiazepines ❓

Reports are inconsistent: benzodiazepines can cause serum phenytoin levels to rise (chlordiazepoxide, clobazam, clonazepam, diazepam), occasionally resulting in toxicity; or fall (clonazepam, diazepam); or remain unaltered (alprazolam, clonazepam). One manufacturer of temazepam predicts that serum phenytoin levels may be increased or decreased by temazepam. In addition phenytoin may cause a fall in the

B

serum levels of clobazam, clonazepam, diazepam, and oxazepam. Zopiclone is predicted to be similarly affected.

Warn the patient to be alert for indicators of phenytoin toxicity (blurred vision, nystagmus, ataxia or drowsiness). Take phenytoin levels as necessary. One manufacturer of temazepam states that phenytoin levels may need to be monitored during temazepam withdrawal, and for phenytoin adverse effects. Be aware that the benzodiazepine may be less effective than expected; consider a dose increase if required.

Benzodiazepines + Pregabalin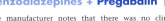

The manufacturer notes that there was no clinically relevant pharmacokinetic interaction between pregabalin and lorazepam, and that concurrent use caused no clinically important effect on respiration. However, they note that pregabalin may potentiate the effects of lorazepam (presumably sedation). All benzodiazepines seem likely to increase sedation when given with pregabalin.

The degree of impairment will depend on the individual patient. However, warn all patients of the potential effects, and counsel against driving or undertaking other skilled tasks.

Benzodiazepines + Probenecid

Probenecid reduces the clearance of adinazolam, lorazepam and nitrazepam. Increased therapeutic and adverse effects (sedation) may be expected. There seems to be no direct information of an interaction with other benzodiazepines, but those that are metabolised like lorazepam and nitrazepam may also interact.

Monitor the outcome of concurrent use for increased sedation and decrease the benzodiazepine dose if this becomes troublesome. Limited evidence suggests that temazepam does not interact.

Benzodiazepines + Protease inhibitors

Midazolam and Triazolam

The protease inhibitors appear to dramatically increase the levels and effects of midazolam and triazolam. Increased and prolonged sedation is expected to occur.

The concurrent use of *oral* midazolam and protease inhibitors is contraindicated. The US manufacturers of the protease inhibitors generally contraindicate *intravenous* midazolam, whereas the UK manufacturers state that it may be used with close monitoring within an intensive care unit or similar setting so that the appropriate management of respiratory depression is available. They also suggest that dose reductions should be considered. The authors of one study suggest that continuous intravenous midazolam doses should be reduced by 50%, but do not consider dose adjustments to single intravenous doses necessary. Triazolam would be expected to interact in the same way as midazolam, and therefore the UK and US manufacturers generally contraindicate its use.

Other benzodiazepines

Interactions between other protease inhibitors and benzodiazepines are variable, although the levels of alprazolam, clorazepate, diazepam, estazolam, flurazepam, zolpidem and zopiclone are most commonly predicted to be increased.

Clorazepate, diazepam, estazolam, and flurazepam are contraindicated by the UK manufacturer of ritonavir and indinavir, but cautioned by the US manufacturer of ritonavir. Alprazolam is contraindicated by the UK and US manufacturers of indinavir, but cautioned by the manufacturers of saquinavir and the US manufacturer of fosamprenavir. Note that the manufacturer of ritonavir also cautions alprazolam during initial use, before induction of alprazolam metabolism develops. The US manufacturer of fosamprenavir and the UK and US manufacturers of saquinavir also suggest the possibility of an interaction with clorazepate, diazepam and flurazepam, and suggest that careful monitoring is needed, with dose adjustments as required. The manufacturer of ritonavir notes that zolpidem may be given concurrently with careful monitoring for excessive sedative effects and consideration of reducing the dose of zolpidem. Zopiclone may be similarly affected.

Benzodiazepines + **Proton pump inhibitors**

Gait disturbances (attributed to benzodiazepine toxicity) occurred in 2 patients given triazolam, and lorazepam or flurazepam, with omeprazole. Another patient taking diazepam and omeprazole became wobbly and sedated. Diazepam plasma levels are increased by esomeprazole but the clinical relevance of this is unknown.

Information is limited, but what is currently known suggests that patients given omeprazole, and possibly esomeprazole, with diazepam may experience increased benzodiazepine effects (sedation, unstable gait etc.). Lansoprazole, pantoprazole, or rabeprazole appear not to interact with diazepam to a clinically relevant extent.

Benzodiazepines + **Rifampicin (Rifampin)**

Rifampicin causes a very marked increase in the metabolism of diazepam (4-fold increase in clearance), midazolam (AUC reduced by 96%), nitrazepam (83% increase in clearance), triazolam (AUC reduced by 95%), zaleplon (AUC reduced by 80%), zolpidem (AUC reduced by 73%) and zopiclone (AUC reduced by 82%). Benzodiazepines that are metabolised similarly (e.g. chlordiazepoxide, flurazepam) are expected to interact in the same way.

The effects of these benzodiazepines may be almost completely abolished if rifampicin is given. Temazepam appears to be a non-interacting alternative. Those benzodiazepines that, like temazepam, undergo glucuronidation (e.g. lorazepam, oxazepam) are not expected to be affected by rifampicin to such an extent as those metabolised primarily by hepatic microsomal oxidation, and may be useful alternatives, although they may still interact to some extent.

Benzodiazepines + **SSRIs**

Fluvoxamine

The metabolism of some benzodiazepines such as alprazolam, bromazepam and diazepam (and also possibly midazolam and triazolam) may be reduced by fluvoxamine.

> The doses of alprazolam, bromazepam and diazepam should be reduced, probably by half, in the presence of fluvoxamine to avoid adverse effects (drowsiness, reduced psychomotor performance and memory). Furthermore, some US manufacturers recommend avoiding the use of fluvoxamine with diazepam as substantial diazepam accumulation could occur.

Other SSRIs

On the whole, no clinically significant interaction appears to occur between the SSRIs and the benzodiazepines or related drugs, such as cloral hydrate or zaleplon. There is some evidence to support the suggestion that sedation is likely to be increased by the concurrent use of SSRIs and benzodiazepines. Rare cases of hallucinations have been seen with zolpidem and some SSRIs.

> No particular action is necessary but remember that the degree of sedation will depend on the individual patient and drug combination. Warn all patients of the potential effects, and counsel caution with driving or undertaking other skilled tasks.

Benzodiazepines + **Theophylline**

Xanthines including theophylline antagonise the sedative effects of some benzodiazepines. This is due to their mutually opposing effects, so it is likely all benzodiazepines will interact similarly, although the extent of the interaction will depend on the benzodiazepine used, the dose used, and the individual patient.

> The extent to which these xanthines actually reduce the anxiolytic effects of the benzodiazepines remains uncertain but be alert for reduced benzodiazepine effects.

Benzodiazepines + **Tricyclics**

The concurrent use of tricyclic antidepressants and benzodiazepines is not uncommon, and normally appears to be uneventful. However, there have been reports of increased drowsiness and incoordination following the use of the combination.

> No particular action is necessary but remember that the degree of sedation will depend on the individual patient and drug combination. Warn all patients of the potential effects, and counsel caution with driving or undertaking other skilled tasks.

Beta blockers

B

Beta blockers + Bupropion

Bupropion is predicted to decrease the metabolism of metoprolol; a case report describes patient taking metoprolol developed bradycardia and hypotension when bupropion was also given.

> The manufacturers of bupropion recommend that if metoprolol is added to existing treatment with bupropion, doses at the lower end of the range should be used. If bupropion is added to existing treatment with metoprolol, decreased doses of metoprolol should be considered. These precautions seem prudent, especially in patients with heart failure, where raised beta blocker levels seem most likely to cause an adverse effect.

Beta blockers + Calcium-channel blockers

Diltiazem

The cardiac depressant effects of diltiazem and beta blockers are additive, although concurrent use can be beneficial. A number of patients, usually those with pre-existing ventricular failure or conduction abnormalities, have developed serious and potentially life-threatening bradycardia. Note that additive hypotensive effects are likely, see antihypertensives, page 89, but in most cases this is likely to be desirable.

> Monitor the outcome of concurrent use for additive haemodynamic effects (e.g. bradycardia, hypotension or heart failure). Note that an interaction has been reported to occur from within a few hours of starting treatment to after 2 years of concurrent use.

Nifedipine or Nisoldipine ❓

Isolated cases of severe hypotension and heart failure have been seen in patients taking beta blockers with nifedipine or nisoldipine. Patients with impaired left ventricular function (which is a caution for the use of nifedipine) and/or those taking high-dose beta blockers are most at risk. Note that all cases of an interaction involved short-acting nifedipine (which is now considered unsuitable in angina or hypertension) or when extended-release nifedipine was crushed. Note that additive hypotensive effects are likely, see antihypertensives, page 89, but in most cases this is likely to be desirable.

> Be aware that concurrent use may result in additive haemodynamic effects (e.g. hypotension or heart failure). However, the combination of a dihydropyridine-type calcium-channel blocker and a beta blocker is generally beneficial.

Verapamil

The cardiac depressant effects of verapamil and beta blockers are additive, and although concurrent use can be beneficial, serious cardiodepression (bradycardia, asystole, sinus arrest) sometimes occurs. An adverse interaction can occur even with beta blockers given as eye drops. Note that additive hypotensive effects are likely, see antihypertensives, page 89.

> Concurrent use should only be undertaken if the patient can initially be closely

monitored. The doses should be carefully titrated to effect. It has been suggested that verapamil injections should not be given to patients recently given beta blockers because of the risk of hypotension and asystole. The UK manufacturer of verapamil contraindicates its intravenous use in those receiving intravenous beta blockers.

Other calcium-channel blockers

The use of beta blockers with felodipine, isradipine, lacidipine, nicardipine, and nimodipine normally appears to be useful and safe. Changes in the pharmacokinetics of the beta blockers and calcium-channel blockers may also occur, but these changes do not appear to be clinically important. Note that additive hypotensive effects are likely, see antihypertensives, page 89, but in most cases this is likely to be desirable.

> Be aware that concurrent use may result in additive haemodynamic effects (e.g. hypotension or heart failure). However, the combination of a dihydropyridine-type calcium-channel blocker and a beta blocker is generally beneficial.

Beta blockers + Ciclosporin (Cyclosporine)

There is some evidence that carvedilol can cause a small to moderate rise in ciclosporin levels. In one study a gradual ciclosporin dose reduction of 20%, over about 3 months, was required to maintain levels within the therapeutic range.

> The manufacturers of carvedilol recommend close monitoring of ciclosporin levels with appropriate dose adjustment when carvedilol is added, which seems prudent. Clinical information about interactions of other beta blockers with ciclosporin seems to be lacking, although metoprolol and atenolol do not appear to interact.

Beta blockers + Clonidine

The use of clonidine with beta blockers can be therapeutically valuable, but a sharp and serious rise in blood pressure (rebound hypertension) can follow the sudden withdrawal of clonidine, which may be worsened by the presence of a beta blocker. Note that additive hypotensive effects are likely, see antihypertensives, page 89.

> Control this adverse effect by stopping the beta blocker several days before starting a gradual withdrawal of clonidine. A successful alternative is to replace the clonidine and the beta blocker with labetalol, which is both an alpha blocker and a beta blocker: the patient may experience tremor, nausea, apprehension and palpitations, but no serious blood pressure rise or headaches occur. If a hypertensive episode develops, re-introduction of oral or intravenous clonidine may be one way to stabilise the situation. It is clearly important to emphasise to patients taking clonidine and beta blockers that they must keep taking both drugs.

Beta blockers + Contraceptives

The blood levels of metoprolol are increased in women taking hormonal contraceptives, but the clinical importance of this is probably very small. Acebutolol, oxprenolol and propranolol pharmacokinetics are minimally affected by contraceptives.

> No action needed. However, be aware that hormonal contraceptives are cautioned or contraindicated in some of the patient groups who may be treated with beta

blockers, and oestrogens (usually in larger doses than those present in combined hormonal contraceptives) can raise blood pressure, which may antagonise the effects of the beta blockers.

Beta blockers + Digoxin ❓

The concurrent use of digoxin and a beta blocker may result in additive bradycardia; one case has been reported in a 91-year-old patient taking digoxin and timolol eye drops. In general there appears to be no pharmacokinetic interaction between digoxin and beta blockers. However, carvedilol appears to increase the bioavailability of digoxin (14% increase in AUC seen in adults, cases suggest a doubling of levels in children).

> Normally uneventful, no immediate action needed. If bradycardia does occur dose adjustment may be necessary, and this seems more likely in children. It has been suggested that the dose of digoxin should be reduced by at least 25% in children given carvedilol, with further adjustments as required.

Beta blockers + Disopyramide ❌

Severe bradycardia has been described after the use of disopyramide with beta blockers including practolol, pindolol and metoprolol. A patient given disopyramide and intravenous sotalol developed asystole (see also drugs that prolong the QT interval, page 277).

> Although an interaction appears rare, fatalities have been reported. The US manufacturers of disopyramide suggest that the combination of disopyramide and beta blockers should generally be avoided, except in the case of life-threatening arrhythmias unresponsive to a single drug.

Beta blockers + Donepezil ❓

The concurrent use of donepezil and a beta blocker may increase the risk of bradycardia.

> Although it appears that the increased risk of bradycardia is probably low, it would be prudent to be alert for bradycardia if a beta blocker is given with donepezil.

Beta blockers + Ergot derivatives ❓

The use of ergot derivatives (e.g. ergotamine) with beta blockers is normally safe and beneficial, but there are a handful of reports of adverse interactions (severe peripheral vasoconstriction and hypertension).

> Interactions seem rare, but it may be prudent to be extra alert for any signs of an adverse response, particularly those suggestive of reduced peripheral circulation (coldness, numbness or tingling of the hands and feet).

Beta blockers + Flecainide ⚠️

The concurrent use of flecainide and beta blockers may have additive cardiac

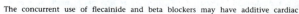

depressant effects. An isolated case of bradycardia and fatal AV block has been reported during the use of flecainide with sotalol, and bradycardia has been reported in a patient taking flecainide and timolol eye drops.

Careful monitoring has been recommended if beta blockers are given with other antiarrhythmics. Monitor for bradycardia.

Beta blockers + Galantamine

The concurrent use of galantamine and a beta blocker may increase the risk of bradycardia.

Although it appears that the increased risk of bradycardia is probably low, it would be prudent to be alert for bradycardia if a beta blocker is given with galantamine.

Beta blockers + H$_2$-receptor antagonists

No clinically significant interaction appears to occur between the beta blockers and cimetidine, although the blood levels of some extensively metabolised beta blockers (labetalol, metoprolol, nebivolol, pindolol and propranolol) can be doubled by cimetidine. Isolated case reports describe bradycardia with atenolol, an irregular heart beat with metoprolol, and hypotension with labetalol, in patients also taking cimetidine.

Normally the beta blockers are considered to have a wide therapeutic range, and so raises in levels are generally well tolerated, even in patients with heart failure. Those with impaired liver function may be more at risk of an interaction with cimetidine. In this type of patient be alert for effects such as hypotension. Note that other H$_2$-receptor antagonists (e.g. famotidine, nizatidine and ranitidine) do not appear to interact and so may be suitable alternatives.

Beta blockers + Hydralazine

Plasma levels of propranolol and other extensively metabolised beta blockers (metoprolol, oxprenolol) are increased by hydralazine, but an increase in adverse effects does not seem to have been reported.

Concurrent use is usually valuable in the treatment of hypertension. Note that additive hypotensive effects are likely, see antihypertensives, page 89. No particular precautions seem to be necessary unless an undesirably large decrease in blood pressure occurs.

Beta blockers + Imatinib ✅

The plasma levels of metoprolol are slightly increased (by about 20%) by imatinib.

The increase in metoprolol levels is small, and no clinically relevant interaction would be expected. Nevertheless, the manufacturer of imatinib recommends monitoring concurrent use because they consider metoprolol to be a drug with a narrow therapeutic index. However, metoprolol is only usually classified as such in patients with heart failure, and even then, increases of this magnitude are not considered clinically relevant. Therefore this advice seems over cautious.

B

Beta blockers + **Inotropes and Vasopressors**

The hypertensive effects of adrenaline (epinephrine) can be markedly increased in patients taking non-selective beta blockers such as propranolol. A severe and potentially life-threatening hypertensive reaction and/or marked bradycardia can develop. Cardioselective beta blockers such as atenolol and metoprolol interact minimally. Dobutamine would be expected to interact in the same way as adrenaline, but some studies and case reports suggest that paradoxical effects may occur. The pressor effects of noradrenaline (norepinephrine) appear to be diminished by the beta blockers. Some evidence suggests anaphylactic shock in patients taking beta blockers may be resistant to treatment with adrenaline (epinephrine).

Patients taking non-selective beta blockers such as propranolol should only be given adrenaline (epinephrine) in very reduced doses because of the marked bradycardia and hypertension that can occur. A less marked effect is likely with the cardioselective beta blockers such as atenolol and metoprolol. Local anaesthetics such as those used in dental surgery usually contain very low concentrations of adrenaline (e.g. 5 to 20 micrograms/mL, i.e. 1:200 000 to 1:50 000) and only small volumes are usually given, so that an undesirable interaction is unlikely. There appears to be less evidence about the other inotropes and vasopressors, but it would seem prudent to monitor blood pressure with both dobutamine and noradrenaline (norepinephrine) titrating doses as necessary.

Beta blockers + **Lidocaine**

The plasma levels of lidocaine can be increased by the concurrent use of propranolol, which has resulted in toxicity in isolated cases. Nadolol possibly interacts similarly, but there is uncertainty about metoprolol. Concurrent use may increase the risk of adverse cardiac effects such as bradycardia.

It would seem prudent to monitor the concurrent use of any beta blocker and lidocaine for cardiac depressant effects.

Beta blockers + **Lumefantrine**

The manufacturer of a preparation containing artemether and lumefantrine notes that *in vitro* lumefantrine significantly inhibits CYP2D6. They therefore contraindicate any drug that is metabolised by CYP2D6, and they name metoprolol.

This seems very restrictive as metoprolol is not contraindicated with proven CYP2D6 inhibitors. Until more is known, it would be prudent to at least monitor the effects of concurrent use. Note that, additive QT-prolonging effects are likely with the artemether component and sotalol, see drugs that prolong the QT interval, page 277.

Beta blockers + **Moxonidine**

Beta blockers can exacerbate the rebound hypertension that follows the withdrawal of clonidine, page 161. Moxonidine is predicted to interact similarly, although there appear to be no reports of an interaction.

Moxonidine is reported to have less affinity for central alpha-receptors than clonidine and therefore would be expected to present less of a risk. However, to be on the safe side the manufacturers advise that any beta blocker should be stopped first, followed by the moxonidine a few days later. Note that additive hypotensive effects are likely, see antihypertensives, page 89.

Beta blockers + NSAIDs ❓

There is evidence to suggest that most NSAIDs can increase blood pressure in patients taking antihypertensives, although some studies have not found the increase to be clinically relevant. However, various small studies have found some evidence of reduced beta blocker effects, either for hypertension or heart failure, particularly with indometacin.

Only some patients are affected. Nevertheless, some have suggested that the use of NSAIDs should be kept to a minimum in patients taking antihypertensives, whereas, others suggest that the interaction is, generally, not clinically relevant. Consider monitoring blood pressure if an NSAID is started or stopped. Note that NSAIDs should generally be avoided in those with heart failure.

Beta blockers + Phenobarbital ❓

The plasma levels and the effects of beta blockers that are mainly metabolised in the liver (e.g. alprenolol, metoprolol, timolol) are reduced by phenobarbital and other barbiturates. The extent of any interaction is likely to vary between different pairs of barbiturates and beta blockers.

A reduced response is possible with the hepatically metabolised beta blockers, although the interaction between phenobarbital and timolol was not clinically significant in one study. Consider an interaction if the response to the beta blocker is less than anticipated. Beta blockers that are mainly excreted unchanged in the urine (e.g. atenolol, nadolol) would not be expected to be affected by the barbiturates and may therefore be suitable alternatives in some cases.

Beta blockers + Pilocarpine ❓

The concurrent use of oral pilocarpine and beta blockers is said to be associated with a risk of conduction disorders (presumably bradycardia). Systemic adverse effects with pilocarpine eye drops are rare, although cardiac adverse effects have been reported with excessive use.

Although palpitations are said to be common with the use of oral pilocarpine there appear to be no published reports to suggest that the concurrent use of a beta blocker presents an additional risk.

Beta blockers + Propafenone

Plasma metoprolol and propranolol levels can be markedly raised (2- to 5-fold) by propafenone. Toxicity may develop. Propafenone and the beta blockers have negative inotropic effects, which could be additive and result in unwanted cardiodepression.

Information is limited. Anticipate the need to reduce the dose of metoprolol and propranolol. Monitor closely. It is possible that other beta blockers that undergo liver metabolism will interact similarly but not those largely excreted unchanged in the urine (e.g. atenolol, nadolol). With all combinations, consider the potential for adverse cardiac effects.

Beta blockers + Protease inhibitors

Ritonavir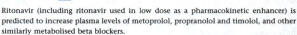

Ritonavir (including ritonavir used in low dose as a pharmacokinetic enhancer) is predicted to increase plasma levels of metoprolol, propranolol and timolol, and other similarly metabolised beta blockers.

It may be prudent to monitor for symptoms such as shortness of breath, hypotension and bradycardia, and reduce the dose of the beta blocker, or withdraw it, as appropriate. The interaction is most likely to be of significance in patients with heart failure.

Tipranavir

Tipranavir (with ritonavir) may significantly increase metoprolol levels. Serious adverse effects such as bradycardia and arrhythmias may occur.

It may be prudent to monitor for symptoms such as shortness of breath, hypotension and bradycardia, and reduce the dose of metoprolol or withdraw the beta blocker as appropriate. Note that concurrent use is contraindicated when metoprolol is used for heart failure.

Beta blockers + Quinidine

Isolated reports describe marked bradycardia and orthostatic hypotension in patients given a beta blocker with quinidine. Quinidine can raise plasma metoprolol, propranolol, and timolol levels, but the clinical relevance of this is uncertain. Additive QT-prolonging effects are likely with sotalol, see drugs that prolong the QT interval, page 277 .

Beta blockers are considered to have a wide therapeutic range, and increases in levels are generally well tolerated. However, patients with heart failure may be more at risk of adverse effects (e.g. shortness of breath, bradycardia, hypotension). Care is advised as both quinidine and the beta blockers have negative inotropic effects, which could be additive and result in unwanted cardiodepression. Note that, additive QT-prolonging effects are likely with quinidine and sotalol, see drugs that prolong the QT interval, page 277 .

Beta blockers + Rifampicin (Rifampin)

Rifampicin increases the clearance of bisoprolol, carvedilol, celiprolol, metoprolol, propranolol and tertatolol, and reduces their plasma levels. Similar but smaller effects have been seen when atenolol is given with rifampicin, but a case report suggests that occasionally the effects may be large enough to be of clinical relevance. The effects of rifampicin on propranolol appear more pronounced.

The significance of this interaction is unclear, but bear it in mind in case of an unexpected response to treatment. Consider increasing the dose of the beta blocker if there is any evidence that the therapeutic response is inadequate.

Beta blockers + **Rivastigmine**

The concurrent use of rivastigmine and a beta blocker may increase the risk of bradycardia.

> Although it appears that the increased risk of bradycardia is probably low, it would be prudent to be alert for bradycardia if a beta blocker is given with rivastigmine.

B

Beta blockers + **SSRIs**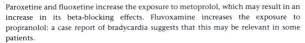

Paroxetine and fluoxetine increase the exposure to metoprolol, which may result in an increase in its beta-blocking effects. Fluvoxamine increases the exposure to propranolol: a case report of bradycardia suggests that this may be relevant in some patients.

> The clinical significance of these potential interactions is unclear, but they seem more likely to be important in those given metoprolol for heart failure; in which case the manufacturers of paroxetine suggest avoiding concurrent use. It would seem prudent to monitor any patient given metoprolol with fluoxetine or paroxetine, and any patient given propranolol with fluvoxamine for hypotension and bradycardia. Pharmacokinetic interactions may occur between other combinations of beta blockers and SSRIs, but any effect is generally modest, and there is no evidence to suggest that clinically relevant adverse effects occur as a result. However, consider an interaction as a cause if bradycardia or undesirable hypotension develop.

Beta blockers + **Tacrine**

The concurrent use of tacrine and a beta blocker may increase the risk of bradycardia.

> Although it appears that the increased risk of bradycardia is probably low, it would be prudent to be alert for bradycardia if a beta blocker is given with tacrine.

Beta blockers + **Terbinafine**

In vitro studies suggest that terbinafine is an inhibitor of CYP2D6. It may therefore be expected to increase the plasma levels of other drugs that are substrates of this enzyme. The manufacturers suggest that the levels of some beta blockers may be raised. Carvedilol, metoprolol, nebivolol, propranolol and timolol are all metabolised, at least in part, by CYP2D6.

> Until more is known it would seem wise to be aware of the possibility of an increase in adverse effects if any of these drugs is given with terbinafine and consider a dose reduction if necessary. The interaction is most likely to be of clinical significance when drugs such as metoprolol are given for heart failure.

Beta blockers + **Triptans**

No clinically important interaction occurs between most triptans and beta blockers, but the plasma levels of rizatriptan are almost doubled by propranolol.

> If propranolol is also given the manufacturers recommend a dose reduction to 5 mg of rizatriptan, with a maximum of two or three doses in 24 hours. In the UK it

is additionally recommended that dosing should be separated by 2 hours, but the basis for this is unclear, as a study found that this does not modify the interaction.

B

Bexarotene

Due to the low systemic exposure to bexarotene after topical use, any increases that occur with CYP3A4 inhibitors are unlikely to be sufficient to result in adverse effects with a low to moderate intensity topical bexarotene regimen.

Bexarotene + Contraceptives

The manufacturer suggests that bexarotene may theoretically increase the metabolism of contraceptive steroids, thereby reducing both their levels and their efficacy.

The manufacturer advises that additional non-hormonal contraception (such as a barrier method) should be used to avoid the risk of contraceptive failure. They point out that this is particularly important because if contraceptive failure were to occur, the foetus might be exposed to the teratogenic effects of bexarotene.

Bexarotene + Corticosteroids

The manufacturers say that, in theory, dexamethasone may reduce bexarotene levels.

This interaction does not appear to have been studied in patients, so the clinical importance of this prediction is unknown. However note that clinically relevant interactions occurring as a result of dexamethasone inducing CYP3A4 appear rare.

Bexarotene + Fibrates

A population analysis of patients with cutaneous T-cell lymphoma found that gemfibrozil substantially increased the plasma levels of oral bexarotene.

The manufacturers state that concurrent use should be avoided.

Bexarotene + Grapefruit juice

The manufacturers say that, in theory, grapefruit juice may raise bexarotene levels.

This interaction does not appear to have been studied in patients, so the clinical importance of this prediction is unknown.

Bexarotene + Macrolides

The manufacturers say that, in theory, clarithromycin and erythromycin may raise bexarotene levels.

This interaction does not appear to have been studied in patients, so the clinical importance of this prediction is unknown. If this prediction is clinically relevant other macrolides may also interact, although it seems unlikely that they all will, see macrolides, page 361.

Bexarotene + **Phenobarbital** ?

The manufacturers say that, in theory, phenobarbital (and therefore probably primidone) may reduce bexarotene levels.

This interaction does not appear to have been studied in patients, so the clinical importance of this prediction is unknown.

Bexarotene + **Phenytoin** ?

The manufacturers say that, in theory, phenytoin (and therefore probably fosphenytoin) may reduce bexarotene levels.

This interaction does not appear to have been studied in patients, so the clinical importance of this prediction is unknown.

Bexarotene + **Protease inhibitors** ?

The manufacturers say that, in theory, protease inhibitors may raise bexarotene levels.

This interaction does not appear to have been studied in patients, so the clinical importance of this prediction is unknown.

Bexarotene + **Rifampicin (Rifampin)** ?

The manufacturers say that, in theory, rifampicin may reduce bexarotene levels.

This interaction does not appear to have been studied in patients, so the clinical importance of this prediction is unknown.

Bexarotene + **Vitamin A** ⚠

Bexarotene is related to vitamin A.

In patients taking bexarotene vitamin A supplements should be limited to 15 000 units or less daily to avoid potentially additive toxic effects.

Bicalutamide

Bicalutamide + **Warfarin and other oral anticoagulants** ?

The manufacturers state that bicalutamide might interact with warfarin by displacing it from its protein binding sites, a mechanism that, as a sole cause of interactions, has now largely been discredited. To date, there appear to be no published or confirmed cases of an interaction.

> Despite this, the manufacturer of bicalutamide recommends that the prothrombin time be carefully monitored when it is given with coumarins, adjusting the dose when necessary.

Bisphosphonates

Bisphosphonates + Food

The absorption of the bisphosphonates is reduced by food.

> Recommendations on the timing of administration of bisphosphonates in relation to food and other drugs vary. Alendronate should be taken with plain (not mineral) water, after an overnight fast, at least 30 minutes before the first food of the day. Clodronate should be given at least 1 hour before or after food. Ibandronate should be given with plain water on an empty stomach at least 30 minutes to 1 hour before the first food of the day. Risedronate should be given at least 30 minutes before the first food or drink of the day or at least 2 hours from any food or drink during the day, and at least 30 minutes before bedtime. Etidronate and tiludronate should be given on an empty stomach at least 2 hours before or after food.

Bisphosphonates + Iron

The oral absorption of bisphosphonates is significantly reduced by aluminium/magnesium hydroxide. Other polyvalent cations, such as iron, are expected to interact similarly.

> Bisphosphonates should be prevented from coming into contact with iron. Recommendations on the timing of administration of bisphosphonates in relation to food and other drugs varies. Alendronate should be taken with plain (not mineral) water, after an overnight fast at least 30 minutes before taking the first dose of iron. Clodronate should probably be taken at least 1 hour before or after iron. Ibandronate should be taken with plain water on an empty stomach at least 30 minutes to 1 hour before iron. Risedronate should be taken at least 30 minutes before taking the first dose of iron or at least 2 hours from any iron doses during the rest of the day, and at least 30 minutes before bedtime. Etidronate and tiludronate should be taken on an empty stomach at least 2 hours apart from iron.

Bisphosphonates + NSAIDs

There is conflicting information as to whether the concurrent use of NSAIDs in patients taking alendronate increases the risk of gastrointestinal adverse effects. In clinical studies, no increased risk has been reported with concurrent use of NSAIDs with ibandronate. Indometacin increases tiludronate bioavailability about 2-fold.

NSAIDs may exacerbate the renal impairment sometimes seen with clodronate; zoledronate is predicted to interact similarly.

> Guidance regarding alendronate is conflicting: some consider that it should not be given to patients taking NSAIDs, others urge caution and others say that there is no evidence of increased gastrointestinal toxicity on concurrent use. It would seem sensible to monitor the concurrent use of alendronate and NSAIDs carefully. The manufacturer of ibandronate advises caution if it is given with an NSAID. The manufacturer advises that indometacin and tiludronate should be given 2 hours apart. Some bisphosphonates alone may cause renal impairment. Renal function should be assessed before giving a bisphosphonate and this would seem particularly important in those taking NSAIDs.

Bisphosphonates + Zinc

The oral absorption of bisphosphonates is significantly reduced by aluminium/magnesium hydroxide. Other polyvalent cations, such as zinc, are expected to interact similarly.

> Bisphosphonates should be prevented from coming into contact with zinc. Recommendations on the timing of administration of bisphosphonates in relation to food and other drugs varies. Alendronate should be taken with plain (not mineral) water, after an overnight fast at least 30 minutes before taking the first dose of zinc. Clodronate should probably be taken at least 1 hour before or after zinc. Ibandronate should be taken with plain water on an empty stomach at least 30 minutes to 1 hour before zinc. Risedronate should be taken at least 30 minutes before taking the first dose of zinc or at least 2 hours from any zinc doses during the rest of the day, and at least 30 minutes before bedtime. Etidronate and tiludronate should be taken on an empty stomach at least 2 hours apart from zinc.

Bupropion

Bupropion + Carbamazepine

Carbamazepine decreases the maximum plasma levels and AUC of bupropion by about 81 to 96%. The AUC of the active metabolite of bupropion, hydroxybupropion, is increased by 50%.

> Monitor for any evidence of reduced efficacy (which is likely) and/or increased toxicity (due to the increased exposure to the metabolite). Note that bupropion is contraindicated in patients with seizure disorders.

Bupropion + Clopidogrel

Clopidogrel increases the AUC of bupropion by 60% and decreases the AUC of its active metabolite, hydroxybupropion, by about 50%.

> The clinical relevance of these modest changes is unclear. It would seem prudent

to monitor for increased bupropion adverse effects (lightheadedness, gastrointestinal effects) and/or efficacy, adjusting the dose as necessary.

B

Bupropion + Dextromethorphan ?

Bupropion may reduce the metabolism of dextromethorphan in some patients.

Dextromethorphan is generally considered to have a wide therapeutic range and its dose is not individually titrated; therefore, the interaction with bupropion is unlikely to be clinically relevant. Nevertheless, it is possible that some patients might become more sensitive to the adverse effects of dextromethorphan while taking bupropion. Note that dextromethorphan is widely found in non-prescription preparations such as cough suppressants.

Bupropion + Flecainide ⚠

The manufacturers warn that bupropion may raise flecainide levels (by inhibiting CYP2D6). This seems a reasonable prediction as other CYP2D6 substrates are affected by bupropion in this way.

If flecainide is added to treatment with bupropion, doses at the lower end of the range should be used. If bupropion is added to existing treatment, decreased doses should be considered.

Bupropion + Herbal medicines or Dietary supplements ?

Mania and dystonia have been reported in patients taking St John's wort (*Hypericum perforatum*) and bupropion.

No general conclusions can be drawn from these isolated reports.

Bupropion + Levodopa ⚠

The manufacturer says that the concurrent use of bupropion and levodopa should be undertaken with caution because limited clinical data suggests a higher incidence of undesirable effects (nausea, vomiting, excitement, restlessness, postural tremor).

Good monitoring is advisable and patients should be given small initial bupropion doses, which should be increased gradually.

Bupropion + MAOIs ✕

In theory, bupropion toxicity may be enhanced by the MAOIs and concurrent use could lead to severe hypertension, but there appears to be no evidence to suggest that this occurs in practice.

Some manufacturers state that concurrent use is contraindicated with and for 2 weeks after the use of an MAOI.

Bupropion + Moclobemide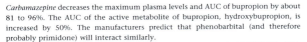

In theory, the concurrent use of bupropion and moclobemide could lead to severe hypertension, but there appears to be no evidence to suggest that this occurs in practice.

Some manufacturers state that concurrent use is contraindicated with and for 24 hours after stopping moclobemide.

B

Bupropion + Phenobarbital

Carbamazepine decreases the maximum plasma levels and AUC of bupropion by about 81 to 96%. The AUC of the active metabolite of bupropion, hydroxybupropion, is increased by 50%. The manufacturers predict that phenobarbital (and therefore probably primidone) will interact similarly.

Monitor for any evidence of reduced efficacy (which is likely) and/or increased toxicity (due to the increased exposure to the metabolite). Note that bupropion is contraindicated in patients with seizure disorders.

Bupropion + Phenytoin

Carbamazepine decreases the maximum plasma levels and AUC of bupropion by about 81 to 96%. The AUC of the active metabolite of bupropion, hydroxybupropion, is increased by 50%. The manufacturers predict that phenytoin (and therefore possibly fosphenytoin) will interact similarly.

Monitor for any evidence of reduced efficacy (which is likely) and/or increased toxicity (due to the increased exposure to the metabolite). Note that bupropion is contraindicated in patients with seizure disorders.

Bupropion + Propafenone

The manufacturers warn that bupropion may raise propafenone levels (by inhibiting CYP2D6). This seems a reasonable prediction as other CYP2D6 substrates are affected by bupropion in this way.

If propafenone is added to treatment with bupropion, doses at the lower end of the range should be used. If bupropion is added to existing treatment, decreased doses should be considered.

Bupropion + Protease inhibitors ⚠

Ritonavir, both at doses used to boost the levels of other protease inhibitors and higher doses, *decreases* the levels of bupropion and its active metabolite: reduced efficacy might be expected. This is the opposite effect to that which was originally predicted.

The extent of reduction in bupropion levels seen suggests that the dose of bupropion might need to be doubled. It would seem prudent to start bupropion at the recommended starting dose and titrate to effect. Nevertheless, because of the original *in vitro* data, the UK manufacturers of bupropion currently state that the recommended doses should not be exceeded.

B

Bupropion + Rifampicin (Rifampin)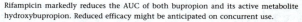

Rifampicin markedly reduces the AUC of both bupropion and its active metabolite hydroxybupropion. Reduced efficacy might be anticipated on concurrent use.

Monitor the efficacy of bupropion in any patient requiring rifampicin, and titrate the bupropion dose as necessary.

Bupropion + SSRIs

In theory, SSRIs that inhibit CYP2D6 (such as paroxetine and fluoxetine) may raise bupropion levels, but studies have not found a clinically relevant effect. However, the concurrent use of bupropion and an SSRI has lead to psychosis, mania, seizures, serotonin syndrome and hypersexuality.

Concurrent use should be well monitored. The manufacturers recommend that drugs that are metabolised by CYP2D6 (most SSRIs are, but fluoxetine, paroxetine and sertraline have been specifically named) should be given with bupropion with caution and initiated at the lower end of the dose range. If bupropion is given to a patient already taking a drug metabolised by CYP2D6, the need to decrease the dose of this drug should be considered. Note that because the SSRIs can reduce the seizure threshold consideration should be given to reducing the dose of bupropion to a maximum of 150 mg daily for smoking cessation.

Bupropion + Ticlopidine

Ticlopidine increases the AUC of bupropion and decreases the AUC of its active metabolite, hydroxybupropion; both by about 85%.

The clinical relevance of these modest changes is unclear. It would seem prudent to monitor for increased bupropion adverse effects (lightheadedness, gastrointestinal effects) and efficacy, adjusting the dose as necessary.

Bupropion + Tricyclics

Bupropion may increase the levels of the tricyclics, including desipramine, imipramine, and nortriptyline. Adverse effects including confusion, lethargy and unsteadiness have been reported with nortriptyline and bupropion. A seizure occurred in two patients given trimipramine or clomipramine with bupropion.

It would be prudent to be alert for increased tricyclic adverse effects if bupropion is also given, reducing the tricyclic dose as necessary. Note that a maximum bupropion dose of 150 mg daily is recommended if it is given with other drugs that reduce the seizure threshold, such as the tricyclics.

Bupropion + Valproate

A study found that the AUC of the active metabolite of bupropion was almost doubled when bupropion was given with valproate. An increase in valproate levels of almost 30% was seen in one patient and visual and auditory hallucinations have been reported in another patient, which resolved when bupropion was stopped.

Monitor for any evidence of increased toxicity (due to the raised bupropion metabolites or valproate). Note that bupropion is contraindicated in patients with seizure disorders.

Buspirone

Buspirone + **Calcium-channel blockers** ⚠

Diltiazem and verapamil inhibit CYP3A4, and they can therefore raise the peak levels of buspirone 3- to 5.5-fold, which increases the likelihood of adverse effects.

The US manufacturers suggest adjusting the buspirone dose according to response, while the UK manufacturers suggest starting with buspirone 2.5 mg twice daily.

Buspirone + **Grapefruit juice** ⚠

Grapefruit juice can significantly increase plasma levels of buspirone (peak level increased more than 4-fold, but a only minor increase in effects seen).

The UK manufacturer recommends a lower dose of buspirone e.g. 2.5 mg twice daily with grapefruit juice whereas the US manufacturer suggests that patients should avoid drinking large quantities of grapefruit juice.

Buspirone + **Herbal medicines or Dietary supplements**

A patient taking buspirone developed marked CNS adverse effects after starting to take herbal medicines including St John's wort (*Hypericum perforatum*), melatonin and *Ginkgo biloba*.Serotonin syndrome, page 454 has been reported in a patient who took buspirone with St John's wort (*Hypericum perforatum*).

The general significance of these cases is unclear, but they highlight the importance of considering the adverse effects of herbal medicines when they are used with conventional medicines.

Buspirone + **Linezolid** ⚠

Linezolid has weak MAO-inhibitory properties and it is therefore possible that it may interact with buspirone in the same way as the non-selective MAOIs (see Buspirone + MAOIs, page 176).

The manufacturers say that unless there are facilities for close observation and monitoring of blood pressure linezolid should not be given with buspirone.

Buspirone + Macrolides

In one study the maximum levels and AUC of buspirone were increased 5-fold and 6-fold, respectively, by erythromycin, which resulted in psychomotor impairment and an increase in adverse effects.

> Monitor the outcome of concurrent use carefully, expecting to need to reduce the buspirone dose. The manufacturers suggest a starting dose of buspirone 2.5 mg twice daily. Other macrolides (such as clarithromycin and telithromycin) may also interact, although it seems unlikely that all macrolides will, see macrolides, page 361.

Buspirone + MAOIs

Elevated blood pressure has been reported in patients taking buspirone with either phenelzine or tranylcypromine. All non-selective MAOIs could, theoretically, interact similarly.

> The manufacturers of buspirone recommend that it should not be used concurrently with any MAOI. One US manufacturer of tranylcypromine contraindicates concurrent use and states that at least 10 days should elapse between stopping the MAOI and starting buspirone.

Buspirone + Protease inhibitors

Ritonavir, and possibly indinavir, are predicted to reduce the metabolism of buspirone. A single case report describes Parkinson-like symptoms attributed to this interaction.

> The UK manufacturer of buspirone recommends that a lower dose of buspirone, 2.5 mg twice daily, should be used with potent inhibitors of CYP3A4, such as ritonavir and other protease inhibitors.

Buspirone + Rifampicin (Rifampin)

Rifampicin can cause a dramatic reduction in the peak levels of buspirone and therefore diminish its effects.

> This interaction would appear to be clinically important. If both drugs are used be alert for the need to use an increased buspirone dose, although the extent of this interaction is so great that this may not be effective.

Buspirone + SSRIs ?

Isolated reports describe the development of serotonin syndrome, page 454 on the concurrent use of buspirone and an SSRI. The combination of buspirone and fluoxetine can be effective, but seizures and worsening of symptoms have been reported. Fluvoxamine may possibly reduce the effects of buspirone.

> The general importance of these adverse reactions is not well understood. There would seem to be little reason for avoiding concurrent use; however, bear them in mind when buspirone is given with an SSRI.

Busulfan

Busulfan + Phenytoin [?]

Phenytoin increases the clearance of busulfan and reduces its AUC by about 20%. Subtherapeutic levels of phenytoin may occur in the presence of busulfan.

The changes in busulfan clearance are relatively small, but nevertheless it has been suggested that phenytoin should be avoided in patients taking busulfan. The UK manufacturer of parenteral busulfan found no evidence that phenytoin increased its clearance whereas another suggests using a benzodiazepine instead of phenytoin for prophylaxis. The US manufacturer of parenteral busulfan gives a dose assuming that phenytoin will also be given, and notes that if other antiepileptics are used instead, the busulfan plasma levels may be increased and monitoring is recommended. If both drugs are given monitor closely to ensure that busulfan remains effective, and that phenytoin levels remain therapeutic.

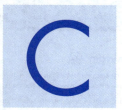

Calcium-channel blockers

Both verapamil and diltiazem are principally metabolised by CYP3A4, and also inhibit this isoenzyme. They are therefore affected by drugs that induce or inhibit CYP3A4, and also themselves affect drugs metabolised by CYP3A4. Many of the dihydropyridine-type calcium-channel blockers are also metabolised by CYP3A4, and are affected by inducers or inhibitors of this isoenzyme. However, they do not generally inhibit CYP3A4 or other isoenzymes to a clinically relevant extent. The exception is perhaps nicardipine, which may cause a clinically relevant inhibition of CYP3A4.

Calcium-channel blockers + Calcium-channel blockers ⚠

Plasma levels of both nifedipine and diltiazem are increased by concurrent use and blood pressure is reduced accordingly. Verapamil is predicted to interact similarly with nifedipine. Amlodipine levels are raised by diltiazem (and therefore possibly verapamil). There are isolated reports of intestinal occlusion attributed to the concurrent use of nifedipine and diltiazem. If nimodipine is used with another calcium-channel blocker, additive reductions in blood pressure are likely.

> Monitor blood pressure on concurrent use and adjust the dose or stop one calcium-channel blocker as appropriate. The clinical use of two calcium-channel blockers is rarely justified and consideration should be given to stopping one or other of the drugs, as appropriate.

Calcium-channel blockers + Carbamazepine

Diltiazem or Verapamil ⚠

Case reports describe raised carbamazepine levels, sometimes accompanied by toxicity, in patients also given diltiazem or verapamil.

> Monitor carbamazepine levels and adjust the dose accordingly. A 50% reduction in the dose of carbamazepine has been suggested if diltiazem is to be used. Indicators of carbamazepine toxicity include nausea, vomiting, ataxia and drowsiness.

Nimodipine ⊗

Nimodipine levels are decreased by 85% by carbamazepine.

The manufacturers contraindicate concurrent use.

Other calcium-channel blockers ⚠

Felodipine, nifedipine and nilvadipine levels are decreased by carbamazepine, probably as a result of CYP3A4 induction. All calcium-channel blockers are metabolised by CYP3A4, and carbamazepine would therefore be expected to decrease their levels to some extent.

Monitor the outcome of concurrent use, being aware that the dose of the calcium-channel blocker may need to be raised. Oxcarbazepine interacts to a lesser extent and may be suitable alternative in some patients.

Calcium-channel blockers + Ciclosporin (Cyclosporine)

Lercanidipine ⊗

The plasma levels of lercanidipine were raised 3-fold by ciclosporin, and the ciclosporin AUC was raised by 21% by lercanidipine. Combined use of calcium-channel blockers and ciclosporin increases the risk of gingival overgrowth.

The manufacturers contraindicate or advise against concurrent use.

Other calcium-channel blockers ⚠

Diltiazem, nicardipine and verapamil markedly raise serum ciclosporin levels but also appear to possess kidney protective effects. Amlodipine has modestly increased ciclosporin levels in some studies, but not in others, and it may also have kidney protective properties. A single case describes elevated ciclosporin levels caused by nisoldipine. Nifedipine normally appears not to interact, but rises and falls in ciclosporin levels have been seen in a few patients. Combined use of calcium-channel blockers and ciclosporin increases the risk of gingival overgrowth.

Ciclosporin levels and/or effects (e.g. on renal function) should be well monitored (especially with diltiazem, nicardipine and verapamil) and dose reductions made as necessary. With diltiazem and verapamil the ciclosporin dose can apparently be reduced by about 25 to 50%.

Calcium-channel blockers + Cilostazol

Diltiazem or Verapamil ⚠

Diltiazem increases the AUC of cilostazol by about 40%. Verapamil would be expected to interact similarly.

Monitor concurrent use for cilostazol adverse effects (such as headache and diarrhoea). The manufacturers suggest reducing the cilostazol dose to 50 mg twice daily.

Other calcium-channel blockers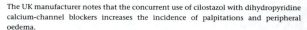

The UK manufacturer notes that the concurrent use of cilostazol with dihydropyridine calcium-channel blockers increases the incidence of palpitations and peripheral oedema.

Monitor the outcome of concurrent use for an increase in these adverse effects.

Calcium-channel blockers + Colchicine

Verapamil may markedly increase colchicine levels, which led to neuromyopathy in one man.

Although this is an isolated case, it is in line with the way both drugs interact with other substances. Therefore it would seem prudent to suspect an interaction in the case of otherwise unexplained colchicine toxicity. Note that concurrent use is contraindicated in renal or hepatic impairment.

Calcium-channel blockers + Corticosteroids

Diltiazem increases the AUC of intravenous and oral methylprednisolone.

The clinical significance of this interaction is unclear. It has been suggested that patients should be monitored for methylprednisolone adverse effects (e.g. fluid retention, hypertension and hyperglycaemia), and this seems a prudent precaution.

Calcium-channel blockers + Darifenacin

Erythromycin almost doubles the AUC of darifenacin by inhibiting its metabolism by CYP3A4. Other moderate inhibitors of CYP3A4 such as diltiazem and verapamil are expected to interact similarly.

The UK manufacturer recommends an initial dose of darifenacin 7.5 mg daily in those taking moderate CYP3A4 inhibitors, increasing the dose to 15 mg daily if the dose is well tolerated. However the US manufacturers suggest that no dose adjustments are necessary with these calcium-channel blockers. Bear in mind the possibility of an interaction if antimuscarinic effects (dry mouth, constipation, drowsiness) are increased.

Calcium-channel blockers + Digoxin

Diltiazem

Serum digoxin levels were found to be unchanged by diltiazem in a number of studies but other studies describe increases ranging from 20 to 85%. Additive bradycardia and heart block may also occur with concurrent use.

All patients taking digoxin with diltiazem should be well monitored for signs of over-digitalisation or additive adverse effects (e.g. bradycardia), and digoxin dose reductions should be made if necessary.

Verapamil

Serum digoxin levels are increased by about 40% by verapamil 160 mg daily, and by about 70% by verapamil 240 mg daily. Digoxin toxicity may develop if the dose is not reduced. Deaths have occurred as a result of this interaction. There is a risk of additive bradycardia and conduction disturbances when cardiac glycosides are given with verapamil.

> An initial 30 to 50% digoxin dose reduction has been recommended. The interaction develops within 2 to 7 days, approaching or reaching a maximum within 14 days or so. Monitor digoxin levels and for signs of digoxin toxicity (such as nausea, vomiting, visual disturbances, confusion) as well as cardiac conduction disorders during this period.

Other calcium-channel blockers

Felodipine, lacidipine, lercanidipine, nicardipine and nisoldipine cause small increases in digoxin levels (maximum rise seen was about 30%, which was not considered clinically significant). The situation with nitrendipine is uncertain but it possibly causes only a small rise in digoxin levels. Serum digoxin levels are normally unchanged or increased only to a small extent by the concurrent use of nifedipine. However, one isolated study indicated that a 45% rise could occur.

> Bear this interaction in mind if patients are treated with digoxin and one of these calcium-channel blockers. The possibility of a serious interaction seems small, but if undesirable bradycardia or other symptoms of over-digitalisation occur consider taking digoxin levels.

Calcium-channel blockers + Disopyramide

Profound hypotension and collapse has occurred in a small number of patients taking verapamil with disopyramide.

> The UK manufacturer warns about giving disopyramide with verapamil (because of additive negative inotropic effects), although in some specific circumstances the combination may be beneficial. However, the US manufacturer advises that until more data is available, disopyramide should not be given within 48 hours before or 24 hours after verapamil. If concurrent used is necessary, monitor closely.

Calcium-channel blockers + Diuretics

Mild to moderate inhibitors of CYP3A4 (such as diltiazem and verapamil) cause up to a 3-fold increase in eplerenone levels, which increases the risks of hyperkalaemia.

> It is generally recommended that the dose of eplerenone should not exceed 25 mg daily in patients taking diltiazem or verapamil. Note that additive hypotensive effects are likely when calcium-channel blockers are given with any diuretic, see antihypertensives., page 89

Calcium-channel blockers + Donepezil ?

The risk of adverse effects, including bradycardia, may be increased if a centrally-acting anticholinesterase is given with a calcium-channel blocker. Although not specifically stated, only the calcium-channel blockers that have effects on heart rate (that is, diltiazem and verapamil) would be expected to be implicated.

> Be alert for bradycardia on the concurrent use of donepezil and diltiazem or verapamil and adjust treatment if necessary.

Calcium-channel blockers + Dutasteride

In one study diltiazem and verapamil were found to decrease the clearance of dutasteride by 44% and 37%, respectively. However, this was not thought to be clinically significant due to the wide therapeutic range of dutasteride.

> No action needed, although bear this interaction in mind if dutasteride adverse effects are troublesome. If this occurs, consider decreasing the dosing frequency of dutasteride.

Calcium-channel blockers + Flecainide

Although flecainide and verapamil have been used together successfully, serious and potentially life-threatening cardiogenic shock and asystole have been seen in a few patients. This is probably because the cardiac depressant effects of the two drugs can be additive.

> This interaction may not be of clinical significance in most patients, however those with poor cardiac reserve may be more susceptible. If both drugs are used, monitor the outcome carefully.

Calcium-channel blockers + Food

Some modified-release preparations of felodipine, nifedipine, and nisoldipine show markedly increased levels when given with food, particularly high-fat food. The bioavailability of lercanidipine is markedly increased and the absorption of manidipine is improved by food. Food modestly decreases the rate and extent of absorption of nimodipine capsules and food also modestly decreases the peak level of nicardipine.

> The manufacturers of *Vascalpha* (felodipine), *Adalat CC* (nifedipine) and *Sular* (nisoldipine) recommend that they are taken on an empty stomach or with a light meal, avoiding high-fat meals. Because of the potential increase in peak plasma concentrations, the manufacturers of lercanidipine advise giving it before meals (at least 15 minutes before has been recommended). The US manufacturer of nimodipine capsules recommends taking them not less than one hour before or 2 hours after meals. It has been recommended that manidipine and *Cardene SR* (nicardipine) should be taken with food. Consider also Grapefruit juice, page 183.

Calcium-channel blockers + Galantamine

The risk of adverse effects, including bradycardia, may be increased if a centrally-acting anticholinesterase is given with a calcium-channel blocker. Although not specifically stated, only the calcium-channel blockers that have effects on heart rate (that is, diltiazem and verapamil) would be expected to be implicated.

> Be alert for bradycardia on the concurrent use of galantamine and diltiazem or verapamil and adjust treatment if necessary.

Calcium-channel blockers + Grapefruit juice

Grapefruit juice very markedly increases the bioavailability of felodipine, manidipine, and nisoldipine, and alters their haemodynamic effects. The bioavailability of nicardipine, nifedipine, nimodipine, nitrendipine or verapamil is increased without significantly altering haemodynamic effects (some ECG changes were seen with verapamil), whereas the bioavailability of amlodipine and diltiazem is only minimally affected.

> The manufacturers of felodipine say that it should not be taken with grapefruit juice. It has been suggested that whole grapefruit or products made from grapefruit peel such as marmalade should also be avoided in patients taking felodipine. The manufacturers of lercanidipine and verapamil also contraindicate grapefruit juice, although this interaction is normally of little relevance with most calcium-channel blockers in the majority of patients. However it would be worth checking the diet of any patient who complains of increased or excessive adverse effects with any calcium-channel blocker (e.g. hypotension, headache, flushing, oedema).

Calcium-channel blockers + H$_2$-receptor antagonists

The plasma levels of diltiazem, felodipine, isradipine, lacidipine, nifedipine, nimodipine, nisoldipine, nitrendipine and possibly verapamil and lercanidipine, are increased by cimetidine.

> If cimetidine is given with a calcium-channel blocker monitor for an increase in the calcium-channel blocker effects (such as hypotension, flushing, headache, peripheral oedema). If necessary, a dose reduction should be considered and the following dose adjustments have been suggested, in general, 30 to 50% decreases have been suggested, but any decrease should be based on patient response. In theory, all calcium-channel blockers may interact similarly, although some evidence suggests that amlodipine does not interact.

Calcium-channel blockers + Herbal medicines or Dietary supplements

St John's wort (*Hypericum perforatum*) reduces the bioavailability of verapamil by 80% and nifedipine by 45%. Other calcium-channel blockers would be expected to interact similarly.

> Patients taking St John's wort with nifedipine or verapamil should have their blood pressure and heart rate monitored to ensure the calcium-channel blocker is still effective, and the dose should be adjusted if needed. There appears to be no information about other calcium-channel blockers, but as they are all metabolised

by CYP3A4, to a greater or lesser extent, it would seem prudent to monitor concurrent use carefully. If an interaction occurs it may be prudent to use an alternative class of drugs (ACE inhibitors, angiotensin II receptor antagonists and beta blockers are not known to be affected by CYP3A4), or advise against the use of St Johnâ s wort.

Calcium-channel blockers + Imatinib

A man taking nifedipine developed a gallstone after starting imatinib. Imatinib is predicted to increase levels of dihydropyridine-type calcium-channel blockers, which are CYP3A4 substrates. This seems reasonable, as imatinib raises the levels of the CYP3A4 substrate *simvastatin*, page 336.

Monitor concurrent use for an increase in calcium-channel blocker adverse effects, such as hypotension, headache, flushing, and oedema.

Calcium-channel blockers + Lithium

The concurrent use of lithium and verapamil can be uneventful, but neurotoxicity (ataxia, movement disorders, tremors) with unchanged lithium levels has been reported in a few patients. Reduced and increased lithium levels have also occurred with verapamil. An acute parkinsonian syndrome and marked psychosis has been seen in at least one patient taking lithium and diltiazem. Reduced lithium clearance, and one possible case of increased lithium levels have been reported with nifedipine.

The clinical significance of this interaction is unclear, as there is good evidence of uncomplicated treatment. Given the unpredictable changes in levels it may be prudent to consider monitoring lithium in patients also given verapamil, and considering an interaction as a possible cause if unexpected adverse effects develop with diltiazem or nifedipine.

Calcium-channel blockers + Macrolides

Lercanidipine

Because potent inhibitors of CYP3A4 have raised lercanidipine levels 15-fold the manufacturers predict that erythromycin will raise lercanidipine levels.

Concurrent use is contraindicated. Other macrolides may also interact, although it seems unlikely that they all will, see macrolides, page 361.

Other calcium-channel blockers

Erythromycin markedly increases the bioavailability of felodipine. Isolated reports describe increased felodipine, nifedipine or verapamil effects and toxicity in patients when given erythromycin, clarithromycin or telithromycin. Note that the calcium-channel blockers are all metabolised by CYP3A4, so all have the potential to interact.

Monitor concurrent use. Anticipate the need to reduce the calcium-channel blocker dose if erythromycin or clarithromycin, or possibly also telithromycin, is added and adverse effects become troublesome (such as hypotension, dizziness, flushing and palpitations).

Calcium-channel blockers + **Magnesium**

Pregnant women have developed bilateral hand contractures or muscular weakness and then paralysis, after receiving intravenous magnesium sulfate with nifedipine. Profound hypotension occurred in two women when nifedipine was added to magnesium sulfate and methyldopa. However a retrospective study did not find an increase in risk of neuromuscular effects or of hypotension on concurrent use. Other calcium-channel blockers would be expected to interact similarly, but this has not been studied.

> If concurrent use is essential be aware of this possible reaction. If problems occur, note that in the two cases of paralysis the interaction resolved rapidly when magnesium was stopped.

Calcium-channel blockers + **NNRTIs**

Efavirenz decreases the bioavailability of diltiazem by increasing its metabolism by CYP3A4; other calcium-channel blockers are expected to interact similarly. Delavirdine is predicted to inhibit the metabolism of the calcium-channel blockers.

> Monitor the outcome of concurrent use (e.g. blood pressure) and adjust the calcium-channel blocker dose as necessary. If dose titration of the calcium-channel blocker proves difficult it may be prudent, where possible, to try an alternative class of drugs. ACE inhibitors, angiotensin II receptor antagonists and beta blockers are not known to be affected by CYP3A4 and therefore may be suitable alternatives in some cases.

Calcium-channel blockers + **NSAIDs**

There is evidence that most NSAIDs can increase blood pressure in patients taking antihypertensives, although some studies have not found the increase to be clinically relevant. Individual patients may experience more significant effects. Some small pharmacokinetic interactions may occur, but they do not appear to be clinically relevant.

> Only some patients are affected. Nevertheless, some have suggested that the use of NSAIDs should be kept to a minimum in patients taking antihypertensives, whereas others suggest that the interaction is, generally, not clinically relevant. Consider monitoring blood pressure if an NSAID is started or stopped.

Calcium-channel blockers + **Phenobarbital**

Nimodipine or Isradipine

Nimodipine levels are decreased by 85% by phenobarbital. Isradipine is expected to be similarly affected by phenobarbital. Note that primidone is metabolised to phenobarbital and it therefore may interact in the same way as phenobarbital.

> The UK manufacturer of nimodipine contraindicates concurrent use with phenobarbital and the UK manufacturer of isradipine advises against concurrent use. If concurrent use is necessary, monitor the outcome, being aware that the dose of the calcium-channel blocker may need to be raised.

Other calcium-channel blockers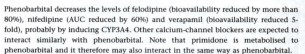

Phenobarbital decreases the levels of felodipine (bioavailability reduced by more than 80%), nifedipine (AUC reduced by 60%) and verapamil (bioavailability reduced 5-fold), probably by inducing CYP3A4. Other calcium-channel blockers are expected to interact similarly with phenobarbital. Note that primidone is metabolised to phenobarbital and it therefore may also interact in the same way as phenobarbital.

> Monitor the outcome of concurrent use, being aware that the dose of calcium-channel blocker may need to be raised. Given the size of the reductions seen it may be prudent to consider alternatives (ACE inhibitors, angiotensin II receptor antagonists and beta blockers are not known to be affected by CYP3A4).

Calcium-channel blockers + **Phenytoin**

Diltiazem or Nifedipine

Case reports describe phenytoin toxicity in patients given diltiazem or nifedipine.

> The general importance of this interaction is unknown, but bear it in mind in case of an unexpected response to treatment. Indicators of phenytoin toxicity include blurred vision, nystagmus, ataxia or drowsiness.

Isradipine, Nimodipine or Nisoldipine

Phenytoin (with carbamazepine) reduces nimodipine levels by 85% and phenytoin reduces the AUC of nisoldipine 10-fold. Fosphenytoin, a prodrug of phenytoin, may interact similarly. A man taking carbamazepine and phenytoin developed neuro-logical toxicity while also taking isradipine. Isradipine levels are also likely to be reduced by phenytoin.

> The manufacturers contraindicate the concurrent use of nimodipine or nisoldipine with phenytoin. The manufacturers of isradipine advise against its use with phenytoin.

Other calcium-channel blockers

Phenytoin reduces the levels of verapamil and felodipine (bioavailability reduced by more than 90%). Other calcium-channel blockers are expected to be similarly affected. Fosphenytoin, a prodrug of phenytoin, may also interact similarly.

> Monitor the outcome of concurrent use, being aware that the dose of calcium-channel blocker may need to be raised. Given the size of the reductions seen it may be prudent to consider alternatives.

Calcium-channel blockers + **Protease inhibitors**

The protease inhibitors, particularly ritonavir, are predicted to increase the levels of the calcium-channel blockers, to varying degrees: case reports describe adverse effects (hypotension, oedema, acute renal failure) on the concurrent use of a number of different protease inhibitor calcium-channel blocker pairs.

> If a protease inhibitor and a calcium-channel blocker are given, monitor for toxicity, such as hypotension, dizziness, flushing, oedema and palpitations,

reducing the dose of the calcium-channel blocker if necessary. Note that the UK manufacturer of lercanidipine contraindicates the concurrent use of strong inhibitors of CYP3A4; this would include most, if not all protease inhibitors. The initial dose of diltiazem should be reduced by 50% with subsequent dose titration and ECG monitoring when given with atazanavir. Consider alternative antihypertensives, such as ACE inhibitors and diuretics, which are primarily eliminated renally.

C

Calcium-channel blockers + Quinidine

Verapamil

Verapamil reduces the clearance of quinidine and in one patient the serum quinidine levels doubled and quinidine toxicity developed. Concurrent use has resulted in dizziness, blurred vision, atrioventricular block and a significant lowering of blood pressure.

A reduction in the dosage of quinidine (of up to 50%) may be needed to avoid toxicity. Monitor for an increase in quinidine adverse effects (e.g. nausea, diarrhoea, tinnitus).

Other calcium-channel blockers

The quinidine levels of a number of patients have increased when nifedipine was stopped, but no interaction has occurred in others. One study even suggests that quinidine serum levels may be slightly raised by nifedipine. Nifedipine levels may be modestly raised by quinidine. One study with diltiazem found that it did not interact with quinidine, whereas another found that diltiazem increased the quinidine AUC by 51%, with resulting significant increases in QTc and PR intervals, and a significant decrease in heart rate and diastolic blood pressure.

Monitor for quinidine adverse effects (e.g. nausea, diarrhoea, tinnitus) and, with nifedipine, for nifedipine adverse effects (e.g. hypotension, flushing, oedema). Adjust the doses of both drugs as necessary.

Calcium-channel blockers + Ranolazine

Verapamil and diltiazem increase ranolazine levels 2.2-fold and 2.4-fold, respectively, which increases the risk of QT prolongation and potentially life-threatening arrhythmias. However, concurrent use may be beneficial.

The UK manufacturer states that lower ranolazine doses and careful dose titration may be needed. The US manufacturer recommends that the dose of ranolazine should be limited to 500 mg twice daily. Monitor for adverse effects (nausea, dizziness) and reduce the dose of ranolazine if needed.

Calcium-channel blockers + Rifampicin (Rifampin)

The plasma levels of diltiazem, nifedipine, nilvadipine, verapamil and possibly those of barnidipine, isradipine, lercanidipine, manidipine, nicardipine, nimodipine, and nisoldipine are markedly reduced by rifampicin. They may become therapeutically ineffective unless their doses are raised. All calcium-channel blockers would be expected to be affected by rifampicin.

> Increase the frequency of blood pressure monitoring and adjust the antihypertensive dose, or use an alternative drug, as necessary. Note that some manufacturers of nifedipine and nimodipine contraindicate their use with rifampicin, and some manufacturers of diltiazem and isradipine advise avoiding concurrent use.

Calcium-channel blockers + Rivastigmine

The risk of adverse effects, including bradycardia, may be increased if a centrally-acting anticholinesterase is given with a calcium-channel blocker. Although not specifically stated, only the calcium-channel blockers that have effects on heart rate (that is, diltiazem and verapamil) would be expected to be implicated.

> Be alert for bradycardia on the concurrent use of rivastigmine and diltiazem or verapamil and adjust treatment if necessary.

Calcium-channel blockers + Sirolimus

The maximum serum levels of sirolimus are raised by diltiazem (43%) and verapamil (over 2-fold). Nicardipine is predicted to interact similarly. Sirolimus modestly increases verapamil levels.

> The manufacturers recommend monitoring and possible sirolimus dose adjustments if these calcium-channel blockers are used concurrently. The clinical relevance of the modest increase in verapamil levels is uncertain, but bear it in mind if an increase in verapamil adverse effects occurs (e.g. hypotension, flushing and oedema).

Calcium-channel blockers + Statins

Marked rises in statin plasma levels have been seen when lovastatin was given with diltiazem, and when simvastatin was given with diltiazem or verapamil. Isolated cases of rhabdomyolysis have been seen when atorvastatin or simvastatin were given with diltiazem or verapamil. Amlodipine appears to increase simvastatin levels by about 40%, and also increases the exposure to simvastatin acid. The UK manufacturer states that concurrent use of amlodipine with simvastatin 80 mg daily (but not 40 mg daily) increases the risk of myopathy. However, it seems that problems with combinations of statins and calcium-channel blockers (particularly the dihydropyridine-type) are rare.

> The manufacturers recommend a maximum simvastatin dose of 20 mg in patients taking verapamil and 40 mg in patients taking diltiazem, and a maximum dose of 40 mg of lovastatin in patients taking verapamil. With amlodipine, the UK manufacturer recommends a maximum dose of simvastatin 40 mg daily, with higher doses only given if the clinical benefit outweighs the risk. Patients should be told to be alert for any signs of possible rhabdomyolysis (i.e. otherwise unexplained muscle tenderness, pain or weakness or dark coloured urine). Fluvastatin, pravastatin and rosuvastatin appear less likely to interact with diltiazem or verapamil.

Calcium-channel blockers + **Tacrine**

The risk of adverse effects, including bradycardia, may be increased if a centrally-acting anticholinesterase is given with a calcium-channel blocker. Although not specifically stated, only the calcium-channel blockers that have effects on heart rate (that is, diltiazem and verapamil) would be expected to be implicated.

> Be alert for bradycardia on the concurrent use of tacrine and diltiazem or verapamil and adjust treatment if necessary.

Calcium-channel blockers + **Tacrolimus**

Nifedipine causes a moderate rise in serum tacrolimus levels and also appears to be kidney protective. Diltiazem and felodipine also appear to elevate tacrolimus levels. Nicardipine, verapamil, and possibly nilvadipine, are predicted to interact similarly.

> Tacrolimus levels and/or effects (e.g. on renal function) should be monitored as a matter of routine, but consider increasing monitoring if one of these calcium-channel blockers is started or stopped.

Calcium-channel blockers + **Theophylline**

Giving calcium-channel blockers to patients taking theophylline normally has no adverse effect on the control of asthma, despite the small or modest alterations that occur in theophylline levels with diltiazem, felodipine, nifedipine and verapamil. However, there are isolated case reports of unexplained theophylline toxicity in 2 patients given nifedipine and 2 patients given verapamil.

> In general no adverse interaction would be expected, however it would be prudent to be aware of the possibility of an interaction when these drugs are given.

Calcium-channel blockers + **Tricyclics**

Diltiazem and verapamil can increase imipramine levels, possibly accompanied by undesirable ECG changes. Two isolated reports describe increased nortriptyline and trimipramine levels in 2 patients given diltiazem. It has been suggested that the postural hypotension that may occur in patients taking tricyclics could be exacerbated by the use of antihypertensives.

> The general importance of this interaction is unclear, but bear it in mind in case of an unexpected response to treatment. Warn patients about the possibility of postural hypotension.

Calcium-channel blockers + **Valproate**

In a group of patients taking sodium valproate, the AUC of nimodipine was found to be about 50% higher than in a control group not taking sodium valproate.

> Monitor concurrent use carefully, bearing in mind it may be necessary to adjust the dose of nimodipine.

Capecitabine

Capecitabine + Folates

A patient died after treatment with capecitabine possibly because the concurrent use of folic acid enhanced capecitabine toxicity. The maximum tolerated dose of capecitabine is decreased by folinic acid.

> The UK manufacturers say that the maximum tolerated capecitabine dose when used alone in the intermittent regimen is 3 g/m^2, but it is reduced to 2 g/m^2 if folinic acid 30 mg twice daily is also given. Consider the use of folate supplements as a contributory factor in the case of troublesome capecitabine adverse effects.

Capecitabine + Phenytoin

Phenytoin toxicity occurred in a patient given capecitabine. Fosphenytoin, a prodrug of phenytoin, may interact similarly.

> As the interaction of capecitabine with phenytoin is in line with the way fluorouracil interacts, it would seem prudent to warn the patient to monitor for signs of phenytoin toxicity (blurred vision, nystagmus, ataxia or drowsiness). Take phenytoin levels and adjust the dose as necessary.

Capecitabine + Warfarin and other oral anticoagulants

Capecitabine has been reported to markedly increase the anticoagulant effects of phenprocoumon and warfarin: in one study the INR in response to warfarin was almost doubled by capecitabine. The interaction may occur within several days or even after months of concurrent use.

> The INR should be more frequently monitored in patients taking capecitabine with these and other coumarins. Note that, from a disease perspective, when treating venous thromboembolic disease in patients with cancer, warfarin is generally inferior (higher risk of major bleeds and recurrent thrombosis) to low-molecular-weight heparins.

Carbamazepine

Carbamazepine is extensively metabolised by CYP3A4 to the active 10,11-epoxide metabolite, which is then further metabolised. Concurrent use of CYP3A4 inhibitors or inducers may therefore lead to toxicity or reduced efficacy. However, importantly, carbamazepine also induces CYP3A4 and so induces its own metabolism (auto-induction). Because of this, it is important that drug interaction studies are multiple-dose and carried out at steady state. Auto-induction also means that moderate inducers of CYP3A4 may have less effect on steady-state carbamazepine levels than expected. Carbamazepine can also act as an inhibitor of CYP2C19.

Carbamazepine + Caspofungin

Population pharmacokinetic data suggests that carbamazepine may reduce caspofungin levels.

> The manufacturers say that consideration should be given to increasing the dose of caspofungin from 50 mg daily to 70 mg daily in adults and to 70 mg/m^2 daily (maximum 70 mg daily) in children.

Carbamazepine + Ciclosporin (Cyclosporine)

Carbamazepine has caused reductions of 50% or more in ciclosporin levels. This has occurred within 3 days of concurrent use.

> Ciclosporin levels and/or effects (e.g. on renal function) should be monitored as a matter of routine, but it may be prudent to increase monitoring and adjust the ciclosporin dose as needed if carbamazepine is stopped, started, or the dose altered.

Carbamazepine + Clopidogrel

On the basis of the interaction with the proton pump inhibitors, page 227, some predict that carbamazepine may theoretically inhibit the conversion of clopidogrel to its active metabolite by CYP2C19.

> The manufacturers advise that concurrent use should be avoided.

Carbamazepine + Contraceptives

Combined hormonal contraceptives, oral progestogen-only contraceptives and probably emergency hormonal contraceptives are less reliable during treatment with carbamazepine. Breakthrough bleeding and spotting can take place and unintended pregnancies have occurred. Controlled studies have shown that carbamazepine can reduce contraceptive steroid levels (both oestrogens and progestogens).

> Because of the consequences of an unwanted pregnancy, especially with drugs that may cause foetal abnormalities, adjustments should be made. For general advice on the use of enzyme inducers, such as carbamazepine, and contraceptives, see contraceptives, page 233.

Carbamazepine + Corticosteroids

The clearance of methylprednisolone and prednisolone is increased in patients taking carbamazepine. Dexamethasone clearance is also increased, and therefore the results of the dexamethasone adrenal suppression test may be invalid in those taking carbamazepine. More study is needed but it is likely that other corticosteroids such as hydrocortisone and prednisone may also be affected.

> Patients taking carbamazepine are likely to need increased doses of dexamethasone, methylprednisolone or prednisolone. Prednisolone is less affected than methylprednisolone and may therefore be preferred in some situations.

Carbamazepine + **Danazol** ⚠️

Serum carbamazepine levels can be doubled by danazol and carbamazepine toxicity may occur.

Consider monitoring carbamazepine levels and adjust the dose if necessary. Carbamazepine toxicity may present as nausea, vomiting, ataxia or drowsiness.

Carbamazepine + **Darifenacin** ⚠️

Carbamazepine (a CYP3A4 inducer) is predicted to decrease darifenacin levels. As CYP3A4 inhibitors raise darifenacin levels, this seems likely.

Monitor the outcome of concurrent use to ensure that darifenacin is effective.

Carbamazepine + **Diuretics** ❌

Because St John's wort (*Hypericum perforatum*) decreases the AUC of eplerenone by 30% the manufacturers say that more potent enzyme inducers (such as carbamazepine) may have a greater effect on eplerenone.

Concurrent use is not recommended by the manufacturers.

Carbamazepine + **Ethosuximide** ❓

Some, but not all studies suggest that carbamazepine reduces ethosuximide levels by about 20% and reduces its half-life by about 50%.

The concurrent use of antiepileptics is common and often advantageous and a clinically relevant interaction seems unlikely in most patients. Nevertheless, consider monitoring concurrent use for potential ethosuximide toxicity and to ensure adequate seizure control.

Carbamazepine + **Exemestane** ⚠️

Rifampicin (*rifampin*) reduces the AUC and maximum serum levels of exemestane by 54% and 41%, respectively. Carbamazepine is predicted to interact similarly.

Monitor concurrent use for exemestane efficacy. The manufacturers suggest doubling the exemestane dose to 50 mg daily.

Carbamazepine + **Gestrinone**

The manufacturers warn that carbamazepine may increase the metabolism of gestrinone and thereby reduce its effects.

The clinical significance of this warning is unclear. There appear to be no reports of an interaction in practice.

Carbamazepine + Grapefruit juice

Grapefruit juice increases carbamazepine levels by about 40%. A case of possible carbamazepine toxicity has been seen in a man taking carbamazepine after he started to eat grapefruit.

> The manufacturers advise monitoring levels and adjusting the dose of carbamazepine as necessary. If monitoring is not practical, or regular intake of grapefruit is not desired, it would seem prudent to avoid grapefruit or grapefruit juice.

Carbamazepine + H$_2$-receptor antagonists

The serum levels of those taking long-term carbamazepine may transiently increase, possibly accompanied by an increase in adverse effects, for the first few days after starting to take cimetidine, but these adverse effects rapidly disappear.

> An increase in carbamazepine adverse effects (nausea, headache, dizziness, fatigue, drowsiness, ataxia, an inability to concentrate, a bitter taste) may be seen, and patients should be warned. However, because the serum levels are only transiently increased the adverse effects normally disappear by the end of a week. Ranitidine appears to be a non-interacting alternative to cimetidine, and oxcarbazepine appears to be a non-interacting alternative to carbamazepine.

Carbamazepine + Herbal medicines or Dietary supplements

St John's wort (*Hypericum perforatum*) modestly increased the clearance of single-dose carbamazepine in one study, but had no effect on multiple-dose carbamazepine in another study.

> Before the publication of these studies the CSM in the UK had advised that patients taking carbamazepine should not take St John's wort. This advice was based on predicted pharmacokinetic interactions. In the light of the above studies, this advice may no longer apply, although concurrent use should probably still be monitored to ensure adequate carbamazepine levels and efficacy.

Carbamazepine + HRT

Enzyme-inducing drugs (such as carbamazepine), which increase the metabolism of contraceptive steroids, may reduce the efficacy of HRT.

> This effect is most noticeable where HRT is prescribed for menopausal vasomotor symptoms, but might be difficult to detect where the indication is osteoporosis. Any interaction may be less likely with transdermal HRT. However, as yet the clinical significance of any interaction is unclear.

Carbamazepine + Imatinib

In a study, the AUC of imatinib was about 70% lower in patients taking enzyme-inducing antiepileptics (including carbamazepine) than patients not taking these drugs.

> The manufacturers suggest that concurrent use should be avoided. However, if this

is not possible it would be prudent to monitor the outcome of concurrent use, and increase the imatinib dose (a 50% increase has been suggested) as necessary.

Carbamazepine + Isoniazid

Carbamazepine levels are markedly and very rapidly increased by isoniazid, and toxicity can occur. *Rifampicin (rifampin)* has been reported both to augment and negate this interaction. Limited evidence suggests that carbamazepine may potentiate isoniazid hepatotoxicity.

Carbamazepine toxicity can develop quickly (within 1 to 5 days) and also seems to disappear quickly if isoniazid is withdrawn. Monitor concurrent use and reduce the carbamazepine dose as necessary. Carbamazepine toxicity may present as nausea, vomiting, ataxia or drowsiness.

Carbamazepine + Lamotrigine

Most studies have found that lamotrigine has no effect on the pharmacokinetics of carbamazepine or its active epoxide metabolite. However, some studies have found that lamotrigine raises the serum levels of carbamazepine-epoxide. Carbamazepine reduces lamotrigine levels. Toxicity has been seen irrespective of changes in levels.

Patients should be well monitored if lamotrigine is added, and the carbamazepine dose reduced if CNS adverse effects occur. Carbamazepine induces the metabolism of lamotrigine, and the recommended starting dose and long-term maintenance dose of lamotrigine in patients already taking carbamazepine is twice that of patients receiving lamotrigine monotherapy. However, if they are also taking valproate in addition to carbamazepine, the lamotrigine dose should be reduced.

Carbamazepine + Levothyroxine

Clinical hypothyroidism can occur in patients stabilised taking levothyroxine when they start carbamazepine.

Be alert for any evidence of changes in thyroid status if carbamazepine is added or withdrawn from patients taking levothyroxine. Monitor thyroid hormone levels if an interaction is suspected.

Carbamazepine + Lithium

Although the combined use of lithium and carbamazepine is beneficial in many patients, mild to severe neurotoxicity is reported to have developed in some, and possibly sinus node dysfunction in others.

Monitor the outcome of concurrent use carefully, but note that signs of toxicity have developed even with lithium levels within the normal range. If severe neurotoxicity develops the lithium treatment should be discontinued promptly, whatever the lithium level. Risk factors appear to be a history of neurotoxicity with lithium therapies and compromised medical or neurological functioning.

Carbamazepine + Macrolides

Erythromycin or Telithromycin

Erythromycin raises carbamazepine levels by as much as 5-fold, which has resulted in toxicity in several cases. Telithromycin is predicted to interact similarly.

Avoid the concurrent use of carbamazepine and erythromycin unless carbamazepine levels can be closely monitored and suitable dose reductions made. Symptoms commonly begin within 24 to 72 hours of starting erythromycin. In most cases toxicity resolves within 5 days of stopping the erythromycin. Carbamazepine toxicity may present as nausea, vomiting, ataxia or drowsiness. The manufacturers of telithromycin recommend avoiding concurrent use during and for up to 2 weeks after carbamazepine treatment. If concurrent use is essential monitor carbamazepine levels and adjust the dose as necessary.

Other macrolides

Clarithromycin raises carbamazepine levels by 20 to 50%, despite dose reductions of up to 40%. Several cases of toxicity have been seen.

Monitor carbamazepine levels and adjust the dose accordingly. It has been recommended that carbamazepine doses are reduced by 30 to 50% and patients monitored within 3 to 5 days of starting clarithromycin. Carbamazepine toxicity may present as nausea, vomiting, ataxia or drowsiness.

Carbamazepine + MAOIs

MAOIs and carbamazepine have been used together, uneventfully and successfully, and there appear to be no reports of an interaction. However, because carbamazepine is structurally related to the tricyclics, page 376, which should be avoided with MAOIs, the manufacturers of carbamazepine suggest avoiding concurrent use.

Avoid concurrent use. MAOIs should be discontinued at least 2 weeks before carbamazepine is started, although this may be over-cautious. Note that, rarely, the MAOIs have been seen to cause convulsions and they should therefore be used cautiously in patients with epilepsy.

Carbamazepine + Mebendazole

Carbamazepine appears to lower the plasma levels of mebendazole.

When treating systemic worm infections it may be necessary to increase the mebendazole dose in patients taking carbamazepine. Monitor the outcome of concurrent use. This interaction is of no importance when mebendazole is used for intestinal worm infections where its action is a local effect on the worms in the gut.

Carbamazepine + Melatonin

One manufacturer predicts that carbamazepine may increase the metabolism of melatonin (by inducing CYP1A2), thereby decreasing its levels. However, note that carbamazepine is not a particularly potent inducer of this isoenzyme.

No action needed.

Carbamazepine + **Methylphenidate**

Limited evidence suggests that carbamazepine may decrease methylphenidate levels.

It would seem wise to monitor the response to methylphenidate treatment carefully in patients taking carbamazepine. Note that the manufacturer states that methylphenidate should be used with caution in patients with epilepsy, as it can, rarely, cause an increase in seizure frequency. If seizure frequency increases, methylphenidate should be discontinued.

Carbamazepine + **Mirtazapine**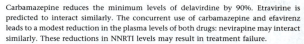

Carbamazepine decreases the AUC and maximum plasma levels of mirtazapine, by 63% and 44%, respectively. Mirtazapine does not appear to affect the pharmacokinetics of carbamazepine.

Monitor concurrent use to assess mirtazapine efficacy, and adjust the dose accordingly. Note that, mirtazapine can lower the seizure threshold, and therefore its use should be carefully considered in patients with epilepsy.

Carbamazepine + **NNRTIs**

Carbamazepine reduces the minimum levels of delavirdine by 90%. Etravirine is predicted to interact similarly. The concurrent use of carbamazepine and efavirenz leads to a modest reduction in the plasma levels of both drugs: nevirapine may interact similarly. These reductions in NNRTI levels may result in treatment failure.

The use of an NNRTI with carbamazepine is not recommended, or should be undertaken with caution. Use an alternative to carbamazepine if possible or monitor NNRTI plasma levels (where possible) and ensure antiviral efficacy. Note that efavirenz may itself cause seizures and caution is recommended in patients with a history of convulsions.

Carbamazepine + **Opioids**

Dextropropoxyphene (Propoxyphene)

Dextropropoxyphene has caused rises in trough serum carbamazepine levels of around 70 to 600%. Several cases of toxicity have been seen.

Monitor carbamazepine levels and adjust the dose if necessary. Consider using a non-interacting analgesic as an alternative. Carbamazepine toxicity may present as nausea, vomiting, ataxia or drowsiness.

Other opioids

Carbamazepine appears to reduce the serum levels of fentanyl (48 to 144% dose increase needed), methadone (opiate withdrawal seen), and tramadol. Buprenorphine is predicted to be similarly affected.

Be alert for the need to increase opioid doses. It may be necessary to give methadone twice daily to prevent withdrawal symptoms towards the end of the day. One UK manufacturer of buprenorphine and one US manufacturer of tramadol advises avoiding the concurrent use of carbamazepine. Note that tramadol should be avoided in patients with a history of epilepsy.

Carbamazepine + **Phenobarbital**

Carbamazepine serum levels are reduced to some extent by phenobarbital, but the levels of its active metabolite are raised; seizure control remains unaffected. In children, phenobarbital clearance is decreased by carbamazepine. Primidone seems to interact similarly.

This interaction seems to be of little clinical importance as seizure control is not affected. However, it would be prudent to monitor phenobarbital levels in children also given carbamazepine as changes in clearance may affect dose requirements.

Carbamazepine + **Phenytoin**

Some reports describe rises in serum phenytoin levels, with toxicity, whereas others describe falls in phenytoin levels. Genetic differences in the metabolism of these drugs may be an explanation for the differences. Falls in carbamazepine levels, sometimes with rises in carbamazepine-epoxide levels, have been described. Fosphenytoin is a prodrug of phenytoin and therefore it may interact similarly.

Monitor antiepileptic levels during concurrent use (where possible including carbamazepine-epoxide, the active metabolite of carbamazepine) so that steps can be taken to avoid the development of toxicity or lack of efficacy. Not all patients appear to have an adverse interaction, and, at present, it does not seem possible to identify those potentially at risk.

Carbamazepine + **Phosphodiesterase type-5 inhibitors**

Carbamazepine is predicted to reduce the levels of phosphodiesterase type-5 inhibitors, because other inducers of CYP3A4 have been shown to do so. For example, sildenafil levels are reduced by about 60% by *bosentan* and tadalafil levels are reduced by 88% by *rifampicin* (*rifampin*). Vardenafil is also metabolised by CYP3A4, and therefore its levels may possibly be lowered by carbamazepine.

If these phosphodiesterase type-5 inhibitors are not effective in patients taking carbamazepine, it would seem sensible to try a higher dose with close monitoring.

Carbamazepine + **Praziquantel**

Carbamazepine markedly reduces the exposure to praziquantel by 90%, but whether this results in neurocysticercosis treatment failures is unclear; one study found that concurrent use was still effective.

When treating systemic worm infections such as neurocysticercosis some authors have advised increasing the praziquantel dose from 25 to 50 mg/kg if carbamazepine is being taken, but in one study this dose was not effective. Note that the manufacturers current recommended dose of praziquantel for neurocysticercosis is 50 mg/kg daily in 3 divided doses. The interaction with carbamazepine is of no importance when praziquantel is used for intestinal worm infections (where its action is a local effect on the worms in the gut).

Carbamazepine + **Protease inhibitors**

Case reports suggest that ritonavir markedly increases carbamazepine levels and toxicity. Cases have also been reported with ritonavir-boosted lopinavir, and nelfinavir. Ritonavir-boosted darunavir also appears to increase the levels of carbamazepine. Carbamazepine reduces indinavir levels and efficacy, reduces tipranavir levels, and would also be expected to decrease the levels of other protease inhibitors.

> Avoid concurrent use where possible (mainly because of the risk of antiviral treatment failure): some manufacturers contraindicate concurrent use. If carbamazepine and a protease inhibitor must be used then extremely close monitoring of both protease inhibitor levels/efficacy and carbamazepine levels/toxicity is warranted. Indicators of carbamazepine toxicity include nausea, vomiting, ataxia and drowsiness. The authors of one report suggest that amitriptyline or gabapentin would be possible alternatives for carbamazepine when used for pain, or valproic acid or lamotrigine for carbamazepine when used for seizures. However, note that ritonavir may raise the levels of some tricyclics, page 440.

Carbamazepine + **Ranolazine**

Rifampicin (rifampin) reduces ranolazine levels by 95%, and loss of efficacy is expected. Carbamazepine is predicted to interact in the same way as rifampicin.

> The manufacturers recommend avoiding concurrent use. In the absence of any information on the magnitude of the effect of carbamazepine on ranolazine levels, this seems prudent.

Carbamazepine + **Sirolimus**

The manufacturers predict that carbamazepine may lower the serum levels of sirolimus, probably because *rifampicin (rifampin)*, another CYP3A4 inducer, has been shown to do so.

> The extent of any change in sirolimus levels is uncertain, but it would seem prudent to increase the frequency of monitoring of sirolimus levels during concurrent use and adjust the sirolimus dose as necessary.

Carbamazepine + **Solifenacin**

The manufacturers predict that potent CYP3A4 inducers (e.g. carbamazepine) will decrease solifenacin levels.

> Be alert for a reduction in the efficacy of solifenacin in patients taking carbamazepine.

Carbamazepine + **SSRIs**

Fluvoxamine or Fluoxetine

Case reports indicate that carbamazepine levels can be increased by fluoxetine (by up to 60%) and fluvoxamine (levels doubled). Toxicity may develop. The use of carbamazepine with an SSRI has, rarely, led to effects such as hyponatraemia, serotonin syndrome, and parkinsonism.

> It would be prudent to monitor carbamazepine levels and be alert for the need to reduce the carbamazepine dose with fluoxetine or fluvoxamine. Carbamazepine toxicity may present as nausea, vomiting, ataxia or drowsiness. The manufacturers of fluoxetine suggest that carbamazepine should be started at or adjusted towards the lower end of the dose range in those taking fluoxetine, and caution is needed if fluoxetine has been taken during the previous 5 weeks. Note that SSRIs can reduce the seizure threshold and so should be used with caution in patients with epilepsy.

Other SSRIs

Citalopram, paroxetine and sertraline levels may be reduced by carbamazepine. The use of carbamazepine with an SSRI has, rarely, led to effects such as hyponatraemia, serotonin syndrome, and parkinsonism.

> Be aware that some SSRIs may be less effective in the presence of carbamazepine and consider a dose increase if necessary. Note that SSRIs can reduce the seizure threshold and so should be used with caution in patients with epilepsy.

Carbamazepine + Statins

Carbamazepine reduces the levels of simvastatin and its active metabolite by around 80%.

> A simvastatin dose increase seems likely to be necessary. Monitor concurrent use to check that simvastatin is effective. Statins metabolised by the same route as simvastatin may also have their levels reduced, at least modestly, see statins, page 457.

Carbamazepine + Tacrolimus

Phenytoin has decreased tacrolimus levels in a few cases, and has been used to reduce tacrolimus levels after an overdose. Other CYP3A4 inducers such as carbamazepine are predicted to interact similarly.

> No interaction is established, but based on the known metabolism of these drugs it would be prudent to monitor tacrolimus levels in a patient given carbamazepine and adjust the dose as necessary.

Carbamazepine + Tetracyclines

Doxycycline levels are reduced and may fall below the accepted therapeutic minimum in patients taking carbamazepine long-term.

> It has been suggested that the doxycycline dose could be doubled to counteract this interaction. Other tetracyclines appear not to interact and may therefore be suitable alternatives.

Carbamazepine + Theophylline

Two case reports describe a marked fall in theophylline levels when carbamazepine was given. Another single case report and a pharmacokinetic study describe a fall in carbamazepine levels when theophylline was given.

The general importance of these reports is uncertain. Concurrent use need not be avoided, but it would be prudent to check that the effects of each drug (and possibly their levels) do not become subtherapeutic.

Carbamazepine + Tiagabine

The plasma concentrations of tiagabine may be reduced 1.5- to 3-fold by carbamazepine.

The manufacturers recommend that tiagabine 30 to 45 mg (in divided doses) should be given to patients taking enzyme-inducing antiepileptics such as carbamazepine. A lower maintenance dose of 15 to 30 mg should be given to patients who are not taking enzyme-inducing drugs.

Carbamazepine + Topiramate

Topiramate levels may be reduced by about 40% by carbamazepine. Carbamazepine levels are not affected by topiramate. However, one report suggests that the toxicity seen when topiramate was added to the maximum tolerated doses of carbamazepine may respond to a reduction in the carbamazepine dose.

Topiramate dose adjustments are unlikely to be needed. Reduce the carbamazepine dose should any carbamazepine adverse effects occur. Indicators of carbamazepine toxicity include nausea, vomiting, ataxia, drowsiness.

Carbamazepine + Toremifene

Carbamazepine can reduce the serum levels of toremifene.

The manufacturers of toremifene suggest that its dose may need to be doubled in the presence of carbamazepine.

Carbamazepine + Trazodone ❓

A single case report describes a moderate rise in carbamazepine levels in a patient given trazodone. Carbamazepine may moderately decrease trazodone levels.

Monitor trazodone efficacy and increase the dose as needed. The clinical significance of the rise in carbamazepine levels is likely to be small. However, if indicators of carbamazepine toxicity (nausea, vomiting, ataxia, drowsiness) develop, consider an interaction as a possible cause.

Carbamazepine + Tricyclics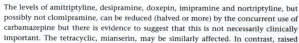

The levels of amitriptyline, desipramine, doxepin, imipramine and nortriptyline, but possibly not clomipramine, can be reduced (halved or more) by the concurrent use of carbamazepine but there is evidence to suggest that this is not necessarily clinically important. The tetracyclic, mianserin, may be similarly affected. In contrast, raised clomipramine levels have been seen in patients taking carbamazepine and an isolated report describes carbamazepine toxicity in a patient shortly after starting desipramine.

> Bear this interaction in mind in case of a reduced response to a tricyclic. Note that the tricyclics can lower the convulsive threshold and should therefore be used with caution in patients with epilepsy.

Carbamazepine + Vaccines

Carbamazepine levels rose modestly 14 days after influenza vaccination in one study. A case report describes carbamazepine toxicity and markedly increased carbamazepine levels in a teenager 13 days after influenza vaccination.

> The moderate increase in carbamazepine levels seen in the study is unlikely to have much clinical relevance. However, the case report of markedly increased carbamazepine levels introduces a note of caution. Carbamazepine toxicity may present as nausea, vomiting, ataxia or drowsiness.

Carbamazepine + Valproate

The levels of carbamazepine are usually only slightly affected by sodium valproate, valproic acid or valpromide although a moderate to marked rise in the levels of its active epoxide metabolite may occur. Carbamazepine may reduce the levels of sodium valproate by 60% or more. Concurrent use may possibly increase the incidence of sodium valproate-induced hepatotoxicity.

> Monitor valproate levels, and adjust the dose if necessary. Also monitor for carbamazepine toxicity (due to raised carbamazepine-epoxide levels), which may present as nausea, vomiting, ataxia or drowsiness.

Carbamazepine + Vitamin D

The long-term use of *phenytoin* can disturb vitamin D and calcium metabolism, which may result in osteomalacia. There are a few reports of patients taking vitamin D supplements who responded poorly to vitamin replacement while taking *phenytoin*. Limited evidence suggests that carbamazepine may interact similarly.

> Monitor the outcome of concurrent use. Larger doses of vitamin D may be needed.

Carbamazepine + Warfarin and other oral anticoagulants

The anticoagulant effects of warfarin can be markedly reduced (by around 50% in many reports) by carbamazepine. Cases of this interaction have been seen with phenprocoumon and acenocoumarol.

> Monitor the INR if carbamazepine is added to warfarin therapy. Continue monitoring until the carbamazepine dose is stabilised. Also monitor the INR if carbamazepine is withdrawn as the effects of warfarin may become excessive within a week. Similar precautions would be prudent with the other coumarins.

Carbamazepine + Zonisamide ❓

Carbamazepine can cause a small to moderate reduction in the levels of zonisamide, and zonisamide has been reported to cause increases, decreases or no changes to carbamazepine serum levels.

> The clinical importance of this interaction is unknown, but be aware of the possibility of changes in the levels of both drugs if they are given together.

C

Carbimazole

Carbimazole + Digoxin ⚠

Carbimazole slightly lowers digoxin levels in euthyroid subjects. However, the drug-disease interaction that also occurs is probably of more importance. Hyperthyroid subjects are relatively resistant to the effects of digoxin and so need higher doses. As treatment with carbimazole progresses and they become euthyroid, the dose of digoxin will need to be decreased.

> Monitor digoxin levels and for digoxin adverse effects (such as bradycardia, nausea, vomiting), adjusting the digoxin dose as necessary, until the patient is euthyroid.

Carbimazole + Theophylline ⚠

Thyroid status may affect the rate at which theophylline is metabolised. In hyperthyroidism it is increased, and so patients require higher theophylline doses. As thyroid function is corrected (e.g. with carbimazole) theophylline metabolism decreases and so smaller doses are needed. Two case reports describe theophylline toxicity in patients being treated for hyperthyroidism. Aminophylline would be expected to interact similarly.

> Monitor the outcome of resolving hyperthyroidism, checking for theophylline adverse effects (headache, nausea, palpitations). Monitor theophylline levels and adjust the dose as necessary.

Carbimazole + Warfarin and other oral anticoagulants ⚠

Hyperthyroidism increases the metabolism of the clotting factors. Correction of hyperthyroidism therefore alters anticoagulant requirements. Increased coumarin requirements have been seen in patients given carbimazole.

> Close monitoring of the INR is advisable for any patient taking an oral anticoagulant until their thyroid hormone levels are stabilised.

Caspofungin

Caspofungin + **Ciclosporin (Cyclosporine)**

Ciclosporin increases the AUC of caspofungin by 35% and may cause increases in liver enzymes (AST and ALT of up to 3-fold in one study).

> The manufacturer advises that ciclosporin and caspofungin should only be used if the benefits outweigh the risks of treatment, and if they are used, close monitoring of liver enzymes is recommended.

Caspofungin + **NNRTIs**

Population pharmacokinetic data suggests that efavirenz and nevirapine may reduce caspofungin levels.

> The manufacturers say that consideration should be given to increasing the dose of caspofungin from 50 mg daily to 70 mg daily in adults and to 70 mg/m^2 daily (maximum 70 mg daily) in children.

Caspofungin + **Phenytoin**

Population data suggests that phenytoin may reduce caspofungin levels. Although the mechanism for this effect is not fully understood it would seem prudent to expect fosphenytoin, a prodrug of phenytoin, to interact similarly.

> The manufacturers say that consideration should be given to increasing the dose of caspofungin from 50 mg daily to 70 mg daily in adults and to 70 mg/m^2 daily (maximum 70 mg daily) in children.

Caspofungin + **Rifampicin (Rifampin)**

Rifampicin initially increases the trough levels of caspofungin by 170%, but after 2 weeks the trough levels of caspofungin decrease, and are about 30% lower than in patients not receiving rifampicin. Antifungal treatment failure has been seen in a patient taking rifampicin with caspofungin (70 mg on the first day then 50 mg daily).

> The manufacturers say that consideration should be given to increasing the dose of caspofungin from 50 mg daily to 70 mg daily in adults and to 70 mg/m^2 daily (maximum 70 mg daily) in children. However, close monitoring is still required because of the isolated report of treatment failure even at the higher dose.

Caspofungin + **Tacrolimus**

Caspofungin slightly decreases trough tacrolimus levels by 26%. Tacrolimus does not affect the pharmacokinetics of caspofungin.

> Tacrolimus levels and/or effects (e.g. on renal function) should be monitored as a

matter of routine, but it is advisable to increase monitoring if caspofungin is started or stopped, and adjust the dose of tacrolimus if required.

Cephalosporins

Cephalosporins + Ciclosporin (Cyclosporine)

Isolated reports suggest that ceftazidime and ceftriaxone may increase ciclosporin levels, whereas one report suggested they did not, although ceftazidime caused a deterioration in some measures of renal function.

Information about these cephalosporins is very limited. The general relevance of these reports is uncertain, but bear them in mind in the event of declining renal function.

Cephalosporins + Contraceptives

A few anecdotal cases of combined hormonal contraceptive failure have been reported with the cephalosporins. The interaction (if such it is) appears to be very rare indeed.

It is possible that the anecdotal cases of contraceptive failure with antibacterials are indistinguishable from the normal accepted failure rate and no special precautions are required. However, for simplicity, some suggest that caution should be taken with short courses of any antibacterial (non-enzyme inducing). For guidance on the use of antibacterials with contraceptives, see contraceptives, page 233.

Cephalosporins + H₂-receptor antagonists

Ranitidine and famotidine modestly reduce the bioavailability of cefpodoxime proxetil. Ranitidine (with sodium bicarbonate) reduces the bioavailability of cefuroxime axetil, but not if it is taken with food. As it is thought that a change in gastric pH is responsible for this interaction it would seem likely that all H₂-receptor antagonists will interact similarly.

The clinical importance of the interaction with cefpodoxime has not been studied, but the manufacturer recommends that it should be given at least 2 hours before H₂-receptor antagonists. As long as cefuroxime is taken with food (as is recommended), any interaction is minimal.

Cephalosporins + Probenecid

Overall, probenecid reduces the clearance, raises the serum levels and sometimes prolongs the half-lives of some, but not all, cephalosporins.

No special precautions are normally needed. However, be aware that elevated serum levels of some cephalosporins (such as cefaloridine and cefalotin) might possibly increase the risk of nephrotoxicity.

Cephalosporins + Proton pump inhibitors

Ranitidine and *famotidine* modestly reduce the bioavailability of cefpodoxime proxetil. *Ranitidine* (with sodium bicarbonate) reduces the bioavailability of cefuroxime axetil, although not if taken with food. As it is thought that a change in gastric pH is responsible for this interaction it would seem likely that the proton pump inhibitors will interact similarly.

The clinical relevance of these effects are unclear. However, as long as cefuroxime is taken with food (as is recommended), any interaction is minimal.

Cephalosporins + Warfarin and other oral anticoagulants

Cephalosporins and related beta lactams with an N-methylthiotetrazole or similar side-chain can occasionally cause bleeding when they are used alone. These effects could therefore be additive with those of the coumarins. The cephalosporins implicated include cefaclor, cefalotin, cefamandole, cefazolin, cefixime, cefonicid, and ceftriaxone. Isolated case reports describe over-anticoagulation in patients taking a coumarin or indanedione and a cephalosporin that does not possess an N-methylthiotetrazole side chain.

Severe bleeding events have been seen with some cephalosporins. As this usually occurs after about 3 days it would seem prudent to monitor the INR at this point and adjust the anticoagulant dose accordingly. If dose alterations are needed further INR monitoring will be required when the cephalosporin is stopped.

Chloramphenicol

Chloramphenicol + Ciclosporin (Cyclosporine)

Case reports describe marked rises in ciclosporin levels in patients also given chloramphenicol. A small study supports these findings.

Ciclosporin levels and/or effects (e.g. on renal function) should be monitored as a matter of routine, but it may be prudent to increase monitoring if chloramphenicol is started or stopped. Adjust the dose of ciclosporin as necessary. It seems doubtful that there will be enough chloramphenicol absorbed from eye drops to interact with ciclosporin, but this needs confirmation.

Chloramphenicol + Clopidogrel ✖

On the basis of the interaction with the proton pump inhibitors, some predict that chloramphenicol may theoretically inhibit the conversion of clopidogrel to its active metabolite by CYP2C19.

The manufacturers advise that concurrent use should be avoided.

Chloramphenicol + **Contraceptives**

One or two cases of combined hormonal contraceptive failure have been reported with chloramphenicol. These isolated cases are anecdotal and unconfirmed, and the interaction (if such it is) appears to be very rare indeed.

It is possible that the anecdotal cases of contraceptive failure with antibacterials are indistinguishable from the normal accepted failure rate and no special precautions are required. However, for simplicity, some suggest that caution should be taken with short courses of any antibacterial (non-enzyme inducing). For guidance on the use of antibacterials with contraceptives, see contraceptives, page 233.

Chloramphenicol + **Iron**

In addition to the serious and potentially fatal bone marrow depression that can occur with chloramphenicol, it may also cause a milder, reversible bone marrow depression, which can oppose the treatment of anaemia with iron.

It has been suggested that chloramphenicol doses of 25 to 30 mg/kg are usually adequate for treating infections without running the risk of elevating serum levels to 25 micrograms/mL or more, which is when this type of marrow depression can occur. Monitor the effects of using iron concurrently. Where possible it would be preferable to use a different antibacterial.

Chloramphenicol + **Paracetamol (Acetaminophen)**

Although there is limited evidence to suggest that paracetamol may affect chloramphenicol pharmacokinetics its validity has been criticised. Evidence of a clinically relevant interaction appears lacking.

No action needed. It would seem prudent to be aware of the potential for interaction, especially in malnourished patients, but routine monitoring would appear unnecessary without further evidence.

Chloramphenicol + **Phenobarbital**

Studies in children show that phenobarbital can markedly reduce chloramphenicol levels. An isolated case describes markedly increased phenobarbital levels in an adult caused by the use of chloramphenicol. Note that primidone is metabolised to phenobarbital and therefore may interact similarly.

Concurrent use should be well monitored to ensure that chloramphenicol levels are adequate. Make appropriate dose adjustments as necessary. The case of raised phenobarbital levels is of uncertain importance.

Chloramphenicol + **Phenytoin**

Phenytoin levels can be raised two- to fourfold by the concurrent use of systemic chloramphenicol, and phenytoin toxicity may occur. Evidence from children suggests that phenytoin may reduce or raise chloramphenicol levels. Fosphenytoin, a prodrug of phenytoin, may interact similarly.

> Monitor concurrent use for phenytoin toxicity (blurred vision, nystagmus, ataxia or drowsiness), monitoring levels and reducing the dose of phenytoin as necessary. The use of a single prophylactic dose of phenytoin or fosphenytoin may be an exception to this. Also monitor for chloramphenicol efficacy and toxicity. It is doubtful if enough chloramphenicol is absorbed from eye drops or ointments for an interaction to occur.

Chloramphenicol + Rifampicin (Rifampin)

Case reports describe markedly reduced chloramphenicol levels in children also given rifampicin. There is a risk that chloramphenicol levels will become subtherapeutic.

> It is unclear if a dose increase of chloramphenicol is appropriate as some consider that increasing the chloramphenicol dose may possibly expose the patient to a greater risk of bone marrow aplasia. It has been suggested that rifampicin prophylaxis should be delayed in patients with invasive *Haemophilus influenzae* infections until the end of chloramphenicol treatment.

Chloramphenicol + Tacrolimus

A marked rise in tacrolimus levels has been reported in several patients also given systemic chloramphenicol.

> Tacrolimus levels and/or effects (e.g. on renal function) should be monitored as a matter of routine, but it may be prudent to increase monitoring if systemic chloramphenicol is started or stopped. It seems doubtful if a clinically relevant interaction will occur with topical chloramphenicol because the dose and the systemic absorption is small, but this needs confirmation.

Chloramphenicol + Vitamin B$_{12}$

In addition to the serious and potentially fatal bone marrow depression that can occur with systemic chloramphenicol, it may also cause a milder, reversible bone marrow depression, which can oppose the treatment of anaemia with iron or vitamin B$_{12}$.

> It has been suggested that chloramphenicol doses of 25 to 30 mg/kg are usually adequate for treating infections without running the risk of elevating serum levels to 25 micrograms/mL or more, which is when this type of marrow depression can occur. Monitor the effects of using iron or vitamin B$_{12}$ concurrently. Where possible it would be preferable to use a different antibacterial.

Chloramphenicol + Warfarin and other oral anticoagulants

Some limited, and poor quality evidence suggests that the anticoagulant effects of acenocoumarol can be increased by oral chloramphenicol. An isolated report attributes a marked INR rise in a patient taking warfarin to the use of chloramphenicol eye drops.

> This interaction is not established but it would be prudent to be aware that increases in INR are possible and consider increasing the frequency of INR monitoring. The interaction with chloramphenicol eye drops seems unlikely to be generally relevant.

C

Chloroquine

Chloroquine + Ciclosporin (Cyclosporine)

Three patients had rapid rises in ciclosporin levels, with evidence of nephrotoxicity in two of them, when they were given chloroquine. Note that hydroxychloroquine may interact similarly.

> Ciclosporin levels and/or effects (e.g. on renal function) should be monitored as a matter of routine, but it may be prudent to increase monitoring if chloroquine or hydroxychloroquine is started or stopped. Adjust the dose of ciclosporin as necessary. When low-dose ciclosporin is given for rheumatoid arthritis, neither chloroquine nor hydroxychloroquine appear to contribute to the known adverse effects of ciclosporin on creatinine and renal function.

Chloroquine + Digoxin

The levels of digoxin were found to be markedly increased by 70% in two elderly patients when they took hydroxychloroquine. A similar increase has been seen with chloroquine in *dogs*.

> The clinical significance of this interaction is uncertain, but it would seem sensible to be aware of this potential interaction if both drugs are used.

Chloroquine + H$_2$-receptor antagonists

Cimetidine reduces the metabolism and halves the clearance of chloroquine. Hydroxychloroquine is expected to be similarly affected.

> The clinical importance of this interaction is uncertain, but it would seem prudent to be alert for any signs of chloroquine of hydroxychloroquine toxicity during concurrent use. Ranitidine may be a suitable alternative as it does not appear to interact with chloroquine.

Chloroquine + Kaolin

Kaolin can reduce the absorption of chloroquine by about 30%. Hydroxychloroquine is predicted to interact similarly.

> The clinical significance of this reduction is unclear, but one way to minimise any

possible effect on chloroquine absorption is to separate the doses of chloroquine and kaolin as much as possible (at least 2 to 3 hours) to minimise the interaction. One manufacturer recommends that the chloroquine dose should be separated from kaolin by at least 4 hours. Hydroxychloroquine dosing should also be separated from kaolin by at least 4 hours. Be alert for any signs of reduced chloroquine efficacy.

Chloroquine + Lanthanum

The manufacturers of lanthanum predict that the absorption of drugs that are affected by gastric pH will be altered by lanthanum. They name chloroquine and hydroxychloroquine, but note that these drugs appear to interact due to altered absorption rather than changes in gastric pH.

The manufacturers recommend separating dosing by at least 2 hours.

Chloroquine + Leflunomide

The manufacturers say that the concurrent use of leflunomide and chloroquine or hydroxychloroquine has not yet been studied, but it would be expected to increase the risk of serious adverse reactions (haematological toxicity or hepatotoxicity).

The manufacturers advise avoiding concurrent use. As the active metabolite of leflunomide has a long half-life of 1 to 4 weeks a washout with colestyramine or activated charcoal is recommended by the manufacturers if patients are to be switched to other DMARDs.

Chloroquine + Mefloquine

In theory there is an increased risk of convulsions if mefloquine is given with chloroquine, but no cases appear to have been reported. The manufacturers suggest that concurrent use increases the risks of ECG abnormalities. Note that hydroxychloroquine may interact similarly.

The manufacturers suggest that concurrent use should be avoided. It has been suggested that patients initially given intravenous quinine for 2 to 3 days should delay mefloquine until at least 12 hours after the last dosing of quinine to minimise interactions leading to adverse events.

Chloroquine + Penicillamine

The concurrent use of chloroquine and penicillamine may result in increased toxicity, possibly as a result of increased penicillamine levels.

If problems occur consider this drug interaction as a possible cause. Note that chloroquine, hydroxychloroquine and penicillamine are associated with serious haematological adverse effects, and therefore the US manufacturer suggests that the use of penicillamine with either of these drugs should be avoided.

Chloroquine + **Praziquantel** ⚠

Chloroquine reduces the bioavailability of praziquantel, which would be expected to reduce its efficacy in systemic worm infections such as schistosomiasis. Note that hydroxychloroquine may interact similarly.

> It has been suggested that an increased dose of praziquantel should be considered in the presence of chloroquine, particularly in anyone who does not respond to initial treatment. This interaction is not of importance when praziquantel is used for intestinal worm infections (where its action is a local effect on the worms in the gut).

Ciclosporin (Cyclosporine)

Ciclosporin (Cyclosporine) + **Colchicine** ⚠

A number of cases of serious muscle disorders (myopathy, rhabdomyolysis), a few with multiple organ failure, have been seen when colchicine and ciclosporin were given concurrently. Ciclosporin toxicity has also been seen rarely.

> Concurrent use should be carefully monitored and treatment stopped at the earliest signs of myopathy. Patients should be reminded to report any unexplained muscle pain, tenderness or weakness. Note that one UK manufacturer of colchicine contraindicates the concurrent use of ciclosporin in patients with renal or hepatic impairment.

Ciclosporin (Cyclosporine) + **Contraceptives**

Isolated reports describe hepatotoxicity and raised ciclosporin levels in two patients taking ciclosporin when given oral combined hormonal contraceptives. A couple of reports also describe some increase in ciclosporin levels with norethisterone.

> The interactions between ciclosporin and hormonal contraceptives or norethisterone are unconfirmed and of uncertain clinical significance. There is insufficient evidence to recommend increased monitoring, but be aware of the potential for an interaction in case of an unexpected response to treatment.

Ciclosporin (Cyclosporine) + **Corticosteroids** ❓

Some evidence suggests that ciclosporin levels may be raised by corticosteroids (2-fold by methylprednisolone) or reduced (10 to 20% reduction with prednisone). Ciclosporin can moderately increase corticosteroid levels, which may lead to symptoms of overdose (cushingoid symptoms such as steroid-induced diabetes, osteonecrosis of the hip joints). Convulsions have also been described during concurrent use.

> Concurrent use is common and advantageous but be alert for any evidence of increased ciclosporin and corticosteroid effects.

Ciclosporin (Cyclosporine) + **Co-trimoxazole**

A large-scale study has found that co-trimoxazole was effective and well tolerated in patients taking ciclosporin, although a 15% rise in serum creatinine levels was noted. Interstitial nephritis, granulocytopenia and thrombocytopenia have been reported in a few patients.

Serious interactions between ciclosporin and co-trimoxazole seem rare and so no additional monitoring would seem to be necessary, at least for low-dose prophylactic co-trimoxazole. However, the manufacturer recommends close monitoring of renal function with concurrent use; this would seem a prudent precaution.

Ciclosporin (Cyclosporine) + **Danazol**

Marked increases in ciclosporin levels (3-fold in one case) have been seen in patients taking danazol.

Ciclosporin levels and/or effects (e.g. on renal function) should be monitored as a matter of routine, but it may be prudent to increase monitoring if danazol is started or stopped.

Ciclosporin (Cyclosporine) + **Digoxin**

Ciclosporin causes 3- to 4-fold rises in digoxin levels in some patients.

The effects of concurrent use should be monitored very closely for digoxin adverse effects (such as bradycardia, nausea, visual disturbances), and the digoxin dose should be adjusted according to levels.

Ciclosporin (Cyclosporine) + **Diuretics**

Potassium-sparing diuretics

The concurrent use of ciclosporin with potassium-sparing diuretics, such as amiloride, spironolactone and eplerenone, may increase potassium levels and lead to renal impairment in isolated cases.

Monitor potassium levels and renal function if a potassium-sparing diuretic is given. The US manufacturers of eplerenone advise avoiding concurrent use, whereas the UK manufacturers advise caution.

Thiazide diuretics

Isolated cases of nephrotoxicity have been described in patients taking ciclosporin with either amiloride/hydrochlorothiazide or metolazone. The concurrent use of ciclosporin with thiazides may increase serum magnesium levels.

The general importance of these adverse interactions is not clear. It seems likely that routine monitoring will detect any adverse effects.

Ciclosporin (Cyclosporine) + Endothelin receptor antagonists

Ambrisentan

Ciclosporin increases ambrisentan exposure 2-fold. Ambrisentan has no effect on the pharmacokinetics of ciclosporin.

> The manufacturer of ambrisentan advises a maximum dose of 5 mg daily with the concurrent use of ciclosporin. Monitor for an increase in ambrisentan adverse effects such as constipation, flushing, and fluid retention.

Bosentan or Sitaxentan

Bosentan decreases the AUC of ciclosporin by 50%, and ciclosporin increases bosentan levels up to 4-fold. Ciclosporin increases sitaxentan trough levels 6-fold. Sitaxentan does not alter ciclosporin levels.

> Concurrent use is contraindicated.

Ciclosporin (Cyclosporine) + Etoposide

High-dose ciclosporin markedly raises etoposide levels and increases the suppression of white blood cell production. Severe toxicity has been reported in one patient.

> Some have suggested reducing the dose of etoposide by 40 or 50%. The use of high-dose ciclosporin for multidrug resistant tumour modulation remains experimental and should only be used in clinical studies. Concurrent use should be very well monitored.

Ciclosporin (Cyclosporine) + Ezetimibe

Ciclosporin may raise ezetimibe levels as much as 3.4-fold. One study found that ezetimibe slightly increased the AUC of ciclosporin by 15%; however, another study found no change in ciclosporin levels on concurrent use.

> The small increase in the AUC of ciclosporin is not usually considered to be clinically significant in most patients; however, the manufacturers advise monitoring ciclosporin levels. It has been suggested that ezetimibe should be started at 5 mg in patients receiving ciclosporin. Be aware of the potential for increased ezetimibe toxicity (abdominal pain, headache, nausea and rarely myopathy). Patients should be advised to report any muscle pain, tenderness or weakness.

Ciclosporin (Cyclosporine) + Fibrates

The use of bezafibrate with ciclosporin has resulted in significantly increased serum creatinine levels. Reductions, no change, or increased ciclosporin levels have also been seen. The use of fenofibrate has also been associated with reduced renal function and possibly reduced ciclosporin levels. Three studies found no pharmacokinetic interaction between ciclosporin and gemfibrozil while a fourth found gemfibrozil caused a significant reduction in ciclosporin levels and an increase in serum creatinine in some patients.

> Ciclosporin levels and effects (e.g. on renal function) should be monitored as a

matter of routine, but it may be prudent to increase monitoring if a fibrate is started or stopped. Adjust the dose of ciclosporin as necessary and stop the fibrate should significant renal impairment occur.

Ciclosporin (Ciclosporine) + Grapefruit juice

A considerable number of single and multiple dose studies have shown that if oral ciclosporin is taken with 150 to 250 mL of grapefruit juice, the trough levels, peak levels and bioavailability of ciclosporin may be increased. Increases in trough levels range from 15 to 85%.

The increases in oral ciclosporin exposure appears to be variable and this interaction is difficult, if not impossible, to control. This is because batches of grapefruit juice vary so much, and also because considerable patient variation occurs with this interaction. The US manufacturers suggest that patients taking ciclosporin should avoid whole grapefruit, as well as the juice. Intravenous ciclosporin does not appear to be affected.

Ciclosporin (Ciclosporine) + Griseofulvin

An isolated case reports that the ciclosporin levels of a man were roughly halved when he took griseofulvin 500 mg daily, despite an approximately 70% increase in the ciclosporin dose. However another case report found no interaction.

This interaction is unconfirmed and of uncertain general significance. There is insufficient evidence to recommend increased monitoring, but be aware of the potential for an interaction in the case of an unexpected response to treatment.

Ciclosporin (Ciclosporine) + H$_2$-receptor antagonists ?

Although some reports suggest that cimetidine and famotidine can rarely increase ciclosporin levels, the majority of the information suggests no interaction occurs. Note that raised creatinine levels have been seen with the concurrent use of ciclosporin and cimetidine or ranitidine, but this does not appear to be related to renal toxicity or reduced renal function. Isolated cases of thrombocytopenia and hepatotoxicity have been reported with ranitidine and ciclosporin.

There is little to suggest that concurrent use should be avoided, but good initial monitoring is advisable.

Ciclosporin (Ciclosporine) + Herbal medicines or Dietary supplements

Alfalfa and/or Black cohosh

An isolated report describes acute rejection and vasculitis when a renal transplant patient taking ciclosporin also took black cohosh and/or alfalfa.

The evidence of for this interaction is limited, but as the effects were so severe in this case it would seem prudent to avoid concurrent use, particularly in patients taking ciclosporin for serious indications such as organ transplantation. For indications such as eczema, psoriasis or rheumatoid arthritis, although avoidance would be prudent, short-term concurrent use is likely to be less hazardous and patients should be counselled about the possible risks (i.e. loss of disease control) should they wish to take alfalfa or black cohosh with ciclosporin.

Geum chiloense

A single report describes a marked (more than 5-fold), rapid increase in the ciclosporin levels of a man who drank an infusion of *Geum chiloense*.

There is insufficient evidence to make any strong recommendations, but be aware of the potential for an interaction.

Red yeast rice (Monascus purpureus)

Red yeast rice has been reported to cause rhabdomyolysis in a kidney transplant patient taking ciclosporin.

Ciclosporin is well known to interact with the statins, and this interaction appeared to be mediated by a statin-like component in the red yeast rice. Patients should report any unexplained muscle pain, tenderness or weakness if they take red yeast rice with ciclosporin.

St John's wort (Hypericum perforatum)

Marked falls in ciclosporin levels (resulting in transplant rejection in some cases) can occur with a few weeks of starting St John's wort.

The advice of the CSM in the UK is that patients taking ciclosporin should avoid or stop taking St John's wort. In the latter situation, the serum ciclosporin levels should be well monitored. Some evidence suggests that monitoring should continue for up to 2 weeks after stopping the St John's wort. It is possible to accommodate this interaction by increasing the ciclosporin dose, although this may be costly and difficult to adequately manage.

Ciclosporin (Cyclosporine) + Lanreotide

Octreotide causes a marked fall in the levels of ciclosporin, and inadequate immunosuppression may result. Lanreotide is predicted to interact similarly.

Ciclosporin levels and effects (e.g. on renal function) should be monitored as a matter of routine, but it may be prudent to increase monitoring if lanreotide is started or stopped.

Ciclosporin (Cyclosporine) + Macrolides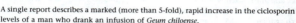

Ciclosporin levels can be markedly raised by clarithromycin (commonly 2- to 3-fold), erythromycin (4- to 5-fold or more, intravenous erythromycin seems to have less effect than oral), josamycin (commonly 2- to 4-fold), and midecamycin (2-fold). Telithromycin is predicted to interact similarly. Although major studies have found no interaction with azithromycin, there have been two isolated case reports of raised ciclosporin levels in patients given azithromycin.

Ciclosporin levels and effects (e.g. on renal function) should be monitored as a matter of routine, but it may be prudent to increase monitoring if macrolides are started or stopped. A ciclosporin dose reduction of about 35% has been suggested when using erythromycin or clarithromycin concurrently. With erythromycin, also consider increased monitoring if the route of administration is changed. Other macrolides may also interact, although it seems unlikely that they all will, see macrolides, page 361.

Ciclosporin (Cyclosporine) + Methotrexate

Previous or concurrent treatment with methotrexate may possibly increase the risk of liver and other toxicity, but effective and valuable concurrent use has also been reported. Ciclosporin causes a moderate rise in methotrexate levels but methotrexate does not appear to affect the pharmacokinetics of ciclosporin.

Both methotrexate and ciclosporin should be closely monitored as a matter of routine, but it may be worth increasing the frequency of this monitoring to aid rapid detection of any adverse effects. The dose of either drug may need to be reduced and drug toxicity (renal and hepatic) may be more common.

Ciclosporin (Cyclosporine) + Metoclopramide

Metoclopramide increases the absorption of ciclosporin and raises its peak levels by almost 50%.

The clinical importance of this interaction is uncertain. Concurrent use should be well monitored to ensure that any increase in ciclosporin peak levels does not increase adverse effects.

Ciclosporin (Cyclosporine) + Modafinil

Ciclosporin levels were reported to be reduced by modafinil in one patient.

This seems to be the only reported case of an interaction between ciclosporin and modafinil, however a modest interaction would be expected as modafinil can induce CYP3A4 by which ciclosporin is metabolised. It would seem prudent to anticipate a reduction in ciclosporin levels if modafinil is used.

Ciclosporin (Cyclosporine) + NNRTIs ⚠

Efavirenz, and to a lesser extent nevirapine, appear to decrease the levels of ciclosporin. The ciclosporin levels of one patient dramatically decreased following the addition of efavirenz. Etravirine is also predicted to interact in this way. In contrast, delavirdine is predicted to inhibit the metabolism of ciclosporin and increase its levels.

Although there is limited information, it is in line with the way these drugs are known to interact. It would seem prudent to closely monitor ciclosporin levels in any patient given an NNRTI, adjusting the ciclosporin dose as necessary.

Ciclosporin (Cyclosporine) + NSAIDs

NSAIDs sometimes reduce renal function in individual patients, which is reflected in serum creatinine level rises and possibly in changes in ciclosporin levels, but concurrent use can also be uneventful. Diclofenac levels can be doubled by ciclosporin.

Concurrent use in rheumatoid arthritis need not be avoided but renal function should be closely monitored. The UK manufacturer of ciclosporin also recommends close monitoring of liver function, because hepatotoxicity is a potential adverse effect of both drugs. It is difficult to generalise about what will or will not happen if any particular NSAID is given. It has been recommended that doses at the lower end of the range for diclofenac should be used initially, and it has been suggested that lower than usual doses should be considered for other NSAIDs.

Ciclosporin (Cyclosporine) + Octreotide

Octreotide causes a marked fall in the levels of ciclosporin, and inadequate immunosuppression may result.

Ciclosporin levels and effects (e.g. on renal function) should be monitored as a matter of routine, but it may be prudent to increase monitoring if octreotide is started or stopped. An increase in the ciclosporin dose of around 50% has been suggested.

Ciclosporin (Cyclosporine) + Orlistat

The absorption of ciclosporin is reduced by orlistat (by more than 50% in some cases) and cases of low levels have been reported with both formulations (*Neoral* and *Sandimmun*). A non-significant episode of acute graft rejection has been reported with *Neoral*.

It has been suggested that the effects of the interaction may be reduced by using the microemulsion formulation of ciclosporin (*Neoral*); however, close monitoring is still required because there is still a risk of subtherapeutic levels. Some recommend avoiding concurrent use. The US manufacturer recommends taking ciclosporin at least 2 hours before or 2 hours after orlistat to reduce the chance of an interaction. However, there is evidence that separation of doses does not avoid the interaction.

Ciclosporin (Cyclosporine) + Phenobarbital

Several cases describe large reductions in ciclosporin levels in patients given phenobarbital, requiring dose increases to keep the levels within the therapeutic range. As primidone is metabolised to phenobarbital it seems likely that it will interact similarly.

Ciclosporin levels and effects (e.g. on renal function) should be monitored as a matter of routine, but it may be prudent to increase monitoring if phenobarbital or primidone are stopped, started, or the dose altered, adjusting the ciclosporin dose as necessary.

Ciclosporin (Cyclosporine) + **Phenytoin**

A study and several case reports describe a reduction in ciclosporin levels (37% reduction in the study) following the addition of phenytoin. Other reports describe the need to make 2- to 4-fold increases in the ciclosporin dose in patients also taking phenytoin in order to keep ciclosporin levels within the therapeutic range. Fosphenytoin, a prodrug of phenytoin, would be expected to interact similarly.

> Ciclosporin levels and effects (e.g. on renal function) should be monitored as a matter of routine, but it may be prudent to increase monitoring if phenytoin is stopped, started, or the dose altered, adjusting the ciclosporin dose as necessary.

Ciclosporin (Cyclosporine) + **Protease inhibitors**

Increased ciclosporin levels have been seen in patients taking protease inhibitors. Large dose decreases (often more than 70%) have been needed to avoid toxicity. Some evidence suggests ciclosporin may increase indinavir, nelfinavir and saquinavir levels.

> Ciclosporin levels should be carefully monitored and the dose adjusted accordingly if protease inhibitors are also given. The general significance of the effects of ciclosporin on some protease inhibitors is unclear, although in one study the effect was not sustained.

Ciclosporin (Cyclosporine) + **Proton pump inhibitors**

Studies suggest that omeprazole 20 mg daily does not usually affect ciclosporin levels, but isolated reports describe doubled ciclosporin levels in one patient, and more than halved ciclosporin levels in another. Both patients were taking omeprazole 40 mg daily.

> This interaction is unlikely to be of general importance, but consider the possibility of an interaction if patients taking higher doses of omeprazole have otherwise unexplained changes in ciclosporin levels.

Ciclosporin (Cyclosporine) + **Quinolones**

Ciclosporin levels are normally unchanged by the use of ciprofloxacin, but increased levels and nephrotoxicity may occur in a small number of patients. Similar results have been found with norfloxacin and levofloxacin.

> No pharmacokinetic interaction usually occurs between ciclosporin and these quinolones, but as very occasionally and unpredictably an increase in serum ciclosporin levels and/or nephrotoxicity occurs it would be prudent to bear these interactions in mind on concurrent use.

Ciclosporin (Cyclosporine) + **Ranolazine**

The concurrent use of ciclosporin and ranolazine may lead to increased levels of both ranolazine and ciclosporin.

> Information is limited, but it would seem prudent to monitor the levels of both

drugs on concurrent use. The manufacturers advise careful dose titration when starting ranolazine. Patients already taking ranolazine and started on ciclosporin should be monitored for adverse effects (nausea, dizziness) and the dose of ranolazine reduced if needed.

Ciclosporin (Cyclosporine) + Rifabutin

A case report suggests that rifabutin increases the clearance of ciclosporin by about 20%.

As information is limited it would be prudent to consider increasing the monitoring of ciclosporin levels and effects (e.g. on renal function) if rifabutin is started or stopped.

Ciclosporin (Cyclosporine) + Rifampicin (Rifampin)

Ciclosporin levels are markedly reduced (in some cases within one day) by the concurrent use of rifampicin. Transplant rejection can rapidly develop if the ciclosporin dose is not increased.

Ciclosporin levels and effects (e.g. on renal function) should be monitored as a matter of routine, but it is essential to increase monitoring if rifampicin is started or stopped. The ciclosporin dose will need to be increased substantially when rifampicin is added (3- to 5-fold increases have been needed in some cases). It has been suggested that other antimycobacterials should be used in patients taking ciclosporin.

Ciclosporin (Cyclosporine) + Sevelamer

Sevelamer did not appear to alter ciclosporin levels in one study; however, a case report describes markedly reduced ciclosporin levels within 6 days of starting sevelamer.

The manufacturers advise that ciclosporin should be taken at least 1 hour before or 3 hours after sevelamer. Consider close monitoring of ciclosporin levels when sevelamer is started or stopped.

Ciclosporin (Cyclosporine) + Sibutramine

One case report describes an increase in ciclosporin levels when a patient was changed from orlistat to sibutramine. The manufacturers predict that ciclosporin will raise sibutramine levels by inhibiting CYP3A4, although note that ciclosporin is only a modest inhibitor of this isoenzyme.

The effect on ciclosporin levels is unconfirmed and no general recommendations can be made. The UK manufacturer of sibutramine recommends caution on the concurrent use of ciclosporin because of the possibility of increased sibutramine levels and adverse effects.

Ciclosporin (Cyclosporine) + **Statins**

Rosuvastatin

The AUC of rosuvastatin is increased 7-fold by ciclosporin. Ciclosporin levels are unaffected.

The UK manufacturer of rosuvastatin contraindicates its use with ciclosporin, whereas the US manufacturer recommends limiting the dose of rosuvastatin to 5 mg daily. If concurrent use is felt necessary, patients should be closely monitored and they should be told to report any unexplained muscle pain, tenderness or weakness or dark coloured urine.

Other statins

Ciclosporin can cause marked rises in the plasma levels of atorvastatin, fluvastatin, lovastatin, pravastatin and simvastatin, and for some of the statins this had led to the development of serious myopathy (rhabdomyolysis) accompanied by renal failure. The plasma levels of ciclosporin appear not to be affected by fluvastatin, lovastatin or pravastatin, but some moderate changes have been seen when atorvastatin or simvastatin were used.

Concurrent use should be very well monitored, a precautionary recommendation being to start (or reduce) the statin at the lowest daily dose, appropriate to the patient's condition. The manufacturers recommend the following maximum statin dose in patients also taking ciclosporin: atorvastatin or simvastatin 10 mg daily, lovastatin 20 mg daily and pravastatin 20 mg daily. Patients should be told to report any unexplained muscle pain, tenderness or weakness or dark coloured urine. If myopathy does occur, withdrawing the statin has been shown to resolve the symptoms. Only simvastatin and atorvastatin appear to affect ciclosporin levels, and it may be prudent to monitor ciclosporin levels more closely if either of these statins is also given.

Ciclosporin (Cyclosporine) + **Sulfinpyrazone**

Sulfinpyrazone can reduce ciclosporin levels (by about 40% in one study), and this has led to transplant rejection in some cases, which developed over a period of several months.

If there is a trend towards decreased ciclosporin levels in patients taking sulfinpyrazone it would be prudent to consider this interaction as a cause and adjust treatment accordingly.

Ciclosporin (Cyclosporine) + **Sulfonamides**

In isolated cases sulfadiazine given orally or sulfadimidine given intravenously with trimethoprim have caused a fall in ciclosporin levels. Sulfametoxydiazine possibly caused a minor fall in ciclosporin levels in one case.

These interactions are not firmly established. Until more information is available it would be prudent to check ciclosporin levels if any sulphonamide is added to established treatment with ciclosporin.

Ciclosporin (Cyclosporine) + **Terbinafine**

Terbinafine causes a small, usually clinically unimportant reduction in ciclosporin levels (maximum levels reduced by 14%).

> This interaction is not usually clinically significant. However, consider monitoring patients whose ciclosporin levels are at the lower end of the therapeutic range.

Ciclosporin (Cyclosporine) + **Ursodeoxycholic acid (Ursodiol)**

Ursodeoxycholic acid unpredictably increases the absorption and raises the levels of ciclosporin in some patients.

> Ciclosporin levels and effects (e.g. on renal function) should be monitored as a matter of routine, but it may be prudent to increase monitoring if ursodeoxycholic acid is started or stopped. Adjust the dose of ciclosporin as necessary.

Ciclosporin (Cyclosporine) + **Vaccines**

The body's immune response is suppressed by ciclosporin. The antibody response to vaccines may be reduced, and the use of live attenuated vaccines may result in generalised infection.

> For many inactivated vaccines even the reduced response seen is considered clinically useful and, in the case of renal transplant patients, influenza vaccination is actively recommended. If a vaccine is given, it may be prudent to monitor the response, so that alternative prophylactic measures can be considered where the response is inadequate. Note that even where effective antibody titres are produced, these may not persist as long as in healthy subjects, and more frequent booster doses may be required. The use of live vaccines is generally considered to be contraindicated. Ideally vaccines should take place before immunosuppressive treatment is started, and live vaccines should not be given for up to 6 months after treatment has stopped.

Ciclosporin (Cyclosporine) + **Vancomycin**

The concurrent use of vancomycin and ciclosporin may increase the risk of nephrotoxicity.

> Renal function should be routinely monitored when either drug is given; however, it may be prudent to increase the frequency of monitoring if both drugs are given.

Ciclosporin (Cyclosporine) + **Warfarin and other oral anticoagulants**

A case report describes reduced ciclosporin levels and reduced warfarin efficacy in patients given both drugs concurrently. A further report describes a rise in ciclosporin levels when an unnamed anticoagulant was given. Other reports describe increased or decreased acenocoumarol effects and decreased ciclosporin levels in 2 patients given both drugs.

Information is limited. In patients taking an anticoagulant with ciclosporin, it may be prudent to consider an increase in the frequency of the standard monitoring of both drugs.

C

Cilostazol

Cilostazol + **Food**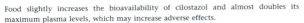

Food slightly increases the bioavailability of cilostazol and almost doubles its maximum plasma levels, which may increase adverse effects.

The manufacturer recommends that cilostazol should be taken 30 minutes before or 2 hours after food.

Cilostazol + **Herbal medicines or Dietary supplements**

A study found no significant increase in the antiplatelet effects of single doses of cilostazol when a single dose of *Ginkgo biloba* was added. However, the bleeding time was significantly increased, although none of the subjects developed any significant adverse effects.

The evidence is too slim to advise patients taking cilostazol to avoid *Ginkgo biloba*. However, as with any two drugs that a affect platelet function some caution (e.g. reporting any evidence of bleeding) would be prudent if *Ginkgo biloba* is used with cilostazol.

Cilostazol + **Macrolides**

Erythromycin increases the maximum plasma level and AUC of cilostazol by 47% and 73%, respectively. Other macrolides may also interact, although it seems unlikely that they all will, see macrolides, page 361.

Increased cilostazol adverse effects (such as headache and diarrhoea) may occur. The manufacturers suggest considering reducing the dose of cilostazol to 50 mg twice daily.

Cilostazol + **Protease inhibitors**

Erythromycin and *ketoconazole* increase the AUC of cilostazol by 47% and almost twofold, respectively. Other drugs that inhibit CYP3A4 (e.g. the protease inhibitors) would be expected to have a similar (probably greater) effect.

Increased cilostazol adverse effects (such as headache and diarrhoea) may occur.

The manufacturers suggest considering reducing the dose of cilostazol to 50 mg twice daily.

Cilostazol + **Proton pump inhibitors** ⚠

Omeprazole increases the AUC of 3,4-dehydro-cilostazol (a metabolite with 4 to 7 times the activity of cilostazol) by about 70%. Esomeprazole may interact similarly.

The manufacturers predict that an increase in cilostazol adverse effects (such as headache and diarrhoea) may occur: consider a cilostazol dose reduction to 50 mg twice daily, depending on efficacy and tolerability.

Cilostazol + **Statins** ⚠

In one study cilostazol increased the AUC of lovastatin and its metabolite, lovastatin acid, by 60% and 70%, respectively. Simvastatin is expected to interact similarly.

It has been suggested that statin dose reductions may be needed on concurrent use, but this seems over-cautious. Patients given a statin should be counselled regarding myopathy (e.g. report any unexplained muscle pain, tenderness or weakness) and it would seem prudent to reinforce this if cilostazol is also given.

Cilostazol + **Warfarin and other oral anticoagulants** ⚠

Cilostazol does not appear to have a clinically relevant effect on the pharmacokinetics or pharmacodynamics of warfarin. Nevertheless, as with other antiplatelet drugs, concurrent use might increase the bleeding risk.

The manufacturers advise that the concurrent use of cilostazol and oral anticoagulants should be monitored because of the increased risk of bleeding.

Cinacalcet

Cinacalcet + **Dextromethorphan**

Cinacalcet very markedly increases dextromethorphan levels.

This is not expected to be of clinical significance as dextromethorphan has a wide therapeutic range and its dose is not individually titrated, but bear this interaction in mind in the case of an unexpected response to treatment. Remember that many non-proprietary cough preparations contain dextromethorphan.

Cinacalcet + **Food**

Cinacalcet absorption is increased by food (AUC increased by 68%).

Cinacalcet should be taken with food or shortly after a meal to maximise absorption.

Cinacalcet + **Macrolides**

Ketoconazole raises cinacalcet levels 2-fold and increased the incidence of cinacalcet adverse effects, probably by inhibiting the metabolism of cinacalcet by CYP3A4. Other potent CYP3A4 inhibitors, such as some macrolides, are predicted to interact similarly, although they differ in their ability to inhibit CYP3A4, see macrolides, page 361.

It may be prudent to monitor parathyroid hormone and serum calcium more frequently if a macrolide that potently inhibits CYP3A4 is started or stopped. The manufacturers specifically mention erythromycin and telithromycin.

Cinacalcet + **Protease inhibitors**

Ketoconazole raises cinacalcet levels 2-fold and increased the incidence of cinacalcet adverse effects, probably by inhibiting the metabolism of cinacalcet by CYP3A4. Other potent CYP3A4 inhibitors, such as the protease inhibitors, are predicted to interact similarly.

It may be prudent to monitor parathyroid hormone and serum calcium more frequently in any patient receiving a protease inhibitor.

Cinacalcet + **Quinolones**

Ciprofloxacin may decrease the clearance (and therefore increase the levels) of cinacalcet, by inhibiting its metabolism by CYP1A2.

It may be prudent to monitor parathyroid hormone and serum calcium more frequently if ciprofloxacin is started or stopped. Note that other quinolones may also interact similarly, although they differ in their ability to inhibit CYP1A2, see quinolones, page 444.

Cinacalcet + **Rifampicin (Rifampin)**

Rifampicin is predicted to decrease cinacalcet levels by inducing its metabolism by CYP3A4. This seems a reasonable prediction as potent CYP3A4 inhibitors raise cinacalcet levels.

It may be prudent to monitor parathyroid hormone and serum calcium more frequently if rifampicin is started or stopped.

Cinacalcet + **SSRIs**

Fluvoxamine may decrease the clearance (and therefore increase the levels) of cinacalcet, by inhibiting its metabolism by CYP1A2.

It may be prudent to monitor parathyroid hormone and serum calcium more frequently if fluvoxamine is started or stopped.

Cinacalcet + Tricyclics

Cinacalcet increases the AUC of desipramine 3.6-fold. Other tricyclics are likely to be similarly affected.

> Dose reductions of the tricyclic are likely to be needed if cinacalcet is also given. If starting a tricyclic in a patient taking cinacalcet it would seem prudent to start at the lowest dose and titrate upwards carefully. Monitor closely for adverse effects such as dry mouth, urinary retention and constipation.

Clindamycin

Clindamycin + Contraceptives

One or two cases of combined oral contraceptive failure have been reported with clindamycin. These isolated cases are anecdotal and unconfirmed, and the interaction (if such it is) appears to be very rare indeed.

> It is possible that the anecdotal cases of contraceptive failure with antibacterials are indistinguishable from the normal accepted failure rate and no special precautions are required. However, for simplicity, some suggest that caution should be taken with short courses of any antibacterial (non-enzyme inducing). For guidance on the use of antibacterials with contraceptives, see contraceptives, page 233.

Clonidine

Clonidine + Inotropes and Vasopressors ❓

Studies suggest that pretreatment with clonidine decreases the blood pressure response to small doses of dopamine and can increase the blood pressure responses to dobutamine, ephedrine and phenylephrine.

> The exact outcome of the concurrent use of clonidine and these drugs is not clear. It has been suggested that the effects may be different at different doses of dopamine. Some suggest that the increase in pressor response is unlikely to be clinically significant. If dobutamine, ephedrine, or phenylephrine are given with clonidine, be aware that they may have a greater than expected effect.

Clonidine + Levodopa ❓

Limited evidence suggests that the control of Parkinson's disease with levodopa may be impaired by clonidine.

> Be alert for a reduction in the control of the Parkinson's disease during concurrent

use. The effects of this interaction appear to be reduced if antimuscarinic drugs are also being used. Be aware that, as with all antihypertensives, additive hypotensive effects may occur with levodopa, see antihypertensives, page 89.

Clonidine + Methylphenidate

Much publicised fears about the serious consequences of using methylphenidate with clonidine appear to be unfounded. There is some evidence to suggest that concurrent use can be both safe and effective.

No action needed.

Clonidine + Tricyclics

The tricyclic antidepressants reduce or abolish the antihypertensive effects of clonidine and a case report describes a hypertensive crisis as a result of this interaction.

This interaction is not seen in all patients. Avoid concurrent use unless the effects on blood pressure can be monitored. Increasing the dose of clonidine seems to be an effective way of managing this interaction.

Clopidogrel

Clopidogrel + Felbamate

On the basis of the interaction with the proton pump inhibitors, page 227, some predict that felbamate may theoretically inhibit the conversion of clopidogrel to its active metabolite by CYP2C19.

The manufacturers advise that concurrent use should be avoided.

Clopidogrel + H$_2$-receptor antagonists

Cimetidine may theoretically inhibit the conversion of clopidogrel to its active metabolite by CYP2C19. However some studies have reported that cimetidine has no significant effect on the antiplatelet effects of clopidogrel.

Until more is known, it may be prudent to use an alternative H$_2$-receptor antagonist, such as ranitidine, which does not affect CYP2C19.

Clopidogrel + Heparin

The antiplatelet effects of clopidogrel are not altered by heparin. Nevertheless, the concurrent use of heparin with antiplatelet drugs such as clopidogrel may increase the risk of bleeding. Furthermore, concurrent use may contribute to the development of epidural or spinal haematoma after epidural anaesthesia.

> The concurrent use of clopidogrel and heparin may be beneficial in specific indications (such as acute coronary syndromes), but it would still be prudent to be aware of the increased risk of bleeding and be alert for any signs of this. Unless specifically indicated, concurrent use should probably be avoided. Extreme caution is needed if concurrent use is considered appropriate in patients undergoing epidural anaesthesia.

Clopidogrel + Herbal medicines or Dietary supplements

Ginkgo biloba alone has been associated with bleeding, platelet and clotting disorders, and there are isolated reports of serious adverse reactions after its concurrent use with clopidogrel. However, a single-dose study found no increase in adverse effects when *Ginkgo biloba* was given with clopidogrel.

> The evidence is too slim to advise patients taking clopidogrel to avoid *Ginkgo biloba*. However, as with any two drugs that affect platelet function some caution (e.g. reporting any evidence of bleeding) would be prudent if *Ginkgo biloba* is used with clopidogrel.

Clopidogrel + Low-molecular-weight heparins

Although in various large clinical studies in patients with acute coronary syndrome or myocardial infarction, most patients received LMWHs and clopidogrel without an obvious difference in the rate of bleeding, concurrent use may increase the risks of bleeding and case reports describe occasional serious bleeding events, including the development of spinal haematoma and retroperitoneal bleeding.

> The concurrent use of clopidogrel and a LMWH may be beneficial in specific indications (such as acute coronary syndromes), but it would still be prudent to be aware of the increased risk of bleeding and be alert for any signs of this. Unless specifically indicated, concurrent use of a LMWH with clopidogrel should probably be avoided because of the possible risk of increased bleeding. Extreme caution is needed if concurrent use is considered appropriate in patients undergoing epidural anaesthesia.

Clopidogrel + Moclobemide

On the basis of the interaction with the proton pump inhibitors, page 227, some predict that moclobemide may theoretically inhibit the conversion of clopidogrel to its active metabolite by CYP2C19.

> The manufacturers advise that concurrent use should be avoided.

Clopidogrel + NRTIs

On the basis of the interaction with the proton pump inhibitors, page 227, some predict that etravirine may theoretically inhibit the conversion of clopidogrel to its active metabolite by CYP2C19. However, note that etravirine is only a weak inhibitor of CYP2C19.

> The manufacturers advise that concurrent use should be avoided.

Clopidogrel + NSAIDs

The risk of faecal blood loss, gastrointestinal haemorrhage and other bleeding is increased by concurrent use of clopidogrel and naproxen or celecoxib. Other NSAIDs may interact similarly.

> The manufacturers advise caution if NSAIDs and clopidogrel are given together. Consider giving additional gastrointestinal prophylaxis such as an H_2-receptor antagonist or a proton pump inhibitor (but see also Clopidogrel + Proton pump inhibitors, below) in patients at risk of gastrointestinal ulceration and bleeding. Note that some NSAIDs (particularly coxibs but also non-selective NSAIDs) are associated with an increased thrombotic/cardiovascular risk, particularly when used at high doses and for long-term treatment. Therefore coxibs are contra-indicated and NSAIDs should generally be avoided in those with ischaemic heart disease, cerebrovascular disease, and peripheral artery disease.

Clopidogrel + Oxcarbazepine

On the basis of the interaction with the proton pump inhibitors, some predict that oxcarbazepine may theoretically inhibit the conversion of clopidogrel to its active metabolite by CYP2C19.

> The manufacturers advise that concurrent use should be avoided.

Clopidogrel + Proton pump inhibitors

High-dose omeprazole almost halves the exposure to the active metabolite of clopidogrel and reduces the antiplatelet action of clopidogrel by 30%. However, preliminary findings from one large clinical study found no reduction in clopidogrel efficacy with omeprazole 20 mg daily. Nevertheless, reduced efficacy has been seen in some, but not all, retrospective analyses. In one controlled study, lansoprazole showed a trend towards a reduction in the antiplatelet action of clopidogrel, whereas in another study, esomeprazole and pantoprazole did not appear to alter clopidogrel antiplatelet effects. Nevertheless, some, but not all, retrospective analyses have shown poorer cardiovascular outcomes in patients taking clopidogrel with these proton pump inhibitors, and also rabeprazole. The mechanism for the interaction between the proton pump inhibitors and clopidogrel is unclear. At present, the most plausible mechanism is that omeprazole inhibits the conversion of clopidogrel to its active metabolite by CYP2C19.

> Consider if concurrent use is necessary, weighing up the patient's other possible risk factors for gastrointestinal bleeding against the possibility of clopidogrel treatment failure. H_2-receptor antagonists have been suggested as an alternative to proton pump inhibitors in this situation, but until the mechanism of any interaction is established, it would be prudent to avoid cimetidine, as it may also inhibit CYP2C19.

Clopidogrel

Clopidogrel + Quinolones ❌

On the basis of the interaction with the proton pump inhibitors, some predict that ciprofloxacin may theoretically inhibit the conversion of clopidogrel to its active metabolite by CYP2C19. However, there do not appear to be any clinically relevant interactions with ciprofloxacin as a result of this mechanism.

> The manufacturers advise that concurrent use should be avoided.

Clopidogrel + SSRIs ❓

The SSRIs may increase the risk of upper gastrointestinal bleeding and the risk may be further increased by the concurrent use of clopidogrel. On the basis of the interaction with the proton pump inhibitors, page 227, some predict that fluoxetine and fluvoxamine may theoretically inhibit the conversion of clopidogrel to its active metabolite by CYP2C19. However, note that fluoxetine does not appear to be a clinically relevant inhibitor of CYP2C19.

> Caution is warranted. Consideration should be given to the prescribing of gastroprotective drugs such as an H_2-receptor antagonist or a proton pump inhibitor (but see also Clopidogrel + Proton pump inhibitors, page 227) in those at high risk of gastrointestinal bleeding, such as elderly patients or those with a history of gastrointestinal bleeding.

Clopidogrel + Statins ✔

Atorvastatin had no clinically relevant effect on the pharmacokinetics or antiplatelet effect of clopidogrel in controlled studies. Similarly, pravastatin, and possibly lovastatin and rosuvastatin, do not to alter the antiplatelet effect of clopidogrel. The data for simvastatin and fluvastatin are limited, with one study showing some reduction in antiplatelet effect. Nevertheless, clinical outcome data from retrospective analysis of large studies does not support an interaction with any of these other statins.

> Although an interaction has been demonstrated in some studies, the anticipated negative effect on clinical outcomes has not been consistently shown. The available data provides insufficient evidence of a negative interaction between clopidogrel and statins to justify stopping any statin during clopidogrel use.

Clopidogrel + Ticlopidine ❌

On the basis of the interaction with the proton pump inhibitors, page 227, some predict that ticlopidine may theoretically inhibit the conversion of clopidogrel to its active metabolite by CYP2C19.

> Until more is known, it may be prudent to use avoid concurrent use. Note that, ticlopidine, like clopidogrel, is a thienopyridine antiplatelet drug, and it is not usually used with clopidogrel because it has the same mechanism of action.

Clopidogrel + Warfarin and other oral anticoagulants ⚠

Clopidogrel does not appear to have a clinically relevant effect on the pharmacokinetics or pharmacodynamics of warfarin. Nevertheless, the concurrent use of clopidogrel, either with warfarin or when given with warfarin and aspirin, increases the bleeding risk.

The concurrent use of warfarin and clopidogrel increases the risk of bleeding and so both drugs should only be given when there is a clear indication for concurrent use. The lowest effective INR should be targeted and the combination used for the shortest duration possible. Monitor for signs of bleeding and check bleeding times as necessary. Consideration should be given to the prescribing of gastroprotective drugs such as an H_2-receptor antagonist or a proton pump inhibitor, but see also Clopidogrel + Proton pump inhibitors, page 227.

Colchicine

Colchicine + Fibrates ❓

Case reports suggest that the current use of fibrates and colchicine can result in rhabdomyolysis or neuromyopathy.

Information is limited, although rhabdomyolysis is associated with both colchicine and the fibrates. Suspect this interaction in any patient taking these drugs who presents with muscle pain or a raised creatinine kinase level.

Colchicine + Macrolides ❓

Several case reports describe acute life-threatening colchicine toxicity caused by the concurrent use of erythromycin or clarithromycin. A retrospective study and individual case reports have identified fatalities associated with the concurrent use of clarithromycin and colchicine.

Information on this interaction is limited, but it appears that erythromycin and clarithromycin can provoke acute colchicine toxicity, at the very least in predisposed individuals. Other macrolides may also interact, although it seems unlikely that they all will, see macrolides, page 361. If any patient is given colchicine and a potentially interacting macrolide be aware of the potential for toxicity, especially in patients with pre-existing renal impairment. Note that one UK manufacturer of colchicine contraindicates the concurrent use of colchicine with clarithromycin or telithromycin in patients with renal or hepatic impairment.

Colchicine + Protease inhibitors ⚠

Several case reports describe acute life-threatening colchicine toxicity caused by the concurrent use of macrolides that are known to inhibit CYP3A4. The manufacturers predict that the protease inhibitors will interact similarly, but to a greater extent.

> If any patient is given colchicine and a protease inhibitor be alert for colchicine adverse effects such as nausea, vomiting, and diarrhoea, especially in patients with pre-existing renal impairment. Colchicine should not be given with any protease inhibitor in patients with hepatic or renal impairment, and is specifically contraindicated by one UK manufacturer of colchicine (they specifically name atazanavir, indinavir and ritonavir). In the US, it is generally recommended that the dose of colchicine be reduced in patients taking protease inhibitors.

- For the treatment of gout, the dose of colchicine should be reduced to a single dose of 600 micrograms, with a further 300-microgram dose one hour later. The dose should not be repeated within 3 days.
- For gout prophylaxis, the dose of colchicine should be reduced to 300 micrograms daily (if the initial dose was 600 micrograms twice daily) or on alternate days (if the initial dose was 600 micrograms daily).
- For familial Mediterranean fever, a maximum total daily dose of colchicine 600 micrograms is recommended.

The guidance for some protease inhibitors varies.

- In patients taking fosamprenavir without ritonavir, the dose of colchicine should be reduced in the treatment of gout to 1.2 mg as a single dose. The dose should not be repeated within 3 days.
- For gout prophylaxis, the dose of colchicine should be halved, from 600 micrograms twice daily to 300 micrograms twice daily, or from 600 micrograms daily to 300 micrograms daily.
- For familial Mediterranean fever, a maximum total daily dose of colchicine 1.2 mg is recommended.

Colchicine + Quinidine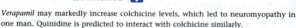

Verapamil may markedly increase colchicine levels, which led to neuromyopathy in one man. Quinidine is predicted to interact with colchicine similarly.

> Consider an interaction in the case of otherwise unexplained colchicine toxicity (e.g. diarrhoea, vomiting). Concurrent use is contraindicated in renal or hepatic impairment.

Colchicine + Statins

Case reports describe myopathy or rhabdomyolysis in patients given colchicine and atorvastatin, fluvastatin, pravastatin or simvastatin. It seems possible that this reaction could occur with colchicine and any statin.

> Although this interaction is rare it is serious. All patients taking statins should be warned about the symptoms of myopathy and told to report muscle pain or weakness. It would be prudent to reinforce this advice if they are given colchicine.

Colestyramine and related drugs

Note that it is generally recommended that other drugs are given one hour before or 4 hours after colestipol, one hour before or 4 to 6 hours after colestyramine, and at least 4 hours before colesevelam. Interactions have therefore only been included where information suggests that different actions may be appropriate.

Colestyramine and related drugs + **Diuretics**

Loop diuretics

The 4-hour diuretic response to furosemide can be reduced by 58% and 77% by colestipol and colestyramine, respectively.

> Furosemide should be given 2 to 3 hours before taking colestyramine or colestipol to minimise this interaction.

Thiazides

The absorption of hydrochlorothiazide and chlorothiazide can be reduced by more than one-third if colestipol is given concurrently. Colestyramine also reduces the absorption of hydrochlorothiazide by more than two-thirds.

> Separating the doses of hydrochlorothiazide and colestyramine by 4 hours can reduce, but not totally overcome the effects of this interaction. Even with a dosing separation, the possibility of this interaction should be considered in patients who have a reduced response to this diuretic.

Colestyramine and related drugs + **Leflunomide**

Studies have shown that colestyramine reduces the levels of the active metabolite of leflunomide by up to 65% after 48 hours.

> Patients taking leflunomide should not be given colestyramine unless it is needed to remove the leflunomide from the body more quickly, such as in overdose or when switching to another DMARD.

Colestyramine and related drugs + Mycophenolate

Colestyramine modestly reduces the AUC of mycophenolic acid after administration of mycophenolate.

> The clinical importance of this reduction has not been assessed but it would seem prudent to confirm that the immunosuppressant effects remain adequate in the presence of colestyramine. Separating the administration is not likely to eliminate this interaction, as colestyramine affects the enterohepatic recirculation of mycophenolate. Note that the US manufacturers of mycophenolate advise avoiding the concurrent use of colestyramine and other drugs that bind to bile acids (e.g. colestipol).

Colestyramine and related drugs + NSAIDs

Giving colestyramine even three or more hours after oral sulindac, piroxicam, or tenoxicam markedly reduced their plasma levels. Colestyramine, given after the NSAID, markedly reduces the levels of *intravenous* meloxicam or tenoxicam.

It is usually recommended that other drugs are given one hour before or 4 to 6 hours after colestyramine. However, meloxicam, piroxicam, sulindac, and tenoxicam undergo enterohepatic recirculation and so the interaction cannot be entirely avoided by separating the doses. Therefore it may be best to avoid using these NSAIDs with colestyramine.

Colestyramine and related drugs + Raloxifene

The manufacturers report that the concurrent use of colestyramine reduced the absorption of raloxifene by about 60%, due to an interruption in enterohepatic cycling.

Separating administration is unlikely to be effective as the interaction is via enterohepatic circulation. It is recommended that these two drugs should not be used concurrently. Other drugs, such as colestipol, are expected to interact similarly.

Colestyramine and related drugs + Valproate

Colestyramine causes a small 20% reduction in the absorption of valproate.

The fall in absorption is small and probably of very limited clinical importance, but the interaction can apparently be totally avoided by separating administration by 3 hours. Note that it is usually recommended that other drugs are given one hour before or 4 to 6 hours after colestyramine. Colesevelam does not appear to interact, and may therefore be a suitable alternative in some patients.

Colestyramine and related drugs + Warfarin and other oral anticoagulants

The anticoagulant effects of phenprocoumon and warfarin can be reduced by colestyramine. An isolated and unexplained report describes a paradoxical increase in the effects of warfarin. Other coumarins are expected to interact similarly. The manufacturers warn that long-term colestyramine or colestipol can reduce vitamin K absorption and can cause hypoprothrombinaemia, and this may affect the anticoagulant effects of both coumarins and indanediones.

If the concurrent use of colestyramine and a coumarin is thought necessary, prothrombin times should be monitored and the dose of the anticoagulant increased appropriately. Giving the colestyramine 4 to 6 hours after the anticoagulant has been shown to minimise the effects of this interaction; however, case reports suggest that, despite a dose separation, an interaction is still possible. Bear in mind that long-term colestyramine and colestipol can reduce vitamin K absorption and can cause hypoprothrombinaemia. This might result in an increased effect of warfarin, but there is little evidence to suggest that this is clinically relevant.

Contraceptives

As HRT contains many of the same hormones as the contraceptives, studies with contraceptives may be applicable to HRT and *vice versa*, although the relative doses should be borne in mind. Similar careful extrapolations may be made between studies with contraceptives and HRT and systemic oestrogens and progestogens. The interaction between the combined hormonal contraceptives and non-enzyme inducing antibacterials is inadequately established and controversial. Almost all of the evidence is anecdotal with no controls. The total number of failures is extremely small when viewed against the number of women worldwide using oral combined hormonal contraceptives; however, this needs to be considered against the personal and ethical consequences of an unwanted pregnancy, which can be serious. For simplicity, and on pragmatic grounds, the UK Faculty of Family Planning and Reproductive Health Care (FFPRHC) Clinical Effectiveness Unit recommends that women taking *combined hormonal contraceptives* should routinely use a second form of contraception, such as condoms, while taking a short course of less than 3 weeks of any antibacterial (non-enzyme inducing), and for 7 days after the antibacterial has been stopped. In addition, if fewer than 7 active pills are left in the pack after the antibacterial has been stopped, the new packet should be started without a pill-free break, omitting any of the inactive tablets. For women using the *combined contraceptive patch*, if the 7 days after the antibacterial has been stopped runs into the usual 7 day patch-free period, a new patch should be applied when it is due to be changed and the patch-free week delayed by 7 days. For women using the *vaginal ring*, if antibacterial use (except amoxicillin) runs beyond the 3 weeks of a ring-cycle, the next ring should be inserted immediately, without having the usual ring-free interval. Combined hormonal contraceptive users who start long-term courses of antibacterials need only use additional contraceptive protection for the first 3 weeks, as after that the gut flora becomes resistant to the antibacterial. Patients who are taking long-term antibacterials for more than 3 weeks who then start a combined hormonal contraceptive do not need any additional contraceptive protection, unless the antibacterial is changed.

- Women taking *combined hormonal contraceptives* (oral or patch) should use an ethinylestradiol dose of at least 50 micrograms daily. The dose may be increased further above 50 micrograms if breakthrough bleeding occurs. Note that, for those using the patch, the use of more than one patch is not recommended. Additional non-hormonal methods of contraception, such as condoms, should also be used by patients using combined hormonal contraceptives, both when taking the liver enzyme inducers and for at least 4 weeks after stopping the drug. Alternatives to all forms of combined hormonal contraceptives should be considered with long-term use of liver enzyme inducers.
- The progestogen-only implant may be continued with *short* courses of enzyme inducers. Additional non-hormonal methods of contraception, such as condoms, should also be used by patients using the progestogen-only implant, both when taking the liver enzyme inducers and for at least 4 weeks after stopping the drug. Alternatives to the progestogen-only implant should be considered with long-term use of liver enzyme inducers.
- The progestogen-only pill is not recommended for use with liver enzyme inducers and alternative methods of contraception are advised.
- The effectiveness of the progestogen-only *emergency* hormonal contraceptive will be reduced in women taking liver enzyme inducers. An increased dose of levonorgestrel 1.5 mg immediately followed by another 1.5-mg dose 12 hours later may be used, although this is unlicensed. A copper IUD may be used as an alternative option.

- Copper or levonorgestrel-releasing intrauterine devices (IUD) and depot progesto-gen-only injections are preferred alternative contraceptive methods, particularly for women requiring hormonal contraception who are likely to be taking the enzyme inducer in the long-term, as these are unaffected by liver enzyme inducers.

Contraceptives + **Co-trimoxazole**

Co-trimoxazole modestly *increases* ethinylestradiol levels and the suppression of ovulation in women taking oral combined hormonal contraceptives. However, there are about 15 anecdotal cases on record of contraceptive failure attributed to co-trimoxazole. There are also isolated cases of contraceptive failure attributed to various sulfonamides, and trimethoprim.

> The pharmacokinetic and pharmacodynamic evidence indicates that co-trimox-azole is not likely to reduce the effectiveness of combined hormonal contracep-tives. It is possible that these case reports of contraceptive failure are coincidental, and fit within the normal failure rate of combined hormonal contraceptives. However, for simplicity, some suggest that caution should be taken with short courses of any antibacterial (non-enzyme inducing). See contraceptives, page 233.

Contraceptives + **Danazol**

There is a theoretical risk that the effects of both danazol and hormonal contraceptives might be altered or reduced on concurrent use.

> The manufacturers state that women of childbearing age taking danazol should use an effective non-hormonal method of contraception.

Contraceptives + **Dapsone**

One or two cases of oral combined hormonal contraceptive failure have been reported with dapsone. These isolated cases are anecdotal and unconfirmed, and the interaction (if such it is) appears to be very rare.

> It is possible that the anecdotal cases of contraceptive failure with antibacterials are indistinguishable from the normal accepted failure rate and no special precautions are required. For simplicity, some suggest that caution should be taken with short courses of any antibacterial (non-enzyme inducing). For general guidance on the use of antibacterials with contraceptives, see contraceptives, page 233.

Contraceptives + **Endothelin receptor antagonists**

Bosentan reduces the levels of ethinylestradiol and norethisterone given as a combined hormonal contraceptive, which may result in contraceptive failure. The contraceptive efficacy of oral progestogen-only contraceptives, the etonogestrel implant and emergency hormonal contraceptives (both progestogen-only and com-bined hormonal preparations) are also expected to be reduced. Sitaxentan *increases* contraceptive steroid levels, and might possibly increase their adverse effects.

> For general advice on the use of enzyme inducers, such as bosentan, and contraceptives, see contraceptives, page 233. With sitaxentan, it would seem

prudent to consider low-dose contraceptives and be cautious about contraceptive adverse effects (e.g. venous thromboembolism).

Contraceptives + **Felbamate**

Felbamate increased the clearance of gestodene from an oral combined hormonal contraceptive in one study, but ovulation remained suppressed.

> What this change means in terms of the reliability of the hormonal contraceptive is not known, but some reduction in its efficacy might be expected. If both drugs are used tell patients to report any changes in bleeding.

Contraceptives + **Fusidic acid**

One or two cases of oral combined hormonal contraceptive failure have been reported with fusidic acid. These isolated cases are anecdotal and unconfirmed, and the interaction (if such it is) appears to be very rare.

> It is possible that the anecdotal cases of contraceptive failure with antibacterials are indistinguishable from the normal accepted failure rate and no special precautions are required. For simplicity, some suggest that caution should be taken with short courses of any antibacterial (non-enzyme inducing). For guidance on the use of antibacterials with contraceptives, see contraceptives, page 233.

Contraceptives + **Gestrinone**

There is a theoretical risk that the effects of both gestrinone and hormonal contraceptives might be altered or reduced on concurrent use. Note that high doses of gestrinone have been shown to be embryotoxic in some *animal* species.

> The manufacturers state that women of childbearing age taking gestrinone should use an effective non-hormonal method of contraception.

Contraceptives + **Griseofulvin**

The effects of oral combined hormonal contraceptives may possibly be disturbed (either inter-menstrual bleeding or amenorrhoea) if griseofulvin is taken concurrently; pregnancies have occurred. Similarly, progestogen-only *emergency* hormonal contraceptives are considered to be less effective in those taking griseofulvin. The situation with progestogen-only oral contraceptives is not clear, but it has been suggested that they are not the contraceptive of choice in those taking griseofulvin because of increased menstrual irregularities.

> As griseofulvin is potentially teratogenic it has been recommended that a barrier method is used during and for 1 month after taking griseofulvin. For general advice on the use of enzyme inducers, such as griseofulvin, and contraceptives, see contraceptives, page 233.

Contraceptives + **Herbal medicines or Dietary supplements** ✗

Both breakthrough bleeding and oral hormonal contraceptive failure have been seen in women taking St John's wort (*Hypericum perforatum*). In two cases the failure of *emergency* hormonal contraception has been attributed to the use of St John's wort, and in one case the contraceptive efficacy of an oral progestogen-only contraceptive was reduced. Etonogestrel implants are also expected to be affected.

> As it is not known who is particularly likely to be at risk, women taking hormonal contraceptives should either avoid St John's wort (the recommendation of the CSM in the UK) or they should use an additional form of contraception. For general advice on the use of enzyme inducers, such as St John's wort, and contraceptives, see contraceptives, page 233.

Contraceptives + **Isoniazid** ⚠

One or two cases of oral combined hormonal contraceptive failure have been reported with isoniazid. However, there is evidence that isoniazid does not cause contraceptive failure when used in combination with other antimycobacterials (without rifampicin (rifampin)). These isolated cases are anecdotal and unconfirmed, and the interaction (if such it is) appears to be very rare.

> It is possible that the anecdotal cases of contraceptive failure with antibacterials are indistinguishable from the normal accepted failure rate and no special precautions are required. For simplicity, some suggest that caution should be taken with short courses of any antibacterial (non-enzyme inducing). For guidance on the use of antibacterials with contraceptives, see contraceptives, page 233.

Contraceptives + **Isotretinoin** ❓

There seems to be no evidence that the reliability of combined hormonal contraceptives is affected by isotretinoin, and they are the contraceptive method of choice with these teratogenic drugs. The adverse effects of isotretinoin on lipids may be additive with those of oral contraceptives, but the importance of this is not known.

> Contraceptives should be started one month before isotretinoin and continued for one month after stopping isotretinoin. In the US, it is standard practice to recommend that a second form of contraception, such as a barrier method, should also be used. This is because, even though hormonal methods of contraception are highly effective, they do, on rare occasions, fail. Note that progestogen-only oral contraceptives are not generally considered reliable enough for use with teratogenic drugs.

Contraceptives + **Lamotrigine** ⚠

In one study, lamotrigine for 2 weeks did not alter the plasma levels of ethinylestradiol and levonorgestrel or the suppression of ovulation in women taking an oral combined hormonal contraceptive. However, another study of 6 weeks' use found a slight reduction in levonorgestrel levels, and some loss in suppression of FSH and LH, but no evidence of ovulation. Combined hormonal contraceptives reduce the levels of lamotrigine, which can lead to a decrease in seizure control.

The manufacturers suggest that reduced contraceptive efficacy cannot be ruled out, and recommend the use of non-hormonal contraceptives. However, the FFPRHC in the UK has found no evidence of reduced contraceptive efficacy and so they suggest that there is no good evidence that non-hormonal methods of contraception are preferable. Lamotrigine can be started as normal in patients already taking hormonal contraceptives. For women already taking lamotrigine and carbamazepine or phenytoin no lamotrigine dose adjustment is necessary when hormonal contraceptives are started, but in the absence of these other antiepileptics the maintenance dose of lamotrigine may need to be increased by as much as twofold, according to clinical response. The manufacturer of lamotrigine suggests that the possibility of decreased contraceptive efficacy cannot be ruled out, but other sources do not agree with this suggestion.

Contraceptives + Macrolides

Controlled studies have not shown the macrolides clarithromycin, dirithromycin, roxithromycin and telithromycin to have any effect on contraceptive steroid levels and/or suppression of ovulation in women given combined hormonal contraceptives. Isolated cases of contraceptive failure have been attributed to erythromycin or spiramycin. Conversely, in two studies of contraceptive failures in dermatology patients, no pregnancies were identified in a total of 74 women taking erythromycin with an oral contraceptive.

The WHO does not recommend any additional precautions while taking macrolides with combined hormonal contraceptives given orally, as the patch, or as the vaginal ring. However, some consider that, for simplicity, precautions should be taken. See contraceptives, page 233.

Contraceptives + MAO-B inhibitors

In a small study, the bioavailability of selegiline was markedly higher (mean of about 20-fold) in women taking oral combined hormonal contraceptives than in those not taking contraceptives.

The manufacturers of selegiline advise avoiding concurrent use. If concurrent use is necessary, monitor for increased selegiline adverse effects (such as nausea, constipation, hypotension and diarrhoea).

Contraceptives + Metronidazole

Isolated cases of oral combined hormonal contraceptive failure have been reported with metronidazole. The interaction (if such it is) appears to be very rare. In a controlled study, metronidazole did not affect contraceptive steroid levels.

It is possible that the anecdotal cases of contraceptive failure with antibacterials are indistinguishable from the normal accepted failure rate and no special precautions are required. For simplicity, some suggest that caution should be taken with short courses of any antibacterial (non-enzyme inducing). For guidance on the use of antibacterials with contraceptives, see contraceptives, page 233.

Contracteptives + **Modafinil**

Modafinil slightly reduced the levels of ethinylestradiol taken as part of a combined hormonal contraceptive; this may reduce contraceptive efficacy. The contraceptive efficacy of oral progestogen-only contracteptives, the etonogestrel implant and emergency hormonal contracteptives (both progestogen-only and combined hormonal preparations) are also expected to be reduced.

> These small changes may be sufficient to cause the failure of combined hormonal contracteptives in rare cases. For additional advice on the use of enzyme inducers, such as modafinil, and contracteptives, see contracteptives, page 233. It is also recommended that additional or alternative methods should be continued for up to 2 cycles after stopping modafinil.

Contracteptives + **Nitrofurantoin**

One or two cases of combined oral contraceptive failure have been reported with nitrofurantoin. These isolated cases are anecdotal and unconfirmed, and the interaction (if such it is) appears to be very rare.

> It is possible that the anecdotal cases of contraceptive failure with antibacterials are indistinguishable from the normal accepted failure rate and no special precautions are required. For simplicity, some suggest that caution should be taken with short courses of any antibacterial (non-enzyme inducing). For guidance on the use of antibacterials with contracteptives, see contracteptives, page 233.

Contracteptives + **NNRTIs**

Efavirenz

In one study efavirenz increased the plasma levels of ethinylestradiol. In another study efavirenz markedly decreased the AUCs of norelgestromin (the principal active metabolite of norgestimate) and levonorgestrel (a secondary active metabolite). The efficacy of emergency hormonal contracteptives and progestogen-only implants or injections may also be reduced by efavirenz.

> The manufacturers recommend using a reliable method of barrier contraception as they cannot rule out the potential for contraceptive failure. Note that this is also advisable to reduce the risk of HIV transmission. As efavirenz is an enzyme inducer the FFPRHC in the UK recommend that their guidance on hormonal contracteptives and liver enzyme inducers is followed. See contracteptives, page 233.

Nevirapine

Nevirapine modestly reduces the plasma concentrations of ethinylestradiol and norethisterone, which could reduce the efficacy of contraception. The efficacy of emergency hormonal contracteptives and progestogen-only implants or injections may also be reduced by nevirapine.

> For general advice on the use of enzyme inducers, such as nevirapine, and contracteptives, see contracteptives, page 233. Note that the manufacturers of nevirapine recommend that combined hormonal contracteptives should not be used as the sole method of contraception in women taking nevirapine.

Contraceptives + **NSAIDs** ❓

A study in women taking ethinylestradiol and norethisterone-containing oral contraceptives found that the addition of etoricoxib increased the steady-state levels of ethinylestradiol by 50 to 60%, but the rise in norethisterone levels was not clinically relevant. Drospirenone may increase the risk of hyperkalaemia if it is given to patients with other drugs which increase potassium levels such as NSAIDs (although this is rare). A few early reports suggest that the very occasional failure of copper IUDs to prevent pregnancy may have been due to an interaction with NSAIDs.

> There would appear to be no reason for avoiding concurrent use but the manufacturers suggest that this increase in ethinylestradiol levels should be considered when choosing a hormonal contraceptive. It may be appropriate to use a contraceptive with a lower dose of ethinylestradiol. It is generally recommended that potassium level are measured during the first cycle of treatment with drospirenone. The evidence is insufficient to justify general precautions if NSAIDs are given to women using IUDs.

Contraceptives + **Orlistat** ⚠

Studies suggest that orlistat does not alter the suppression of ovulation in women taking oral combined hormonal contraceptives. However, isolated pregnancies have occurred with oral contraceptives in women also taking orlistat, and the UK manufacturer says that severe orlistat-induced diarrhoea might be a risk for this.

> The manufacturers recommend additional contraceptive measures (presumably barrier methods) if severe diarrhoea occurs.

Contraceptives + **Oxcarbazepine** ⚠

Combined hormonal contraceptives and possibly oral progestogen-only contraceptives are less reliable during treatment with oxcarbazepine. Breakthrough bleeding and spotting can take place. A pharmacokinetic study suggests that the levels of ethinylestradiol and levonorgestrel are modestly reduced by oxcarbazepine; this may lead to a reduction in contraceptive efficacy. The contraceptive efficacy of the etonogestrel implant and emergency hormonal contraceptives (both progestogen-only and combined hormonal preparations) are also expected to be reduced.

> The increase in failure rate appears small, but because of the consequences of an unwanted pregnancy, especially with drugs that may cause foetal abnormalities, adjustments should be made. For additional advice on the use of enzyme inducers, such as oxcarbazepine, and contraceptives, see contraceptives, page 233.

Contraceptives + **Penicillins** ⚠

Failure of oral combined hormonal contraceptives has been attributed to the concurrent use of penicillins, but the interaction (if such it is) appears to be very rare. Controlled studies have not shown any effect of ampicillin or amoxicillin on contraceptive steroid levels and the suppression of ovulation in women given these contraceptives.

> It is possible that the anecdotal cases of contraceptive failure with antibacterials are indistinguishable from the normal accepted failure rate and no special

precautions are required. For simplicity, some suggest that caution should be taken with short courses of any antibacterial (non-enzyme inducing). For guidance on the use of antibacterials with contraceptives, see contraceptives, page 233.

Contraceptives + Phenobarbital

Combined hormonal contraceptives and possibly progestogen-only oral contraceptives are less reliable during treatment with phenobarbital. Inter-menstrual breakthrough bleeding and spotting can take place, and pregnancies have occurred. Controlled studies have shown that phenobarbital can reduce contraceptive steroid levels. Similarly, emergency hormonal contraceptives are considered to be less effective in those taking phenobarbital. Note that primidone is metabolised to phenobarbital and therefore may interact similarly.

> The increase in failure rate appears small, but because of the consequences of an unwanted pregnancy, especially with drugs that may cause foetal abnormalities, adjustments should be made. For additional advice on the use of enzyme inducers, such as phenobarbital or primidone, and contraceptives, see contraceptives, page 233.

Contraceptives + Phenytoin

Combined hormonal contraceptives and possibly progestogen-only oral contraceptives are less reliable during treatment with phenytoin. Inter-menstrual breakthrough bleeding and spotting can take place, and pregnancies have occurred. Controlled studies have shown that phenytoin can reduce contraceptive steroid levels (both progestogens and oestrogens). Similarly, emergency hormonal contraceptives are considered to be less effective in those taking phenytoin. Fosphenytoin, a prodrug of phenytoin, may interact similarly.

> The increase in failure rate appears small, but because of the consequences of an unwanted pregnancy, especially with drugs that may cause foetal abnormalities, adjustments should be made. For general advice on the use of enzyme inducers, such as phenytoin, and contraceptives, see contraceptives, page 233.

Contraceptives + Protease inhibitors

Ritonavir and nelfinavir, given alone, markedly reduce the levels of ethinylestradiol. Ritonavir-boosted protease inhibitors modestly (atazanavir) to markedly (darunavir, fosamprenavir, lopinavir and tipranavir) reduce ethinylestradiol levels and this might result in reduced contraceptive efficacy. Conversely, atazanavir or amprenavir alone modestly to markedly *increase* the levels of ethinylestradiol and norethisterone. It is possible that the protease inhibitors could reduce the contraceptive efficacy of progestogen-only oral contraceptives containing norethisterone. The efficacy of emergency hormonal contraceptives may also be decreased.

> Guidance from the WHO states that when an oral combined hormonal contraceptive is chosen, a preparation containing a minimum of 30 micrograms of ethinylestradiol should be used. Also, whatever other methods of contraception are being used, barrier methods are always advisable to reduce the risk of HIV transmission, and the WHO notes that this will also compensate for any reduction in the effectiveness of the contraceptive. For additional advice on the use of

enzyme inducers, such as protease inhibitors, and contraceptives, see contraceptives, page 233. If atazanavir and amprenavir are used without ritonavir, the marked *increase* in norethisterone and ethinylestradiol levels suggest some caution is appropriate. The US manufacturer of atazanavir recommends that an oral combined hormonal contraceptive with no more than 30 micrograms of ethinylestradiol be used, whereas the UK manufacturer of atazanavir recommends avoiding oral hormonal contraceptives.

Contraceptives + Quinolones

Ciprofloxacin, moxifloxacin and ofloxacin have been shown not to affect the pharmacokinetics of oral combined hormonal contraceptives in controlled studies. Contraceptive failure does not appear to have been reported, and ovarian suppression is not affected.

It is possible that the anecdotal cases of contraceptive failure with antibacterials are indistinguishable from the normal accepted failure rate and no special precautions are required. However, for simplicity, some suggest that caution should be taken with short courses of any antibacterial (non-enzyme inducing). For guidance on the use of antibacterials with contraceptives, see contraceptives, page 233.

Contraceptives + Rifabutin

Combined hormonal contraceptives and progestogen-only oral contraceptives are considered to be less reliable during treatment with rifabutin. Pharmacokinetic studies suggest that the levels of oestrogens and progestogens are modestly and slightly reduced, respectively, by rifabutin. Emergency hormonal contraceptives are considered to be less effective in those taking rifabutin and the etonogestrel implant is also expected to be less effective.

For general advice on the use of enzyme inducers, such as rifabutin, and contraceptives, see contraceptives, page 233. It has been recommended that an alternative or additional form of contraception should also be used while taking rifabutin, and for 4 to 8 weeks after stopping rifabutin.

Contraceptives + Rifampicin (Rifampin)

Combined hormonal contraceptives are less reliable during treatment with rifampicin. Breakthrough bleeding and spotting are common, and pregnancies have occurred. Pharmacokinetic studies suggest that the levels of oestrogens and progestogens are reduced by rifampicin. Progestogen-only oral contraceptives and emergency hormonal contraceptives are therefore considered to be less effective in those taking rifampicin.

For advice on the use of enzyme inducers, such as rifampicin, and contraceptives, see contraceptives, page 233. It has been recommended that an alternative or additional form of contraception should also be used while taking rifampicin, and for 4 to 8 weeks after stopping rifampicin.

Contraceptives + Sulfonamides

Isolated cases of contraceptive failure have been attributed to various sulfonamides.

It is possible that the anecdotal cases of contraceptive failure with antibacterials are indistinguishable from the normal accepted failure rate and no special precautions are required. However, for simplicity, some suggest that caution should be taken with short courses of any antibacterial (non-enzyme inducing). For guidance on the use of antibacterials with contraceptives, see contraceptives, page 233.

Contraceptives + Tacrolimus

The manufacturers of tacrolimus say that during clinical use ethinylestradiol has been shown to increase tacrolimus levels, and *in vitro* data suggests that gestodene and norethisterone may do the same. Tacrolimus has the potential to interfere with the metabolism of hormonal contraceptives.

The manufacturers suggest that other (presumably non-hormonal) contraceptive measures should be used.

Contraceptives + Tetracyclines

Contraceptive failure has been attributed to a tetracycline in several reported cases, some of which specified long-term antibacterial use. The interaction (if such it is) appears to be very rare. Controlled studies have not found that tetracyclines affect contraceptive steroid levels (from tablets, the patch or the vaginal ring).

It is possible that the anecdotal cases of contraceptive failure with antibacterials are indistinguishable from the normal accepted failure rate and no special precautions are required. However, for simplicity, some suggest that caution should be taken with short courses of any antibacterial (non-enzyme inducing). For guidance on the use of antibacterials with contraceptives, see contraceptives, page 233.

Contraceptives + Tizanidine

Hormonal contraceptives increase the levels of tizanidine up to 4-fold: the blood pressure-lowering effect of tizanidine was increased by 12/8 mmHg.

A clinical response or adverse effect with tizanidine might occur at lower doses of tizanidine in patients taking hormonal contraceptives, therefore during dose titration individual doses should be reduced.

Contraceptives + Topiramate

Ethinylestradiol levels may be modestly reduced by high-dose topiramate, increasing the risk of breakthrough bleeding in women taking oral combined hormonal contraceptives; contraceptive efficacy may be reduced. The contraceptive efficacy of oral progestogen-only contraceptives, the etonogestrel implant and emergency hormonal contraceptives (both progestogen-only and combined hormonal preparations) are also expected to be reduced.

Topiramate is a weak enzyme inducer. However, the potential for contraceptive failure still exists and it has been suggested that an oral combined hormonal contraceptive containing at least 35 micrograms of ethinylestradiol would be suitable for women taking topiramate. The manufacturers advise that patients should be told to report any changes in their bleeding patterns. For general advice on the use of enzyme inducers, such as topiramate, and contraceptives, see contraceptives, page 233.

Contraceptives + **Trimethoprim**

Isolated cases of contraceptive failure have been attributed to trimethoprim.

It is possible that the anecdotal cases of contraceptive failure with antibacterials are indistinguishable from the normal accepted failure rate and no special precautions are required. However, for simplicity, some suggest that caution should be taken with short courses of any antibacterial (non-enzyme inducing). For guidance on the use of antibacterials with contraceptives, see contraceptives, page 233.

Contraceptives + **Ursodeoxycholic acid (Ursodiol)**

Ursodeoxycholic acid does not affect the bioavailability of ethinylestradiol. However, oestrogens may decrease the effectiveness of ursodeoxycholic acid by increasing the elimination of cholesterol in bile.

The manufacturers suggest that concurrent use should be avoided.

Contraceptives + **Warfarin and other oral anticoagulants**

Acenocoumarol dose requirements appear to be about 20% lower during the use of a combined hormonal contraceptive. An isolated report describes a marked increase in the INR of a woman taking warfarin when she was given emergency contraception with levonorgestrel. In contrast, the anticoagulant effects of phenprocoumon were slightly decreased by oral contraceptives.

Direct information is limited. Combined hormonal contraceptives are usually contraindicated in patients with thromboembolic disorders. However, if they are used be aware that the anticoagulant response may be affected.

Corticosteroids

Corticosteroids + **Digoxin**

Corticosteroids can cause potassium loss, which increases the risk of digoxin toxicity.

Monitor concurrent use for digoxin adverse effects (e.g. bradycardia). Consider monitoring potassium levels. No problems of this kind would usually be expected with corticosteroids used topically or by inhalation, because the amounts absorbed are likely to be relatively small.

Corticosteroids + Diuretics

Both loop or thiazide diuretics and corticosteroids can reduce potassium levels, which can lead to life-threatening cardiac arrhythmias. The extent of this interaction will depend on the drugs used and the patient. One study reported hypokalaemia in 31% of patients given a potassium-depleting diuretic and a corticosteroid. Naturally occurring corticosteroids such as cortisone and hydrocortisone cause the greatest potassium loss. Fludrocortisone can also cause hypokalaemia. The synthetic corticosteroids (glucocorticoids) have a less marked potassium-depleting effect and are therefore less likely to cause problems. These include betamethasone, dexamethasone, prednisolone, prednisone and triamcinolone.

> Consider monitoring potassium levels, based on the severity of the patient's condition, the number of potassium-depleting drugs used, and any predisposing disease states.

Corticosteroids + Herbal medicines or Dietary supplements

Constituents of liquorice can delay the clearance of prednisolone and hydrocortisone. Liquorice, if given in large quantities with corticosteroids, may cause additive hypokalaemia.

> The clinical significance of this interaction is unclear however it may be prudent to monitor the concurrent use of liquorice and corticosteroids, especially if liquorice ingestion is prolonged or if large amounts are taken as additive effects on water and sodium retention, and potassium depletion may occur.

Corticosteroids + Macrolides

Clarithromycin and erythromycin can reduce the clearance of methylprednisolone, thereby increasing both its therapeutic and adverse effects. Other macrolides may also interact, although it seems unlikely that they all will, see macrolides, page 361. An isolated case of Cushing's syndrome has been reported in a patient taking long-term clarithromycin after using inhaled budesonide.

> Appropriate methylprednisolone dose reductions (based on symptoms) may be needed to avoid the development of corticosteroid adverse effects. In general concurrent use need not be avoided, but it would be prudent to monitor for corticosteroid adverse effects. In most cases the interaction should be manageable by reducing the corticosteroid dose until the macrolide is withdrawn. Bear the case report in mind should a patient taking inhaled corticosteroids develop otherwise unexpected cushingoid adverse effects. Prednisolone seems to be a non-interacting alternative, except possibly in those also taking enzyme inducers (e.g. phenobarbital, page 245).

Corticosteroids + Methotrexate

Dexamethasone may increase the acute hepatotoxicity of high-dose methotrexate.

> Monitor the outcome of concurrent use: full blood count and liver function tests are likely to already be monitored.

Corticosteroids + **Mifepristone**

The UK manufacturer of mifepristone says that the efficacy of corticosteroids (including inhaled corticosteroids) is expected to be reduced in the 3 to 4 days following the use of mifepristone.

Patients taking corticosteroids should be monitored in the 3 to 4 days following the use of mifepristone, and consideration given to increasing the corticosteroid dose. The US manufacturer contraindicates the use of mifepristone in those receiving long-term corticosteroids.

Corticosteroids + **Nasal decongestants**

Ephedrine increased the clearance of dexamethasone by 40% in one study, but the clinical effect of this is unknown. The manufacturers of betamethasone predict that it will be similarly affected.

Monitor the outcome of concurrent use to ensure dexamethasone efficacy. Adjust the dose as necessary.

Corticosteroids + **NSAIDs**

Corticosteroids may increase the incidence and/or severity of ulceration associated with NSAIDs, and increase the possibility of gastrointestinal bleeding.

Concurrent use need not be avoided, but be aware that the risks are increased. Consider the use of mucosal protectants such as H_2-receptor antagonists or proton pump inhibitors, particularly in at-risk patients (e.g. the elderly).

Corticosteroids + **Phenobarbital**

The therapeutic effects of systemic dexamethasone, hydrocortisone, methylprednisolone, prednisolone and prednisone are decreased by phenobarbital. Primidone and some other corticosteroids probably interact similarly, although direct evidence is lacking. The dexamethasone adrenal suppression test may be expected to be unreliable in those taking phenobarbital.

Prednisone and prednisolone appear to be less affected and therefore may be preferred. Monitor concurrent use to ensure corticosteroid efficacy and increase the corticosteroid dose as necessary.

Corticosteroids + **Phenytoin**

The therapeutic effects of dexamethasone, fludrocortisone, methylprednisolone, prednisolone, prednisone (and probably other glucocorticoids) can be markedly reduced by phenytoin. One study suggested that dexamethasone may increase phenytoin levels, but another study and two case reports suggest that an important *decrease* can occur. The results of the dexamethasone adrenal suppression test may prove to be unreliable in those taking phenytoin. Fosphenytoin, a prodrug of phenytoin, may interact similarly with these corticosteroids.

The significance of the falls in corticosteroid levels will depend on the disease the corticosteroid is prescribed for. Monitor the outcome of concurrent use closely, especially in transplant patients. The interaction can be managed by increasing the steroid dose, changing the steroid to one that is less affected by phenytoin (possibly prednisone or prednisolone) or changing to a non-interacting antiepileptic (e.g. valproate), as appropriate. Consider monitoring phenytoin levels if dexamethasone is given.

C

Corticosteroids + Protease inhibitors

Ritonavir increases the levels of a number of systemic corticosteroids (e.g. prednisone, prednisolone) and other corticosteroids are predicted to interact similarly. Case reports suggest that inhaled corticosteroids may be similarly affected: several cases of Cushing's syndrome have been seen in patients taking inhaled or intranasal fluticasone. Other protease inhibitors are likely to interact similarly, although the extent of any effect is likely to vary between different protease inhibitors. Dexamethasone is predicted to reduce the levels of indinavir, saquinavir, and possibly darunavir.

The concurrent use of corticosteroids with ritonavir or nelfinavir is not recommended unless the benefits outweigh the risks. If concurrent use is necessary, monitor for signs of corticosteroid overdose such as fluid retention, hypertension and hyperglycaemia. The problem may take months to manifest itself with inhaled corticosteroids. Consider changing to inhaled beclometasone, which is less affected. The clinical outcome of the reductions in protease inhibitor levels by dexamethasone is unclear, particularly as dexamethasone rarely appears to cause clinically significant interactions by this mechanism. However it would seem prudent to monitor antiviral efficacy if these combinations are used until further information is available.

Corticosteroids + Rifabutin

The effects of cortisone, dexamethasone, fludrocortisone, hydrocortisone, methylprednisolone, prednisolone and prednisone can be markedly reduced by *rifampicin*. The UK manufacturers and the CSM in the UK suggest that rifabutin may interact similarly, although this is likely to be to a lesser extent.

The significance of the falls in corticosteroid levels will depend on the disease the corticosteroid is prescribed for. Monitor the outcome of concurrent use closely, especially in transplant patients, and increase the dose accordingly. Note that systemic corticosteroids are usually considered as contraindicated, or only to be used with great care, in patients with active or quiescent tuberculosis. Topical preparations are not likely to be affected.

Corticosteroids + Rifampicin (Rifampin)

The effects of cortisone, dexamethasone, fludrocortisone, hydrocortisone, methylprednisolone, prednisolone and prednisone can be markedly reduced by rifampicin.

The significance of the falls in corticosteroid levels will depend on the disease the corticosteroid is prescribed for. Monitor the outcome of concurrent use closely, especially in transplant patients, and increase the dose accordingly. Note that systemic corticosteroids are usually considered as contraindicated, or only to be used with great care, in patients with active or quiescent tuberculosis. Topical preparations are not likely to be affected.

Corticosteroids + **Salbutamol (Albuterol) and related bronchodilators**

Beta$_2$ agonists, such as salbutamol and terbutaline, can cause hypokalaemia. This can be increased by other potassium-depleting drugs such as the corticosteroids. In severe cases the risk of serious cardiac arrhythmias could be increased.

The CSM in the UK advises monitoring potassium in severe asthma, because of the probability of multiple potassium-depleting drugs being used, and because some conditions predispose these patients to hypokalaemia (e.g. hypoxia). Consider monitoring based on the severity of the patient's condition, and the number of potassium-depleting drugs used. Note that the combined use of beta$_2$-agonists and corticosteroids in asthma is usually beneficial.

Corticosteroids + **Tacrolimus**

Tacrolimus levels are said to have been increased, decreased and unaltered by methylprednisolone.

The combination of tacrolimus and corticosteroids is commonly used. The clinical importance of this interaction is therefore probably limited, but if abnormal results occur, remember that this drug combination could perhaps be a cause.

Corticosteroids + **Theophylline**

Theophylline and corticosteroids have established roles in the management of asthma and their concurrent use is common and beneficial. There are isolated reports of increases in theophylline levels (sometimes associated with toxicity) when oral or parenteral corticosteroids are given, but other studies have found no changes. The general clinical importance of these findings is uncertain. Both theophylline and corticosteroids can cause hypokalaemia, which may be additive.

The CSM in the UK advises monitoring potassium in severe asthma, because of the probability of multiple potassium-depleting drugs being used, and because some conditions predispose these patients to hypokalaemia (e.g. hypoxia). Consider monitoring based on the severity of the patient's condition, and the number of potassium-depleting drugs used.

Corticosteroids + **Vaccines**

Patients who are immunised with live vaccines while receiving immunosuppressive doses of corticosteroids may develop generalised, possibly life-threatening, infections.

It has been recommended that live vaccination should be postponed for at least 3 months after high-dose corticosteroids are stopped. Adult patients taking the equivalent of 40 mg of prednisolone daily for more than one week would generally be considered to be immunosuppressed.

Corticosteroids + **Warfarin and other oral anticoagulants**

Only small increases or decreases in anticoagulation normally occur when low to moderate doses of corticosteroids are given with oral anticoagulants. However, some patients have shown very marked prothrombin time increases when given high-dose corticosteroids.

> Monitor the anticoagulant effect if corticosteroids are started or stopped in patients taking oral anticoagulants. Note that corticosteroids are associated with a weak increase in peptic ulceration and gastrointestinal bleeding, and the risk of this could theoretically be increased if over-anticoagulation occurs.

Co-trimoxazole

Co-trimoxazole is a combination product containing sulfamethoxazole and trimethoprim.

Co-trimoxazole + **Dapsone**

The levels of both dapsone and trimethoprim are possibly raised by concurrent use. Both increased efficacy and, rarely, dapsone toxicity have been seen. Note that co-trimoxazole contains trimethoprim.

> Be alert for evidence of dapsone toxicity (methaemoglobinaemia). No adverse effects would be expected if topical dapsone is used in a patient taking oral trimethoprim.

Co-trimoxazole + **Digoxin**

Digoxin levels can be increased by about 22% by trimethoprim, but some individuals may show a much greater rise.

> Monitor for digoxin adverse effects (such as bradycardia, nausea, vomiting) if trimethoprim is given, and consider measuring digoxin levels, particularly in the elderly. Adjust the dose as necessary. Trimethoprim is a constituent of co-trimoxazole but it is not known whether prophylactic doses of co-trimoxazole (160 mg of trimethoprim a day from a 960-mg dose of co-trimoxazole) will interact to a clinically significant degree. An interaction would seem likely with high-dose co-trimoxazole, and care is needed in the elderly with any co-trimoxazole dose.

Co-trimoxazole + **Methotrexate**

Several cases of severe bone marrow depression (some of which were fatal) have been reported in patients given low-dose methotrexate and co-trimoxazole. Pancytopenia has also been reported in a few patients given co-trimoxazole shortly after stopping methotrexate.

> Low-dose co-trimoxazole is commonly given without problem to patients taking methotrexate as prophylaxis of pneumocystis pneumonia. This type of patient should be having regular blood monitoring as a matter of course. However, the situation with higher doses of either drug is potentially more hazardous. Some have recommended avoiding the combination. If both drugs must be used, the haematological picture should be very closely monitored because the outcome can be life-threatening.

Co-trimoxazole + Phenytoin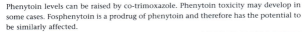

Phenytoin levels can be raised by co-trimoxazole. Phenytoin toxicity may develop in some cases. Fosphenytoin is a prodrug of phenytoin and therefore has the potential to be similarly affected.

> The risk of toxicity appears small and is most likely in those with phenytoin levels at the top end of the range. Monitor phenytoin levels and adjust the dose accordingly. Indicators of phenytoin toxicity include blurred vision, nystagmus, ataxia or drowsiness.

Co-trimoxazole + Procainamide

Trimethoprim causes a marked increase in the plasma levels of procainamide and its active metabolite, *N*-acetylprocainamide. Note that co-trimoxazole contains trimethoprim.

> Anticipate the need to reduce the procainamide dose if trimethoprim is given to patients taking procainamide.

Co-trimoxazole + Pyrimethamine

Serious pancytopenia and megaloblastic anaemia have occasionally occurred in patients given pyrimethamine and co-trimoxazole.

> Caution should be used in prescribing the combination, especially in the presence of other drugs (e.g. methotrexate, phenytoin) or disease states that may predispose to folate deficiency. Note that the manufacturer of sulfadoxine with pyrimethamine recommends that the concurrent use of sulfonamides (including co-trimoxazole) should be avoided. If both drugs are given, consider folinic acid supplementation.

Co-trimoxazole + Rifampicin (Rifampin)

Rifampicin reduces the AUCs of trimethoprim and sulfamethoxazole by 56% and 28%, respectively, in HIV-positive subjects, but apparently has no effect on trimethoprim in healthy subjects. Co-trimoxazole can increase rifampicin levels in patients with tuberculosis.

> The efficacy of co-trimoxazole prophylaxis may be reduced in HIV-positive patients taking rifampicin. Bear this in mind when using the combination. The risk of hepatotoxicity may be increased due to raised rifampicin levels; however,

liver function tests should already be closely monitored so no additional precautions seem necessary.

Co-trimoxazole + **Warfarin and other oral anticoagulants** ⚠

The anticoagulant effects of warfarin, acenocoumarol, and phenprocoumon are increased by co-trimoxazole. Bleeding may occur if the anticoagulant dose is not reduced appropriately.

The incidence of the interaction with co-trimoxazole appears to be high. If bleeding is to be avoided the INR should be well monitored and the warfarin, acenocoumarol, or phenprocoumon dose should be reduced accordingly. A pre-emptive warfarin dose reduction of about 10 to 20% has been suggested. However, others suggest that co-trimoxazole should be avoided. Consider using an alternative non-interacting antibacterial if appropriate.

Cyclophosphamide

Cyclophosphamide + **Digoxin** ⚠

Treatment with cyclophosphamide (as part of antineoplastic regimens) appears to damage the lining of the intestine so that digoxin is much less readily absorbed when given in tablet form.

In one of the studies this interaction was overcome by giving the digoxin in liquid or liquid-in-capsule form. Monitor carefully, adjusting dose, drug or preparation as appropriate.

Cyclophosphamide + **Prasugrel** ❓

Prasugrel may slightly inhibit the metabolism of *bupropion* by CYP2B6 and decrease the levels of its metabolite by 23%. The manufacturers therefore suggest that the metabolism of other substrates of CYP2B6, such as cyclophosphamide, may also be affected.

A clinically significant interaction would seem unlikely. Consider an interaction if any increase in cyclophosphamide adverse effects, such as leucopenia and neutropenia, develop.

Cyclophosphamide + **Vaccines** ✖

The immune response of the body is suppressed by cytotoxic antineoplastics. The effectiveness of vaccines may be poor and generalised infection may occur in patients immunised with live vaccines. In one study the antibody response to pneumococcal vaccination was reduced by 60% in patients receiving antineoplastics including cyclophosphamide, and suboptimal responses to influenza and measles vaccines have been reported.

Live vaccines should not be given to patients who are receiving cytotoxics or other immunosuppressant antineoplastics. In the UK, it is recommended that live vaccines should not be given during or within at least 6 months of such treatment. Monitor the immune response to other types of vaccine. Consider whether vaccination can be carried out before or after cyclophosphamide use.

C

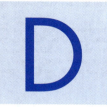

Danazol

Danazol + Sirolimus ⚠

The manufacturers predict that sirolimus levels will be increased by danazol. Note that similar predictions have proven to be true with ciclosporin (cyclosporine) and tacrolimus.

Sirolimus levels and/or effects (e.g. on renal function) should be monitored as a matter of routine, but it may be prudent to increase monitoring if danazol is started or stopped.

Danazol + Statins ⚠

Severe rhabdomyolysis and myoglobinuria developed in a man taking lovastatin about 2 months after danazol was added. Other reports describe similar interactions with danazol in another patient taking lovastatin and a man taking simvastatin.

The US manufacturer of lovastatin suggests that the dose should be started at 10 mg daily, and should not exceed 20 mg daily in the presence of danazol. Similarly the US manufacturer of simvastatin suggests that the dose should be started at 5 mg daily and both the US and UK manufacturers state that the dose should not exceed 10 mg daily in the presence of danazol. It would seem prudent to remind patients of the symptoms of myopathy if danazol is given to a patient taking lovastatin or simvastatin, and tell them to report any unexplained muscle pain, tenderness or weakness.

Danazol + Tacrolimus ⚠

An isolated report describes an increase in tacrolimus levels in a patient also given danazol. This is in line with the way other similarly metabolised drugs are known to interact.

Tacrolimus levels and/or effects (e.g. on renal function) should be monitored as a matter of routine, but it may be prudent to increase monitoring if danazol is started or stopped. Adjust the dose of tacrolimus as necessary.

Danazol + Warfarin and other oral anticoagulants

Increased anticoagulant effects and bleeding have been seen when danazol was given to patients taking warfarin. Other coumarins may interact similarly.

It would seem prudent to increase the frequency of INR monitoring if danazol is started in a patient taking any coumarin. Some recommend reducing the dose of the anticoagulant (halved has been suggested) when danazol is started, but this has been disputed.

Dapsone

D

Dapsone + Probenecid

Dapsone levels can be raised by about 50% by probenecid.

The extent of the rise and evidence that the haematological toxicity of dapsone may be dose-related suggests that this interaction may be clinically important. Monitor concurrent use for dapsone adverse effects.

Dapsone + Rifabutin

Rifabutin increases the clearance of dapsone, but may also increase its toxicity (methaemoglobinaemia).

Concurrent use should be well monitored to confirm that treatment is effective. It may be necessary to raise the dose of dapsone but note that this may increase its toxicity; therefore be alert for any evidence of methaemoglobinaemia.

Dapsone + Rifampicin (Rifampin)

Rifampicin increases the excretion of dapsone, lowers its serum levels, but increases the risk of toxicity (methaemoglobinaemia) by raising dapsone metabolite levels.

Concurrent use should be well monitored to confirm that treatment is effective. It may be necessary to raise the dose of dapsone but note that this may increase its toxicity; therefore be alert for any evidence of dapsone toxicity (methaemoglobinaemia).

Dapsone + Trimethoprim

The levels of both dapsone and trimethoprim are possibly raised by concurrent use. Both increased efficacy and dapsone toxicity have been seen.

Concurrent use appears to be an effective form of treatment, but be alert for evidence of apparently rare cases of increased dapsone toxicity (methaemoglobinaemia).

Darifenacin

Darifenacin + Flecainide ⚠

Darifenacin increases the levels of CYP2D6 substrates such as the tricyclics (imipramine AUC increased by 70%). The manufacturers of darifenacin therefore advise caution with some other CYP2D6 substrates, and specifically name flecainide.

The clinical importance of this potential interaction does not appear to have been assessed, but be alert for the need to reduce the flecainide dose if darifenacin is added.

Darifenacin + Macrolides ⚠

Erythromycin almost doubles the AUC of darifenacin by inhibiting its metabolism by CYP3A4. Other macrolides, such as clarithromycin and telithromycin, are considered to be more potent CYP3A4 inhibitors and so they may have a greater effect on darifenacin levels.

Bear in mind the possibility of an interaction if antimuscarinic effects (dry mouth, constipation, drowsiness) are increased. The US manufacturer of darifenacin suggests that no dose adjustments are necessary with erythromycin, whereas the UK manufacturer suggests starting darifenacin at a dose of 7.5 mg daily, increasing to 15 mg daily according to tolerability. In addition, the UK manufacturer contraindicates the concurrent use of potent CYP3A4 inhibitors (which may be expected to include clarithromycin and telithromycin) whereas the US manufacturer recommends that the dose of darifenacin is limited to 7.5 mg daily.

Darifenacin + Phenobarbital ⚠

Phenobarbital (a CYP3A4 inducer) is predicted to decrease darifenacin levels. Primidone, which is in part metabolised to phenobarbital, would be expected to interact similarly.

As CYP3A4 inhibitors raise darifenacin levels this predicted interaction between darifenacin and phenobarbital or primidone seems likely. Monitor the outcome of concurrent use to ensure that darifenacin is effective.

Darifenacin + Phenytoin ⚠

Phenytoin (a CYP3A4 inducer) is predicted to decrease darifenacin levels. Fosphenytoin, a prodrug of phenytoin, would be expected to interact similarly.

As CYP3A4 inhibitors raise darifenacin levels this predicted interaction between darifenacin and phenytoin or fosphenytoin seems likely. Monitor the outcome of concurrent use to ensure that darifenacin is effective.

Darifenacin + Quinidine

Paroxetine increases the AUC of darifenacin by a modest 33%. Quinidine is predicted to interact similarly (both paroxetine and quinidine are CYP2D6 inhibitors). However, changes of this magnitude seem unlikely to be clinically relevant.

No dose adjustments are recommended by the US manufacturer. The UK manufacturer recommends that the dose of darifenacin should be started at 7.5 mg daily and, if well tolerated, titrated to 15 mg daily. This seems a cautious approach. Bear in mind the possibility of an interaction if antimuscarinic effects (dry mouth, constipation, drowsiness) are increased.

Darifenacin + Rifampicin (Rifampin)

Rifampicin (a CYP3A4 inducer) is predicted to decrease darifenacin levels.

As CYP3A4 inhibitors raise darifenacin levels this predicted interaction between darifenacin and rifampicin seems likely. Monitor the outcome of concurrent use to ensure that darifenacin is effective.

Darifenacin + SSRIs

Paroxetine increases the AUC of darifenacin by a modest 33%, which is unlikely to be clinically relevant.

No dose adjustments are recommended by the US manufacturer. The UK manufacturer recommends that the dose of darifenacin should be started at 7.5 mg daily and, if well tolerated, titrated to 15 mg daily. This seems a cautious approach. Bear in mind the possibility of an interaction if antimuscarinic effects (dry mouth, constipation, drowsiness) are increased.

Darifenacin + Terbinafine

Paroxetine increases the AUC of darifenacin by a modest 33%. Terbinafine is predicted to interact similarly (both paroxetine and terbinafine are CYP2D6 inhibitors). However, changes of this magnitude seem unlikely to be clinically relevant.

No dose adjustments are recommended by the US manufacturer. The UK manufacturer recommends that the dose of darifenacin should be started at 7.5 mg daily and, if well tolerated, titrated to 15 mg daily. This seems a cautious approach. Bear in mind the possibility of an interaction if antimuscarinic effects (dry mouth, constipation, drowsiness) are increased.

Darifenacin + Tricyclics

Darifenacin increases the AUC of imipramine by about 70% and increases the AUC of its active metabolite 2.6-fold. Other tricyclics are similarly metabolised and therefore their levels may also be raised by darifenacin.

Monitor concurrent use for signs of tricyclic adverse effects (dry mouth, constipation, blurred vision).

D

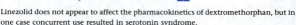

Dextromethorphan

Dextromethorphan + Linezolid

Linezolid does not appear to affect the pharmacokinetics of dextromethorphan, but in one case concurrent use resulted in serotonin syndrome.

It would be prudent to monitor for symptoms of serotonin syndrome, page 454, if concurrent use is necessary.

Dextromethorphan + MAO-B inhibitors

Cases of serotonin syndrome, page 454, have been seen when dextromethorphan has been used with non-selective MAOIs. The likelihood of an interaction with MAO-B inhibitors would appear to be very small, but because of the potential severity of this syndrome, some caution would appear to be prudent.

The manufacturer of rasagiline contraindicates its use with dextromethorphan. Some consider that patients taking selegiline should also try to avoid dextromethorphan.

Dextromethorphan + MAOIs

Two fatal cases of hyperpyrexia and coma (symptoms similar to serotonin syndrome, page 454) have occurred in patients taking phenelzine with dextromethorphan (in overdosage in one case). Three other serious but non-fatal reactions occurred in patients taking dextromethorphan with isocarboxazid or phenelzine.

Concurrent use is generally contraindicated both with and within 14 days of taking an MAOI.

Dextromethorphan + Moclobemide

Moclobemide inhibits the metabolism of dextromethorphan, and isolated cases of severe CNS reactions have occurred in patients given the combination.

Moclobemide is contraindicated with dextromethorphan.

Dextromethorphan + NSAIDs

The manufacturers say that valdecoxib (the pro-drug of parecoxib) caused a 3-fold increase in dextromethorphan levels.

It seems unlikely that normal therapeutic doses of dextromethorphan will cause a problem in most patients taking parecoxib as dextromethorphan has a wide therapeutic range, but be aware that some patients may become more sensitive to its effects.

Dextromethorphan + Quinidine

Quinidine markedly increased dextromethorphan levels in one study. Some of the patients (given dextromethorphan 60 mg) experienced dextromethorphan toxicity (nervousness, tremors, restlessness, dizziness, shortness of breath, confusion etc.).

> It seems unlikely that normal therapeutic doses of dextromethorphan will cause a problem in most patients taking quinidine as dextromethorphan has a wide therapeutic range, but be aware that some patients may become more sensitive to its effects.

Dextromethorphan + Sibutramine

There are no reports of adverse reactions between sibutramine and dextromethorphan but the manufacturers predict that concurrent use may lead to the potentially fatal serotonin syndrome.

> The manufacturers suggest that concurrent use should be avoided. Avoid concurrent use, or monitor closely for symptoms of serotonin syndrome, page 454.

Dextromethorphan + SSRIs

A serotonin-like syndrome has developed in several patients taking SSRIs with dextromethorphan, although in many of these cases the use of other drugs with serotonergic actions may have contributed. Paroxetine and fluoxetine moderately inhibit the metabolism of dextromethorphan.

> It would seem prudent for patients taking any SSRI to be cautious if using dextromethorphan-containing products because serotonin syndrome, page 454, can be serious. The pharmacokinetic interaction between dextromethorphan paroxetine and fluoxetine may increase the risks of this effect.

Digoxin

There is a relatively narrow gap between therapeutic and toxic digoxin levels. Normal therapeutic levels are about one-third of those that are fatal, and serious toxic arrhythmias begin at about two-thirds of the fatal levels. The normal range for digoxin levels is 0.8 to 2 nanograms/mL (or 1.02 to 2.56 nanomol/L). To convert nanograms/mL to nanomol/L multiply by 1.28, or to convert nanomol/L to nanograms/mL multiply by 0.781. Note that micrograms/L is the same as nanograms/mL. If a patient is over-digitalised, signs and symptoms of toxicity are likely to occur, which may include loss of appetite, nausea and vomiting, and bradycardia. These effects are often used as clinical indicators of toxicity, and a pulse rate of less than 60 bpm is usually considered to be an indication of over-treatment. Other symptoms include visual disturbances, headache, drowsiness and occasionally diarrhoea. Death may result from cardiac arrhythmias. Patients treated for cardiac arrhythmias can therefore demonstrate arrhythmias when they are both under- as well as over-digitalised.

Digoxin + Diuretics

Eplerenone ✔

The AUC of digoxin is increased by 16% by eplerenone.

> Changes of this magnitude are unlikely to cause problems in most patients and the US manufacturer states that the pharmacokinetic interaction is not clinically significant. Nevertheless, the UK manufacturer of eplerenone advises caution in patients with digoxin levels near the upper end of the therapeutic range.

Loop or Thiazide diuretics ❓

Hypokalaemia, which can be caused by potassium-depleting diuretics such as the loop or thiazide diuretics, increases the toxicity of digoxin.

> Potassium levels should be routinely monitored during diuretic therapy. However, if symptoms of digoxin toxicity occur (see digoxin, page 257) it may be prudent to re-check potassium levels.

Spironolactone ⚠

Limited evidence suggests that digoxin levels may be increased by about 20% by spironolactone, but because spironolactone or its metabolite, canrenone, can interfere with some digoxin assay methods, the evaluation of this interaction is difficult.

> Monitor digoxin adverse effects (see digoxin, page 257)) and consider taking digoxin levels. Adjust the dose as necessary. Measurement of free digoxin levels or use of a chemiluminescent assay (CLIA) or turbidometric immunoassay for digoxin has been reported to mostly eliminate interference.

Digoxin + Donepezil ⚠

There is no pharmacokinetic interaction between digoxin and donepezil; however, the bradycardic effects of these drugs may possibly be additive.

> It may be prudent to be alert for bradycardia on concurrent use.

Digoxin + Galantamine ⚠

In a study galantamine had no pharmacokinetic effect on digoxin. However, one subject was hospitalised for second-and third-degree heart block and bradycardia.

> It may be prudent to be alert for bradycardia on concurrent use.

Digoxin + Herbal medicines or Dietary supplements

Danshen ⚠

Danshen does not appear to interact with digoxin, but it can falsify the results of serum immunoassay methods.

> These false readings could be eliminated by monitoring the free (i.e. unbound)

digoxin concentrations or using another assay method (such as a chemilumines-
cent assay).

Ginkgo biloba

A small study found that *Ginkgo biloba* leaf extract had no significant effects on the pharmacokinetics of a single dose of digoxin.

No dose adjustment would be expected to be necessary if patients taking digoxin also wish to take ginkgo.

Ginseng

Panax ginseng (Asian ginseng), *Panax quinquefolius* (American ginseng) and *Eleutherococcus senticosus* (Siberian ginseng) may interfere with the results of digoxin assays.

The general significance of this interaction is uncertain, but be aware that ginseng may possibly interfere with digoxin assays, particularly if an unexpected digoxin level is reported.

Liquorice (Kanzo) ?

An isolated case of digoxin toxicity has been reported in an elderly patient attributed to the use of a herbal laxative containing kanzo (liquorice). Excessive use of laxatives containing liquorice or anthraquinones may lead to hypokalaemia which increases the risk of digitalis toxicity.

An interaction is unlikely if these laxatives are used appropriately. However bear the potential for an interaction in mind in patients who regularly use or abuse liquorice or anthraquinone-containing laxatives.

St John's wort (Hypericum perforatum) ✗

There is good evidence that St John's wort can reduce the levels of digoxin by roughly 30%. Digoxin toxicity has occurred in a patient taking digoxin when he stopped taking St John's wort.

Digoxin levels should be well monitored if St John's wort is either started or stopped and appropriate digoxin dosage adjustments made if necessary. The recommendation of the CSM in the UK is that St John's wort should not be taken by patients taking digoxin.

Other herbal medicines ?

A digoxin level of 0.9 nanograms/mL was found in a patient taking an un-named herbal remedy, which contained black cohosh root (*Cimicifuga racemosa*), cayenne pepper fruit (*Capsicum annuum*), hops flowers (*Humulus lupulus*), skullcap herb (*Scutellaria lateriflora*), valerian root (*Valeriana officinalis*) and wood betony herb (*Pedicularis canadensis*), all of which contain digoxin-like compounds which are detected by digoxin antibody immunoassays. Three packaged teas (*Breathe Easy*, blackcurrant, and jasmine) and 3 herbs (pleurisy root, chaparral, peppermint) have been found, in theory, to provide a therapeutic daily dose of digoxin, if 5 cups a day are drunk.

It is apparent that if a patient taking digoxin also consumed these herbal remedies or teas they could develop symptoms of digoxin toxicity. However, theoretical interactions with herbal remedies are not always translated into practice. For example, hawthorn is used in cardiac disorders and the leaves and berries are reported to contain digoxin-like substances, but a study in healthy subjects found no pharmacokinetic or pharmacodynamic interaction between digoxin and an extract of hawthorn leaves and flowers (*Crataegus oxyacantha*). Therefore although these predicted interactions should be borne in mind when using digoxin and herbal remedies they cannot be taken as total proof that an interaction will occur.

D

Digoxin + Levothyroxine

Hypothyroid subjects are relatively sensitive to the effects of digoxin and so need lower doses. As treatment with levothyroxine progresses, and they become euthyroid, the dose of digoxin will need to be increased.

Monitor the outcome of resolving hypothyroidism, checking for to ensure that the effects of digoxin are adequate. Monitor digoxin levels as necessary.

Digoxin + Lithium

No pharmacokinetic interaction seems to occur between digoxin and lithium. However, the addition of digoxin to lithium possibly has a short-term detrimental effect on the control of mania. An isolated report describes severe bradycardia in one patient given both drugs.

The probability of a clinically significant interaction occurring seems low, but bear these cases in mind if both drugs are given.

Digoxin + Macrolides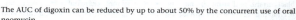

Clarithromycin markedly increases digoxin levels, and numerous cases of digoxin toxicity have been reported. Increases in digoxin levels also occur with telithromycin. Cases of rapid and marked two- to fourfold increases in digoxin levels have also been reported for azithromycin, erythromycin, josamycin and roxithromycin.

Monitor all patients well for signs of increased digoxin effects (see digoxin, page 257) when any macrolide is first given. Measure digoxin levels and reduce the dose as necessary.

Digoxin + Neomycin ▲

The AUC of digoxin can be reduced by up to about 50% by the concurrent use of oral neomycin.

Separating administration does not prevent this interaction. Monitor the response to digoxin treatment and adjust the dose as necessary.

Digoxin + NSAIDs

Indometacin

Rises in digoxin levels and digoxin toxicity have been reported in neonates given digoxin with indometacin. The picture is less clear in adults, as there are studies reporting either no change or increased digoxin levels and there seem to be no examples of a consistent interaction in practice.

In neonates, digoxin levels should be monitored if concurrent use is necessary, and the dose reduced accordingly (50% has been suggested). In adults, bear this interaction in mind if patients are given both drugs and monitor digoxin levels if a problem is suspected.

Other NSAIDs

Studies have found that both diclofenac and etoricoxib can raise digoxin levels by about one-third. Studies suggest that digoxin levels are unchanged by ibuprofen, although some reports suggest increases of up to 60% are possible.

Although rises of this extent (especially with ibuprofen) would be expected to be clinically significant, there appear to be no reports of an interaction in practice. Bear this interaction in mind in patients taking both drugs, and monitor digoxin levels if a problem is suspected.

Digoxin + Opioids

Some UK manufacturers state that digoxin toxicity has occurred rarely during the concurrent use of digoxin and tramadol. There appear to be no published reports of an interaction.

In the absence of any more information, it is difficult to judge the general relevance of these cases.

Digoxin + Penicillamine

Digoxin levels can be reduced by up to about 60% by penicillamine.

The manufacturer of penicillamine advises that digoxin should not be taken within 2 hours of penicillamine. It is unclear whether separating the dose will be successful in managing this interaction. Patients should be monitored for signs of under-digitalisation. Consider checking digoxin levels if an interaction is suspected.

Digoxin + Phenytoin

Phenytoin moderately reduces digoxin levels, but the clinical significance of this is unknown. There are also isolated case reports of marked bradycardia in patients taking digoxin with phenytoin. Fatalities have been reported when phenytoin was used in cases of suspected digoxin toxicity.

It would seem sensible to monitor the effects of concurrent use and consider monitoring digoxin levels if an interaction is suspected. As fosphenytoin is a prodrug of phenytoin it would seem prudent to take similar precautions if it is given to patients taking digoxin. The use of phenytoin in digoxin toxicity appears to be obsolete.

Digoxin + Propafenone

Propafenone can increase digoxin levels by 30 to 90% or more (particularly in children).

Most patients appear to be affected and dose reductions in the range of 15 to 70% were found necessary in one study. The extent of the rise may possibly depend on the propafenone level rather than on the propafenone dose. Monitor digoxin levels and adjust the dose accordingly.

Digoxin + Protease inhibitors

A woman had elevated digoxin levels and signs of toxicity after she was given ritonavir. Pharmacokinetic studies have shown that ritonavir and saquinavir with ritonavir cause modest to marked increases in single-dose digoxin levels. There appears to be a greater effect with intravenous digoxin than with oral digoxin.

It would seem prudent to closely monitor patients taking digoxin when ritonavir is started or stopped. There do not appear to be any reports or studies of the interaction of digoxin with other protease inhibitors; however, most protease inhibitors are inhibitors and/or substrates for P-glycoprotein, so it would seem likely that they may all interact to a greater or lesser degree.

Digoxin + Proton pump inhibitors

A small rise in digoxin levels may occur in patients also given omeprazole, pantoprazole, rabeprazole and possibly lansoprazole. These changes are thought to be within the normal variations of digoxin levels and so are not considered clinically significant. However, one patient developed digoxin toxicity 3 months after starting to take omeprazole.

No action needed. The isolated case of toxicity seems unlikely to be generally significant. Nevertheless, the UK manufacturer of lansoprazole suggests that digoxin levels should be monitored if lansoprazole is started or stopped.

Digoxin + Quinidine

The levels of digoxin in most patients are doubled on average within 5 days of quinidine being added; digoxin toxicity is likely to occur.

Halve the digoxin dose, monitor digoxin levels and further adjust the dose as necessary. Patients with renal impairment may require larger dose reductions. Remember to increase the digoxin dose if quinidine is stopped.

Digoxin + Quinine

The digoxin levels of some but not all patients may rise by more than 60% if they are given quinine, and there is a report of digoxin toxicity in an elderly patient during concurrent use.

Monitor the effects of concurrent use for digoxin adverse effects (see digoxin, page 257) and reduce the digoxin dose where necessary. Some patients may show a substantial increase in digoxin levels whereas others will show only a small or moderate rise.

Digoxin + Ranolazine

Ranolazine increases digoxin levels by 50%.

It would seem prudent to monitor digoxin levels if ranolazine is started, anticipating the need to reduce the digoxin dose.

Digoxin + Rifampicin (Rifampin)

In general, digoxin levels may be modestly reduced by the concurrent use of rifampicin, although cases of greater reductions (up to 80%) have also been reported.

It would seem sensible to monitor the outcome of concurrent use and monitor digoxin levels if an interaction is suspected. It may be that renal impairment increases the extent of this interaction.

Digoxin + Rivastigmine

There is no pharmacokinetic interaction between digoxin and rivastigmine; however, the bradycardic effects of both drugs may possibly be additive.

It may be prudent to be alert for bradycardia on concurrent use.

Digoxin + Salbutamol (Albuterol) and related bronchodilators

In one study, oral salbutamol slightly reduced digoxin levels, by 0.3 nanomol/L. Note that all beta$_2$ agonists (oral and inhaled) can cause hypokalaemia, which could lead to the development of digitalis toxicity.

It may be prudent to monitor potassium levels if beta$_2$ agonists are started, particularly nebulised, oral or intravenous beta$_2$ agonists. If symptoms of digoxin toxicity occur on concurrent use (see digoxin, page 257) it may be prudent to recheck potassium levels.

Digoxin + Statins

Atorvastatin, fluvastatin and simvastatin cause minor increases in digoxin levels.

The small changes seen in the digoxin levels with the statins seem unlikely to be clinically relevant in most patients.

Digoxin + Sucralfate

Sucralfate causes only a small reduction in the absorption of digoxin, but an isolated and unconfirmed report describes a marked reduction in one patient.

The reduction in digoxin levels is small and therefore normally unlikely to be clinically relevant. Nevertheless, consider an interaction if digoxin seems ineffective.

Digoxin + Sulfasalazine ⚠

Digoxin absorption can be reduced by up to 50% by sulfasalazine. Digoxin levels are reduced accordingly. This interaction appears to be dose related.

Monitor to ensure that the effects of digoxin are adequate, and consider measuring digoxin levels if an interaction is suspected. Adjust the dose as necessary.

Digoxin + Tacrine ⚠

The pharmacokinetics of digoxin are unchanged by tacrine, but their bradycardic effects may possibly be additive.

It may be prudent to be alert for bradycardia on concurrent use.

Digoxin + Tizanidine ⚠

The manufacturers state that the concurrent use of digoxin and tizanidine may potentiate bradycardia, but there do not appear to be any reports of problems with concurrent use.

Monitor heart rate and adjust the digoxin dose accordingly.

Digoxin + Topiramate

Topiramate slightly reduces the maximum levels and AUC of digoxin by less than 20%.

The manufacturer suggests good monitoring of digoxin if topiramate is added or withdrawn, but changes of this magnitude are unlikely to be clinically relevant in most patients.

Digoxin + Trimethoprim

Digoxin levels can be increased by about 22% by trimethoprim, but some individuals may show a much greater rise.

Monitor the effects of digoxin (see digoxin, page 257) if trimethoprim is given, and consider measuring digoxin levels, particularly in the elderly. Adjust the dose as necessary.

Dipyridamole

Dipyridamole + H₂-receptor antagonists

The effective disintegration, dissolution and eventual absorption of dipyridamole in tablet or suspension form depends upon having a low pH in the stomach. Drugs that significantly raise the gastric pH (such as the H₂-receptor antagonists) are expected to reduce the bioavailability of dipyridamole tablets. This effect has been seen with famotidine.

> The clinical significance of this interaction is unknown; however, bear it in mind if should any unexpected reduction in dipyridamole efficacy occur. Note that modified-release preparations of dipyridamole (that are buffered) do not appear to be affected.

D

Dipyridamole + Proton pump inhibitors

The effective disintegration, dissolution and eventual absorption of dipyridamole in tablet or suspension form depends upon having a low pH in the stomach. Drugs that significantly raise the gastric pH (such as the proton pump inhibitors) are expected to reduce the bioavailability of dipyridamole tablets. This effect has been seen with lansoprazole.

> The clinical significance of this interaction is unknown; however, bear it in mind should any unexpected reduction in dipyridamole efficacy occur. Note that modified-release preparations of dipyridamole (that are buffered) do not appear to be affected.

Dipyridamole + Warfarin and other oral anticoagulants

Mild bleeding (epistaxis, bruising, haematuria) can sometimes occur if anticoagulants are given with dipyridamole. Note that prothrombin times remain stable and well within the therapeutic range.

> These effects would not be unexpected if an antiplatelet and an anticoagulant are used concurrently. Bear them in mind when considering the combination. There is some evidence that maintaining anticoagulant control at the lower end of the therapeutic range minimises possible bleeding complications.

Disopyramide

Disopyramide + Macrolides ✗

Erythromycin appears to raise disopyramide levels; concurrent use has led to

QT prolongation, cardiac arrhythmias and heart block. The concurrent use of clarithromycin and disopyramide has led to torsade de pointes, ventricular fibrillation and severe hypoglycaemia, and the concurrent use of azithromycin and disopyramide has led to ventricular fibrillation. Disopyramide and some macrolides can prolong the QT interval. See drugs that prolong the QT interval, page 277.

Some of the manufacturers of disopyramide recommend avoiding the combination of disopyramide and macrolides that inhibit CYP3A, and this would certainly be prudent in situations where close monitoring is not possible. If concurrent use of any macrolide is essential, monitor closely for signs of disopyramide toxicity and QT prolongation.

Disopyramide + Phenobarbital ✗

Disopyramide exposure is reduced by about 35% by phenobarbital. Note that primidone is metabolised to phenobarbital and therefore may interact similarly.

The extent to which this interaction would reduce the antiarrhythmic effects of disopyramide is unknown, but monitor disopyramide efficacy and levels (if possible) if phenobarbital is added or withdrawn. One manufacturer suggests avoiding the combination.

Disopyramide + Phenytoin ✗

Disopyramide levels are reduced by phenytoin and may fall below therapeutic levels. Loss of arrhythmic control may occur. Fosphenytoin, a prodrug of phenytoin, may interact similarly.

Monitor disopyramide efficacy and levels (where possible). Adjust the disopyramide dose as necessary. Disopyramide levels appear to return to normal within 2 weeks of withdrawing the phenytoin. Note that one manufacturer of disopyramide recommends avoiding the combination.

Disopyramide + Protease inhibitors

Saquinavir ✗

Both saquinavir and disopyramide have a high risk of prolonging the QT interval, which may lead to the potentially fatal torsade de pointes arrhythmia. Dangerous QT prolongation is likely if they are used together.

Concurrent use is generally considered to be contraindicated. For more information on QT prolongation, see drugs that prolong the QT interval, page 277.

Other protease inhibitors ⚠

Disopyramide levels may be increased by ritonavir, which may increase the risk arrhythmias and other adverse effects. Other protease inhibitors are predicted to interact similarly.

Monitor concurrent use closely for adverse effects, and decrease the disopyramide dose as necessary.

Disopyramide + **Rifampicin (Rifampin)**

Disopyramide levels can be reduced by rifampicin.

It seems likely that the dose of disopyramide will need to be increased in most patients taking rifampicin. Monitor the effects of concurrent use and adjust the dose as necessary.

Disopyramide + **Warfarin and other oral anticoagulants**

Limited data suggests that warfarin requirements can be increased or decreased by disopyramide.

D

There is insufficient evidence to recommend monitoring all patients, but bear this interaction in mind if any unexplained change in anticoagulant control occurs in patients taking warfarin who are given disopyramide.

Disulfiram

Disulfiram + **Isoniazid**

In most patients the use of isoniazid with disulfiram is uneventful, but a number of patients have developed difficulties in co-ordination, changes in affect and behaviour, and drowsiness.

Concurrent use need not be avoided, but if marked changes in mental status occur, or if there is unsteady gait, the manufacturers recommend that the disulfiram should be withdrawn.

Disulfiram + **Metronidazole**

Acute psychoses and confusion can be caused by the concurrent use of metronidazole and disulfiram.

Concurrent use should be avoided or very well monitored. Withdrawing the drugs appears to resolve any adverse effects.

Disulfiram + **Phenytoin**

Phenytoin levels are markedly and rapidly increased by the concurrent use of disulfiram. Phenytoin toxicity has been seen in isolated cases. Fosphenytoin, a prodrug of phenytoin, may interact similarly.

This interaction seems to occur in most patients and develops rapidly. Monitor phenytoin levels and adverse effects (e.g. blurred vision, nystagmus, ataxia or drowsiness) carefully during concurrent use. Phenytoin dose reductions may be needed, but it may be difficult to maintain the balance required. Recovery may take 2 to 3 weeks after the disulfiram is withdrawn.

Disulfiram + Theophylline ⚠

The clearance of theophylline is slightly reduced by disulfiram. Higher doses of disulfiram appear to have a greater effect. As aminophylline is metabolised to theophylline, it would be expected to interact similarly.

Monitor the effects of theophylline if disulfiram is added and consider monitoring levels. Theophylline dose reductions may be needed.

Disulfiram + Warfarin and other oral anticoagulants ⚠

The anticoagulant effects of warfarin are increased by disulfiram, and in some cases bleeding has occurred.

It seems likely that most individuals will demonstrate this interaction. Monitor the INR in response to warfarin and adjust the dose accordingly when adding or withdrawing disulfiram. In patients taking disulfiram consideration should be given to using a smaller warfarin loading dose.

Diuretics

Diuretics + Herbal medicines or Dietary supplements

Germanium ✖

On two occasions severe oedema (12 to 13 kg weight gain) developed over 10 to 14 days in a patient taking furosemide after he also took a preparation containing ginseng and germanium. The effects were attributed to the germanium.

This is an isolated report, and its general significance is unclear. However, note that it has been said that the use of germanium should be discouraged due to its potential to cause renal toxicity.

Liquorice ❓

A patient developed hypokalaemia after taking liquorice and hydrochlorothiazide. This interaction seems possible with liquorice (which can lower potassium levels) and any potassium-depleting diuretic (i.e. thiazides or loop diuretics).

The additive effects of these drugs may result in clinically significant hypokalaemia, but evidence is extremely sparse. Consider this interaction in a case of otherwise unexplained hypokalaemia.

St John's wort (Hypericum perforatum)

St John's wort decreases the AUC of eplerenone by 30%.

Concurrent use is not recommended by the manufacturers because of the possibility of decreased efficacy.

Diuretics + **Lithium**

Amiloride

Some manufacturers suggest that amiloride reduces the renal clearance of lithium, thereby increasing the risk of lithium toxicity. There appears to be no evidence to confirm this alleged interaction and several studies suggesting that no interaction occurs.

No additional monitoring of lithium levels appears to be necessary, but as an interaction has been reported with other potassium-sparing diuretics, it would be prudent to reinforce the symptoms of lithium toxicity (see lithium, page 355) and tell patients to report them if they should occur.

Eplerenone

The concurrent use of eplerenone and lithium has not been studied, but the manufacturers predict that eplerenone may raise lithium levels.

The UK manufacturers state that concurrent use should be avoided or lithium levels closely monitored. Patients taking lithium should be aware of the symptoms of lithium toxicity (see lithium, page 355) and told to report them immediately should they occur.

Loop diuretics

The concurrent use of lithium and a loop diuretic can be safe and uneventful, but serious lithium toxicity has been described. The risk of lithium toxicity is greatly increased during the first month of concurrent use.

Patients taking lithium should be aware of the symptoms of lithium toxicity (see lithium, page 355) and told to report them immediately should they occur. Consider increased monitoring of lithium levels in patients newly started on this combination. Note that, in rare cases lithium has been associated with QT prolongation. In theory, this may be exacerbated by hypokalaemia caused by loop diuretics. For more information, see Drugs that prolong the QT interval, page 277.

Spironolactone

One study found that spironolactone caused the lithium levels to rise from 0.63 to 0.9 mmol/L. However, another study found no interaction.

Evidence for this interaction is sparse, no additional monitoring is necessary, but patients taking lithium should be aware of the symptoms of lithium toxicity (see lithium, page 355) and told to report them immediately should they occur.

Thiazides ⚠

The thiazide and related diuretics can cause a rapid rise in lithium levels, which may lead to lithium toxicity.

Lithium levels should be closely monitored if a thiazide is started or stopped. One UK manufacturer recommends an initial lithium dose reduction, but this does not seem to be in line with most other recommendations. Patients taking lithium should be aware of the symptoms of lithium toxicity (see lithium, page 355) and told to report them immediately should they occur. Note that, in rare cases lithium has been associated with QT prolongation. In theory, this may be exacerbated by hypokalaemia caused by thiazides. For more information, see Drugs that prolong the QT interval, page 277.

Triamterene ⚠

Triamterene appears to increase lithium excretion.

Information is sparse. The reports available do not give a clear indication of the outcome of concurrent use, but some monitoring would seem prudent. Patients taking lithium should be aware of the symptoms of lithium toxicity (see lithium, page 355) and told to report them immediately should they occur.

Diuretics + Macrolides ⚠

Erythromycin increases the AUC of eplerenone 2.9-fold. The manufacturer predicts that clarithromycin and telithromycin will interact to a greater extent. Eplerenone reduced the AUC of erythromycin by 14%, which was not considered clinically relevant.

The manufacturers recommend a maximum eplerenone dose of 25 mg daily in those taking erythromycin. Because they predict a greater effect with clarithromycin and telithromycin they contraindicate the concurrent use of these macrolides. Other macrolides seem less likely to interact, see macrolides, page 361.

Diuretics + NSAIDs

Potassium-sparing diuretics ⚠

The manufacturer advises caution on the concurrent use of NSAIDs and eplerenone because NSAIDs can cause renal impairment, especially in dehydrated or elderly patients. Several cases of acute renal failure have been seen when triamterene was given with NSAIDs.

Patients should be well hydrated and have their renal function checked before starting this combination.

Loop diuretics ❓

The antihypertensive and diuretic effects of loop diuretics appear to be reduced by NSAIDs, although the extent of this interaction largely depends on the individual NSAID. Indometacin appears to cause the most significant effect. The concurrent use of NSAIDs with loop diuretics may exacerbate congestive heart failure and increase the risk of hospitalisation.

> Concurrent use need not be avoided but the effects should be checked and the diuretic dose raised as necessary. Not all patients are affected. Patients at greatest risk are likely to be the elderly with cirrhosis, cardiac failure and/or renal impairment, and they may need to avoid NSAIDs.

Thiazides

There is evidence that most NSAIDs can increase blood pressure in patients taking antihypertensives, including diuretics, although some studies have not found the increase to be clinically relevant. The concurrent use of NSAIDs with thiazide diuretics may exacerbate congestive heart failure and increase the risk of hospitalisation. Diuretics may increase the risk of NSAID-induced acute renal failure.

> Only some patients are affected. Nevertheless, some have suggested that the use of NSAIDs should be kept to a minimum in patients taking antihypertensives, whereas, others suggest that the interaction is, generally, not clinically relevant. Consider monitoring blood pressure if an NSAID is started or stopped. Note that NSAIDs should generally be avoided in those with heart failure.

D

Diuretics + Phenobarbital

St John's wort (*Hypericum perforatum*) decreases the AUC of eplerenone by 30%. The manufacturers therefore predict that more potent enzyme inducers, such as phenobarbital, may have a greater effect. Note that primidone is metabolised to phenobarbital and therefore may interact similarly.

> Concurrent use is not recommended by the manufacturers.

Diuretics + Phenytoin

Furosemide ⚠

The diuretic effects of furosemide can be reduced as much as 50% if phenytoin is taken concurrently.

> The clinical significance of this finding is unclear. However, it may be prudent to consider monitoring the diuretic effects of furosemide if phenytoin is started. Fosphenytoin, a prodrug of phenytoin, may interact similarly.

Eplerenone

St John's wort (*Hypericum perforatum*) decreases the AUC of eplerenone by 30%. The manufacturers therefore predict that more potent enzyme inducers, such as phenytoin, may have a greater effect. Fosphenytoin, a prodrug of phenytoin, may interact similarly.

> Concurrent use is not recommended by the manufacturers.

Diuretics + **Potassium** ✖

The concurrent use of spironolactone or triamterene with potassium supplements can result in severe and even life-threatening hyperkalaemia. Amiloride and eplerenone are expected to interact similarly. Potassium-containing salt substitutes can be as hazardous as potassium supplements.

The manufacturers of eplerenone contraindicate the concurrent use of potassium supplements, but in the US, this contraindication is only in patients given eplerenone for hypertension. If a potassium supplement is given to a patient taking a potassium-sparing diuretic close monitoring of potassium levels, both before and during treatment, is necessary.

Diuretics + **Protease inhibitors** ✖

Saquinavir increases the AUC of eplerenone 2.1-fold. The manufacturer predicts that nelfinavir and ritonavir will interact to a greater extent.

In the UK, the manufacturer recommends that the dose of eplerenone should not exceed 25 mg daily in patients taking saquinavir. In the US, the manufacturer recommends that the starting dose of eplerenone for hypertension should be reduced to 25 mg daily for patients taking these drugs. This seems a sensible precaution. It seems likely that most protease inhibitors will interact similarly; however, because the manufacturers predict a greater effect with nelfinavir and ritonavir they contraindicate the concurrent use of these protease inhibitors.

Diuretics + **Reboxetine** ❓

Reboxetine may reduce potassium levels. Hypokalaemia is therefore possible if reboxetine is used with potassium-depleting diuretics (e.g. loop or thiazide diuretics).

Monitor potassium levels on concurrent use.

Diuretics + **Rifampicin (Rifampin)** ✖

St John's wort (*Hypericum perforatum*) decreases the AUC of eplerenone by 30%. The manufacturers therefore predict that more potent enzyme inducers, such as rifampicin, may have a greater effect.

Concurrent use is not recommended by the manufacturers.

Diuretics + **Salbutamol (Albuterol) and related bronchodilators** ❓

Beta$_2$ agonists, such as salbutamol and terbutaline, can cause hypokalaemia. This can be increased by other potassium-depleting drugs such as the loop or thiazide diuretics. In severe cases the risk of serious cardiac arrhythmias could be increased.

The CSM in the UK advises monitoring potassium in severe asthma, because of the probability of multiple potassium-depleting drugs being used, and because some conditions predispose these patients to hypokalaemia (e.g. hypoxia). Consider monitoring based on the severity of the patient's condition, and the number of potassium-depleting drugs used.

Diuretics + **Sevelamer**

Sevelamer abolished the diuretic effect of furosemide 250 mg twice daily in a haemodialysis patient. Urine output returned to the patient's normal levels 24 hours after sevelamer was stopped, and the reduction in urine output was not seen when the dosing frequency was altered so that furosemide was taken in the morning and sevelamer was taken at lunch and dinnertime.

> If the effect of furosemide seems less than expected, give the furosemide at least 1 hour before or 3 hours after sevelamer.

Diuretics + **Tacrolimus**

The concurrent use of tacrolimus and potassium-sparing diuretics may cause hyperkalaemia.

> The manufacturers suggest that concurrent use should be avoided. If concurrent use is essential potassium levels should be monitored closely.

Diuretics + **Theophylline**

Furosemide is reported to increase, decrease or to have no effect on theophylline levels. Both theophylline and loop or thiazide diuretics can cause hypokalaemia, which may be additive. Aminophylline is expected to interact similarly.

> Be aware for the potential for changes in theophylline levels if furosemide is also given. Consider measuring theophylline levels, and make appropriate dose adjustments as necessary. It may be prudent to monitor potassium levels in any patient given theophylline or aminophylline and a thiazide or loop diuretic.

Diuretics + **Toremifene**

Hypercalcaemia is a recognised adverse effect of toremifene, and the manufacturers suggest that drugs such as the thiazides, which decrease renal calcium excretion, may increase the risk of hypercalcaemia.

> This warning is based on theoretical considerations, and its clinical importance awaits confirmation.

Domperidone

Domperidone + **Dopamine agonists**

Domperidone may reduce the prolactin-lowering effect of bromocriptine. Other dopamine agonists may be similarly affected.

> Consider alternatives to domperidone wherever possible if prolactin levels are to be reduced. Note that domperidone is the antiemetic of choice in Parkinson's disease.

Domperidone + Macrolides

Erythromycin increases the plasma levels of domperidone about 3-fold and further increases the QT prolongation seen with domperidone alone

The manufacturers state that the concurrent use of domperidone with erythromycin should be avoided. This seems to be a very cautious approach, but may be prudent because alternatives to this combination would usually be available.

Donepezil

Donepezil + SSRIs ❓

Two case reports suggest that paroxetine may increase donepezil levels and adverse effects. The manufacturers predict that fluoxetine will also interact, as, like paroxetine, it inhibits CYP2D6.

The general importance of this interaction is unknown, but consider this interaction if adverse effects are troublesome.

Dopamine agonists

Dopamine agonists + Ergot derivatives

Bromocriptine and cabergoline are ergot dopamine agonists and although the manufacturers have no evidence of an interaction with other ergot derivatives, they do not recommend concurrent use, presumably because of the risks of additive adverse effects. It would seem prudent to use similar caution with other dopamine agonists that are ergot derivatives (e.g. lisuride, pergolide), although there appears to be no information available.

Avoid concurrent use.

Dopamine agonists + H₂-receptor antagonists ❓

Cimetidine may reduce the clearance of pramipexole by 35%. *Ciprofloxacin* increases the AUC of ropinirole by 84%. The manufacturers therefore predict that other CYP1A2 inhibitors (they name cimetidine) will interact similarly.

The clinical relevance of these interactions do not appear to have been assessed but it would be prudent to be alert for adverse effects (such as nausea, hypotension, drowsiness). Consider reducing the dose of the dopamine agonist if these become troublesome.

Dopamine agonists + HRT

Population pharmacokinetic analysis of clinical study data showed that oestrogens (from HRT) reduced ropinirole clearance by one-third.

> In women already receiving HRT, ropinirole treatment may be started using the usual dose titration. However, a reduction in the ropinirole dose may be needed if HRT is started, and an increase if it is withdrawn.

Dopamine agonists + Macrolides

Erythromycin markedly increases bromocriptine levels (up to 4.6-fold), and a case of toxicity has been reported. Bromocriptine toxicity has also occurred in a patient given josamycin. Clarithromycin increases the bioavailability of cabergoline about 2- to 4-fold.

D

> Concurrent use should be well monitored if macrolides that affect CYP3A4 are given (e.g. clarithromycin, erythromycin, telithromycin, see macrolides, page 361, for further details). It has been suggested that the bromocriptine dose may need to be reduced by 50% to avoid toxicity. One manufacturer of cabergoline advises avoiding the concurrent use of macrolides, and specifically names erythromycin.

Dopamine agonists + Metoclopramide

Centrally-acting dopamine antagonists (such as metoclopramide) are expected to oppose the effects of the dopamine agonists (reduction in clinical response seen). Metoclopramide would also be expected to reduce the prolactin-lowering effect of bromocriptine.

> Concurrent use should be avoided, or monitored closely to ensure that the dopamine agonist remains effective. Domperidone is the antiemetic of choice in Parkinson's disease.

Dopamine agonists + Nasal decongestants

Post-partum women taking bromocriptine have developed symptoms such as severe headache, marked hypertension, psychosis, or seizures with cerebral vasospasm after also taking phenylpropanolamine or pseudoephedrine.

> Direct information seems to be limited to these cases, but the severity of the reactions suggests that it might be prudent for postpartum patients to avoid these and related drugs while taking bromocriptine. Advise patients to also avoid non-prescription products containing these drugs (often cough and cold remedies). Note that bromocriptine is not recommended for the routine suppression of lactation postpartum.

Dopamine agonists + Quinolones

Ciprofloxacin increases the AUC of ropinirole by 84%.

> The clinical relevance of this pharmacokinetic interaction has not been assessed, but it may be prudent to monitor for an increase in ropinirole adverse effects (such

as nausea, hypotension, drowsiness). The manufacturers suggest that an adjustment of the ropinirole dose may be required in the presence of ciprofloxacin. Other quinolones may also interact, see quinolones, page 444.

Dopamine agonists + SSRIs ⚠

Ciprofloxacin increases the AUC of ropinirole by 84%. The manufacturers therefore predict that other CYP1A2 inhibitors (they name fluvoxamine) will interact similarly.

The clinical relevance of this pharmacokinetic interaction has not been assessed but it may be prudent to monitor for an increase in ropinirole adverse effects (such as nausea, hypotension, drowsiness). The manufacturers suggest that the ropinirole dose may need to be adjusted in patients taking fluvoxamine.

Doripenem

Doripenem + Probenecid ⚠

Probenecid increases the AUC of doripenem by 75%.

The manufacturers do not recommend concurrent use.

Doripenem + Valproate ⚠

The carbapenems reduce valproate levels, which has resulted in seizures. Doripenem is expected to interact similarly.

Monitor valproate levels in any patient given carbapenems. The valproate dose may need to be increased. Consider using another antibacterial, or an alternative to valproate. Limited evidence suggests that carbamazepine and phenytoin are not affected.

Doxapram

Doxapram + Theophylline ⚠

No pharmacokinetic interaction appears to occur between theophylline and doxapram in neonates. However, the manufacturers of doxapram say that clinical data suggests there may be an interaction (not confined to neonates), which is manifested by agitation, muscle fasciculation (twitching) and hyperactivity.

Although this reaction seems rare, it would be prudent to monitor concurrent use for any adverse outcome.

Drugs that prolong the QT interval

The consensus of opinion is that the concurrent use of two or more drugs that prolong the QT interval should generally be avoided because of the risk of additive effects, leading to the possible development of serious and potentially life-threatening torsade de pointes arrhythmias. It is thought that torsade de pointes is unlikely to develop until the corrected QT (QTc) interval exceeds 500 milliseconds, but this is not an exact figure and the risks are uncertain and unpredictable. Because of these uncertainties, many drug manufacturers and regulatory agencies now contraindicate the concurrent use of drugs known to prolong the QT interval, and a 'blanket' warning is often issued because the QT-prolonging effects of the drugs are expected to be additive. The extent of the drug-induced prolongation usually depends on the dosage of the drug and the particular drugs in question. For some drugs QT prolongation is a fairly frequent effect when the drug is used alone, and it is well accepted that use of these drugs requires careful monitoring (e.g. a number of the antiarrhythmics). Pairs of antiarrhythmics should therefore be avoided where possible. For other drugs, QT prolongation is rare, but because of the relatively benign indications for these drugs, the risk-benefit ratio is considered poor, and use of these drugs has been severely restricted or discontinued (e.g. astemizole, terfenadine, cisapride). For others there is less clear evidence of the risk of QT prolongation (e.g. tacrolimus, tamoxifen, tricyclic antidepressants) and therefore the associated risks of combinations of these types of drug are much lower. Drugs known to have a high risk of causing QT-prolongation include:

- Antiarrhythmics (class Ia: disopyramide, procainamide, quinidine)
- Antiarrhythmics (class III: amiodarone, sotalol)
- Antihistamines (possibly mizolastine)
- Antimalarials (artemether, present in co-artemether, and other artemisinin derivatives, halofantrine)
- Antipsychotics (amisulpride, droperidol, haloperidol (high dose and intravenous use), pimozide, sertindole, thioridazine)
- Arsenic trioxide
- Erythromycin (intravenous, but see also, below)
- Ranolazine
- Sparfloxacin (see also, below)

Drugs known to be associated with some risk of causing QT-prolongation include:

- Clomipramine (risk with other tricyclics appears to be mainly in overdose)
- Chlorpromazine
- Lithium (if levels raised)
- Macrolides (clarithromycin, oral erythromycin, (see also, above), spiramycin)
- Methadone (doses greater than 100 mg)
- Quinolones (gatifloxacin, levofloxacin, moxifloxacin, and see also, above)
- Paliperidone (around 12 milliseconds)
- Pentamidine intravenous
- Quinine
- Vardenafil (8 to 10 milliseconds)

Further, hypokalaemia increases the risks of torsade de pointes arrhythmias and so potassium levels should be closely monitored when drugs that can cause hypokalaemia are used with drugs that prolong the QT interval. However, there appear to be very few reports of this interaction. Drugs known to lower potassium levels include:

- Amphotericin B
- Corticosteroids

Drugs that prolong the QT interval

- Loop diuretics
- Salbutamol (Albuterol) and related bronchodilators
- Stimulant laxatives (in abuse or overuse)
- Theophylline
- Thiazide diuretics

Drugs that prolong the QT interval + 5-HT₃-receptor antagonists ⚠️

All available 5-HT$_3$-receptor antagonists (dolasetron, granisetron, ondansetron, palonosetron, tropisetron) have caused small increases (generally not exceeding 15 milliseconds) in the QTc interval. Some consider that these changes are not clinically relevant. Nevertheless, many of the manufacturers give various cautions about using 5-HT$_3$-receptor antagonists together with other drugs that prolong the QT interval, page 277.

> The US manufacturer of dolasetron advises caution with antiarrhythmics and other drugs that may prolong the QT interval. Both the UK and US manufacturers of granisetron advise caution with other drugs known to cause QT prolongation. The UK manufacturer of ondansetron recommends caution in patients treated with antiarrhythmics or beta blockers (presumably sotalol) or other QT prolonging drugs whereas the US manufacturer does not issue any cautions regarding QT-prolongation. The UK manufacturer of palonosetron recommends caution with other drugs that prolong the QT interval; however, on the basis of a controlled study that found that palonosetron did not prolong the QT interval, the US manufacturers have removed this warning. The Australian manufacturer of tropisetron recommends caution with other drugs that increase the QT interval.

Duloxetine

Duloxetine + Flecainide ⚠️

Duloxetine (a moderate inhibitor of CYP2D6) may inhibit the metabolism of flecainide (a substrate for CYP2D6), increasing the risk of flecainide adverse effects.

> The manufacturer advises caution. It would seem prudent to closely monitor for flecainide adverse effects.

Duloxetine + Herbal medicines or Dietary supplements ⚠️

Concurrent use of duloxetine and St John's wort (*Hypericum perforatum*) may lead to serotonin syndrome, page 454. One possible case has been reported.

> The manufacturers advise caution. Monitor concurrent use carefully for symptoms including agitation, confusion and tremor.

Duloxetine + **Lithium**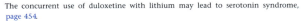

The concurrent use of duloxetine with lithium may lead to serotonin syndrome, page 454.

> The manufacturers advise caution. Monitor concurrent use carefully for symptoms including agitation, confusion and tremor.

Duloxetine + **MAOIs**

The concurrent use of MAOIs and duloxetine may lead to serotonin syndrome, page 454.

> The manufacturers contraindicate the use of duloxetine with non-selective irreversible MAOIs, during and for 14 days after discontinuing an MAOI. At least 5 days should be allowed after stopping duloxetine before starting an MAOI.

D

Duloxetine + **Moclobemide**

There is a possible risk of serotonin syndrome, page 454, if duloxetine is used with moclobemide; one case has been reported.

> The manufacturers advise against concurrent use but give no specific advice about a washout period, but, based on other interactions, it would seem prudent to wait for 5 days after duloxetine is stopped before starting the other drug. It has been suggested that no washout is needed after moclobemide, but others consider a 24-hour washout a prudent measure.

Duloxetine + **Opioids**

The concurrent use of duloxetine with tramadol or pethidine (meperidine) may lead to serotonin syndrome, page 454.

> The manufacturers advise caution. Monitor concurrent use carefully for symptoms including agitation, confusion and tremor.

Duloxetine + **Propafenone**

Duloxetine (a moderate inhibitor of CYP2D6) may inhibit the metabolism of propafenone (a substrate for CYP2D6), increasing the risk of propafenone adverse effects.

> If the combination is used it would be prudent to closely monitor for propafenone adverse effects (such as postural hypotension, bradycardia, urinary retention, etc.).

Duloxetine + **Quinidine**

Inhibitors of CYP2D6 are expected to increase duloxetine levels. This has been seen with *fluoxetine* and is predicted to occur with quinidine.

> The manufacturer advises caution on concurrent use. Monitor for duloxetine adverse effects, which include nausea, dry mouth, and hot flushes.

Duloxetine + **Quinolones** ❌

Potent inhibitors of CYP1A2 are expected to increase duloxetine levels. A 6-fold increase has been seen with *fluvoxamine* and is predicted to occur with quinolones (e.g. ciprofloxacin and enoxacin).

The manufacturer advises that concurrent use should be avoided. Note that the quinolones may interact to varying extents, see quinolones, page 444.

Duloxetine + **SSRIs**

Fluvoxamine ❌

The concurrent use of duloxetine and an SSRI may result in serotonin syndrome, page 454. Fluvoxamine increases duloxetine exposure 6-fold.

The manufacturers contraindicate concurrent use.

Other SSRIs ⚠

The concurrent use of duloxetine and an SSRI may result in serotonin syndrome, page 454. Low-dose paroxetine caused a modest increase in the AUC of duloxetine, and fluoxetine is predicted to interact similarly.

The manufacturers of duloxetine advise caution on the concurrent use of SSRIs. Monitor concurrent use carefully for symptoms including agitation, confusion and tremor.

Duloxetine + **Tricyclics** ⚠

Duloxetine markedly increases the AUC of desipramine. Other tricyclics metabolised by CYP2D6, such as nortriptyline, amitriptyline and imipramine, may interact similarly. The use of duloxetine with other serotonergic drugs, such as the tricyclics, may increase the risk of serotonin syndrome, page 454.

The manufacturer advises caution on concurrent use. Monitor for tricyclic adverse effects (blurred vision, dry mouth, confusion), and for signs of serotonin syndrome. Patients should report symptoms including agitation, confusion and tremor.

Duloxetine + **Triptans** ⚠

Concurrent use of duloxetine and the triptans (e.g. sumatriptan) may lead to serotonin syndrome, page 454.

The manufacturers advise caution. Patients should report symptoms including agitation, confusion and tremor.

Duloxetine + **Tryptophan** ⚠

Concurrent use of duloxetine and tryptophan may lead to serotonin syndrome, page 454.

> The UK manufacturers advise caution with concurrent use (e.g. be alert for symptoms including agitation, confusion and tremor); however, the US manufacturer advises avoiding concurrent use.

Duloxetine + **Warfarin and other oral anticoagulants** ❓

A case report describes a markedly raised INR in a patient taking warfarin when duloxetine was also given, and another case report describes a decrease in INR with acenocoumarol when duloxetine was given. Note that SNRIs alone have, rarely, been associated with bleeding, and there is the theoretical possibility that the risk might be increased when used with warfarin and related drugs.

> Consider increasing INR monitoring if duloxetine is added or withdrawn from treatment with warfarin or any coumarin. Also bear in mind the possibility of increased bleeding risk in the absence of alterations in INR.

Dutasteride

Dutasteride + **Protease inhibitors** ⚠

Moderate CYP3A4 inhibitors increase dutasteride levels by 60 to 80%, which, due to the wide safety margin of dutasteride, is not thought to be clinically significant. However, potent CYP3A4 inhibitors, such as the protease inhibitors (particularly indinavir and ritonavir), would be expected to have a larger effect, which may cause a clinically significant rise in dutasteride levels.

> The manufacturers suggest reducing the dosing frequency if increased dutasteride adverse effects occur.

D

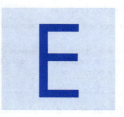

Endothelin receptor antagonists

Endothelin receptor antagonists + Phosphodiesterase type-5 inhibitors ⚠

Bosentan markedly reduces the AUC of sildenafil (by about 70%) and modestly reduces the AUC of tadalafil (by about 40%). Bosentan levels are modestly reduced by sildenafil and not affected to a clinically relevant extent by tadalafil.

> The efficacy of sildenafil and tadalafil might be reduced in patients taking bosentan, and should be closely monitored. Sildenafil might increase the effects of bosentan, therefore patients should be monitored for signs of bosentan adverse effects such as flushing, headache and oedema. Tadalafil is unlikely to have this effect.

Endothelin receptor antagonists + Protease inhibitors ⚠

The protease inhibitors are predicted to inhibit the metabolism of bosentan and markedly increases its levels. The manufacturer of sitaxentan predicts that ritonavir (an OATP inhibitor) may increase sitaxentan levels.

> Concurrent use should be closely monitored for bosentan adverse effects (e.g. oedema, liver function test abnormalities). For indinavir or nelfinavir, reduce the bosentan dose to 62.5 mg daily or on alternate days. For patients already established on other protease inhibitors for at least 10 days, a similar bosentan starting dose is advised. In those already taking bosentan, the bosentan should be stopped for 36 hours before starting protease inhibitor, and restarted after the protease inhibitors has been given for at least 10 days at this reduced dose. The exception to this advice is indinavir and nelfinavir: patients taking these drugs need not stop bosentan, but the dose should be reduced to 62.5 mg daily or on alternate days. The extent and clinical significance of this interaction with sitaxentan is unknown; other OATP inhibitors, such as nelfinavir, have had no significant interaction with sitaxentan whereas ciclosporin significantly increases sitaxentan levels. Until more information is available, patients taking ritonavir with sitaxentan should be closely monitored for an increase in sitaxentan adverse effects (such as peripheral oedema, headache, nasal congestion).

Endothelin receptor antagonists + **Rifampicin (Rifampin)**

Bosentan

Rifampicin may cause transient increases in the trough levels of bosentan, but at steady-state the plasma levels of bosentan are decreased. The UK manufacturer warns that the risk of liver impairment may be increased by concurrent use.

The UK manufacturer recommends that concurrent use should be avoided.

Ambrisentan or Sitaxentan

In a study rifampicin caused a transient (approximately 2-fold) increase in ambrisentan exposure, which resolved after about a week. The manufacturer of sitaxentan predicts that rifampicin (an OATP inhibitor) may increase sitaxentan levels.

Be alert for an increase in ambrisentan adverse effects (such as headache and peripheral oedema) on the initial concurrent use of rifampicin. Any increase in adverse effects would be expected to resolve after the first week. The extent and clinical significance of the interaction between sitaxentan and rifampicin is unknown; other OATP inhibitors, such as *nelfinavir*, have had no significant interaction with sitaxentan whereas *ciclosporin* significantly increases sitaxentan levels. Until more information is available, patients taking sitaxentan with rifampicin should be closely monitored for an increase in sitaxentan adverse effects (such as peripheral oedema, headache, nasal congestion).

E

Endothelin receptor antagonists + **Sirolimus**

The concurrent use of sirolimus with bosentan has not been studied. Based on the information available for ciclosporin, page 212 the manufacturers suggest that an interaction is possible.

The UK manufacturer of bosentan advises against concurrent use, but if this is required, close monitoring of bosentan adverse effects and immunosuppressant levels is recommended.

Endothelin receptor antagonists + **Statins**

Bosentan modestly reduces the AUC of simvastatin (by 34%) and its active metabolite (by 46%), which could lead to a reduction in simvastatin efficacy. Lovastatin may be also affected. The manufacturer of sitaxentan predicts that atorvastatin (an OATP inhibitor) may increase sitaxentan levels.

Monitor the outcome of concurrent use to ensure that these statins are effective. The extent and clinical significance of the interaction between atorvastatin and sitaxentan is unknown; other OATP inhibitors, such as *nelfinavir*, have had no significant interaction with sitaxentan whereas *ciclosporin* significantly increases sitaxentan levels. Until more information is available, patients taking sitaxentan with atorvastatin should be closely monitored for an increase in sitaxentan adverse effects (such as peripheral oedema, headache, nasal congestion).

Endothelin receptor antagonists + **Tacrolimus**

The concurrent use of tacrolimus with bosentan has not been studied. Based on the information available for ciclosporin, page 212 the manufacturers suggest that an interaction is possible.

> The UK manufacturer of bosentan advises against concurrent use, but if this is required, close monitoring of bosentan adverse effects and immunosuppressant levels is recommended.

Endothelin receptor antagonists + **Warfarin and other oral anticoagulants**

Bosentan appears to cause a modest reduction in warfarin levels, which may result in an increase in warfarin requirements in some patients. Sitaxentan inhibits the metabolism of warfarin and a lower dose of warfarin is likely to be needed.

> It is recommended that the INR should be closely monitored in any patient taking warfarin during the period that bosentan is started or stopped, or if the dose is altered. Other coumarins should be similarly monitored until further information is available. If patients taking sitaxentan are started on a coumarin, use the lowest possible dose of the anticoagulant (0.5 mg daily has been suggested) and increases the dose gradually (0.5 mg daily has been suggested) until the target INR is reached. If sitaxentan is started in a patient already taking an anticoagulant, the dose of the anticoagulant should be reduced (80% has been suggested).

Entacapone or Tolcapone

Entacapone or Tolcapone + **Inotropes and Vasopressors**

Entacapone potentiated the increase in heart rate and arrhythmogenic effects of isoprenaline (isoproterenol) and adrenaline (epinephrine) in a study in healthy subjects. Tolcapone would be expected to interact similarly.

> The manufacturers of entacapone and tolcapone suggest caution on the concurrent use of drugs such as adrenaline (epinephrine), dobutamine, dopamine, isoprenaline (isoproterenol) and noradrenaline (norepinephrine). The use of these drugs is usually closely monitored, but be aware that drug levels and effects may be greater than expected.

Entacapone or Tolcapone + **Iron**

Entacapone forms chelates with iron *in vitro*.

> The manufacturer recommends that iron preparations and entacapone are given 2 to 3 hours apart.

Entacapone or Tolcapone + **MAOIs**

In theory, the concurrent use of entacapone or tolcapone and an MAOI may result in hypertension.

Concurrent use is contraindicated.

Entacapone or Tolcapone + **Mirtazapine**

Both COMT inhibitors and drugs with noradrenaline re-uptake inhibitory activity (the manufacturers of tolcapone name mirtazapine) can impair the inactivation of catecholamines, so in theory the effects of catecholamines may be increased by concurrent use. This may lead to increases in blood pressure.

The manufacturers advise caution on concurrent use, but note that studies with the tricyclics, which were predicted to interact similarly, suggest that no adverse interaction occurs.

E

Entacapone or Tolcapone + **Moclobemide**

In a single dose study, there was no adverse effect on heart rate or blood pressure when entacapone was given with moclobemide.

The manufacturers of entacapone and tolcapone recommend caution until further clinical experience is gained.

Entacapone or Tolcapone + **Tricyclics**

Studies suggest that no important interaction occurs between entacapone and imipramine or between tolcapone and desipramine.

Despite these studies, the manufacturer of entacapone recommends caution as there is limited clinical experience of the use of entacapone with a tricyclic antidepressant. Similarly, the manufacturers of tolcapone suggest that caution should be exercised if desipramine is taken concurrently.

Entacapone or Tolcapone + **Venlafaxine**

Both COMT inhibitors and drugs with noradrenaline re-uptake inhibitory activity (the manufacturers of tolcapone name venlafaxine) can impair the inactivation of catecholamines, so in theory the effects of catecholamines may be increased by concurrent use. This may lead to increases in blood pressure.

The manufacturers advise caution on concurrent use, but note that studies with the tricyclics, which were predicted to interact similarly, suggest that no adverse interaction occurs.

Entacapone or Tolcapone + **Warfarin and other oral anticoagulants** ⚠

Entacapone slightly increases *R*-warfarin levels and causes a slight increase in INR of 13%, which is unlikely to be generally relevant. Tolcapone is not expected to interact with warfarin, but this needs confirmation.

The manufacturer of entacapone advises monitoring the INR if patients taking warfarin are given entacapone. Similar advice is given for tolcapone (due to the lack of clinical data).

Enteral feeds

E

Consider also the interactions of food.

Enteral feeds + **Phenytoin** ⚠

A 70% reduction in phenytoin absorption has been described when it is given with enteral feeds (e.g. *Isocal*, *Jevity*) administered via nasogastric or jejunostomy tubes.

This interaction has been managed by giving the phenytoin diluted in water 2 hours after stopping the feed, flushing with 60 mL of water, and waiting another 2 hours before restarting the feed. However, one study found this method unsuccessful. Other suggestions include waiting 6 hours after the phenytoin dose before restarting the feed, stopping continuous feed 1 hour rather than 2 hours before and after phenytoin administration, the use of twice daily phenytoin or the use of intravenous phenytoin. Monitor the outcome carefully. The same problem can also occur when enteral feeds are given by a jejunostomy tube but methods to manage this are not established.

Enteral feeds + **Quinolones** ⚠

The absorption of ciprofloxacin can be as much as halved by enteral feeds such as *Ensure*, *Jevity*, *Osmolite*, *Pulmocare* and *Sustacal*.

No treatment failures have been reported but this interaction is expected to be clinically important. Monitor the outcome of concurrent use carefully.

Enteral feeds + **Sucralfate** ⚠

Sucralfate can interact with the protein component of enteral feeds within the oesophagus to produce an obstructive plug (a bezoar).

The manufacturers recommend separating the administration of sucralfate suspension and enteral feeds given by nasogastric tube by one hour.

Enteral feeds + **Theophylline**

Enteral feeds can significantly affect theophylline levels (a reduction of 50% was seen in one case).

> Avoiding giving enteral feeds for one hour either side of theophylline seems to be an effective way of managing this interaction, but it would still be prudent to monitor the outcome on theophylline levels. Not all preparations of theophylline are necessarily affected, but there is insufficient evidence to identify those that may be a problem.

Enteral feeds + **Warfarin and other oral anticoagulants** ❓

Enteral feeds may contain sufficient vitamin K_1 (commonly about 4 to 10 micrograms per 100 mL) to antagonise the effects of warfarin and other vitamin K antagonists.

E

> Starting or stopping enteral feeds might affect dose requirements of vitamin K antagonists (coumarins and indanediones). It is also possible that there is a local interaction in the gut, as in one case separating the administration of the warfarin and an enteral feed by 3 hours or more was effective. Limited evidence suggests that withholding the enteral feed for a hour before and after warfarin administration might slightly reduce the effect of any interaction. Nevertheless, patients should be advised not to add or substitute dietary supplements such as *Ensure* without increased monitoring of their coagulation status.

Ergot derivatives

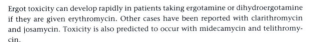

Ergot derivatives + **Macrolides** ❌

Ergot toxicity can develop rapidly in patients taking ergotamine or dihydroergotamine if they are given erythromycin. Other cases have been reported with clarithromycin and josamycin. Toxicity is also predicted to occur with midecamycin and telithromycin.

> The combination of ergot derivatives and macrolides that inhibit CYP3A4 is best avoided. Note that the macrolides differ in their ability to inhibit CYP3A4, see macrolides, page 361.

Ergot derivatives + **NNRTIs**

Delavirdine or Efavirenz

Delavirdine and efavirenz are predicted to inhibit the metabolism of ergot derivatives, which may result in the development of ergotism. However, note that efavirenz is usually considered to be a CYP3A4 *inducer*, and therefore may possibly decrease ergot derivative levels.

The manufacturers generally contraindicate potent CYP3A4 inhibitors.

Nevirapine

Nevirapine is predicted to increase the metabolism of ergot derivatives, and might therefore be expected to reduce their efficacy.

Warn patients that ergot derivatives may be less effective. Consider alternative antimigraine treatments.

Ergot derivatives + Protease inhibitors

A patient taking indinavir rapidly developed ergotism after taking usual doses of ergotamine. Several other patients taking ritonavir with ergotamine have had the same reaction. A patient taking nelfinavir developed peripheral arterial vasoconstriction after taking ergotamine. Other ergot derivatives and protease inhibitors are predicted to interact similarly.

Concurrent use is generally contraindicated.

Ergot derivatives + Reboxetine

The manufacturers suggest that concurrent use of reboxetine and ergot derivatives might result in increased blood pressure, although no clinical data are quoted.

The general significance of this interaction is unclear; however, bear it in mind should a patient develop an increase in blood pressure, particularly when either the ergot derivative or reboxetine is newly started.

Ergot derivatives + Rifampicin (Rifampin)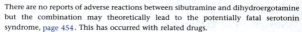

Rifampicin is predicted to increase the metabolism of ergot derivatives, and might therefore be expected to reduce their efficacy. Note that rifampicin has been used as a potent enzyme inducer to reduce ergotamine levels in a patient with ergotism, and was said to play a key role in reducing ergotamine levels.

Monitor the outcome of concurrent use to ensure the effects of ergot derivatives are adequate.

Ergot derivatives + Sibutramine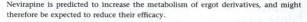

There are no reports of adverse reactions between sibutramine and dihydroergotamine but the combination may theoretically lead to the potentially fatal serotonin syndrome, page 454. This has occurred with related drugs.

The manufacturers contraindicate concurrent use.

Ergot derivatives + SSRIs

Isolated cases of the serotonin syndrome have been seen in patients taking paroxetine (with imipramine), or sertraline, when they were also given dihydroergotamine.

These appear to be isolated cases. Nevertheless they illustrate the potential for the development of serotonin syndrome, page 454, in patients given multiple drugs that affect serotonin receptors. It would seem prudent to monitor closely for symptoms such as agitation, fever, diarrhoea or tremor on concurrent use.

Ergot derivatives + Tetracyclines ?

Several patients taking ergotamine or dihydroergotamine developed ergotism when they were also given doxycycline or tetracycline. Liver impairment may have been a contributory factor.

The general importance of this interaction is uncertain, but it seems likely to be small. Impaired liver function may possibly be a contributory factor in this interaction. It may be prudent to monitor patients with this risk factor more closely for signs of ergotism (such as nausea, vomiting, diarrhoea, cold hands or feet). Note that one of the manufacturers of ergotamine recommends that the concurrent use of tetracycline should be avoided.

Ergot derivatives + Triptans ⊗

Although there is some evidence of safe use, the simultaneous use of ergot derivatives is contraindicated with all triptans because of the theoretical risk of additive vasoconstriction.

In the UK the manufacturers of sumatriptan say that ergotamine should not be given less than 6 hours after taking sumatriptan, and recommend that sumatriptan should not be taken less than 24 hours after taking ergotamine. Similar recommendations are made by the manufacturers of almotriptan, rizatriptan, and zolmitriptan, whereas the manufacturers of eletriptan, frovatriptan and naratriptan recommend that ergot derivatives are not given for a minimum of 24 hours (not just 6 hours) after these triptans. In general, in the US, it is recommended that triptans and ergotamine or ergot-type medication should not be taken within 24 hours of each other.

Ertapenem

Ertapenem + Valproate ⚠

Ertapenem appears to dramatically and rapidly reduce valproate levels resulting in increased seizure frequency.

It would be prudent to monitor valproate levels in any patient given carbapenems. The valproate dose may need to be increased. Consider using another antibacterial, or an alternative to valproate; limited evidence suggests that carbamazepine and phenytoin do not interact. Note that ertapenem should be used with caution in patients with a history of seizures.

Ethosuximide

Ethosuximide + Isoniazid ❓

A single report describes a patient who developed psychotic behaviour and signs of ethosuximide toxicity when concurrently treated with isoniazid.

> The clinical importance of this interaction is unknown, but bear it in mind in case of an unexpected response to treatment. Indicators of ethosuximide toxicity include nausea, vomiting, anorexia and insomnia.

Ethosuximide + Phenobarbital ❓

Primidone modestly lowers ethosuximide levels and possibly shortens its half-life. Similarly, phenobarbital has been reported both to reduce and not affect the half-life of ethosuximide. Phenobarbital levels (derived from primidone) do not appear to be affected by ethosuximide.

> A clinically relevant interaction seems unlikely in most patients; however, consider monitoring the effect of concurrent use and increase the dose of ethosuximide if necessary.

Ethosuximide + Phenytoin ❓

Three cases have occurred in which ethosuximide appeared to have been responsible for increasing phenytoin levels, leading to the development of phenytoin toxicity in 2 patients. Phenytoin may reduce the half-life of ethosuximide but not all studies have found this. Fosphenytoin, a prodrug of phenytoin, may interact similarly.

> Warn the patient to monitor for indicators of phenytoin toxicity (blurred vision, nystagmus, ataxia or drowsiness). Take phenytoin levels as necessary, and monitor the effectiveness of ethosuximide treatment.

Ethosuximide + Valproate ⚠️

Sodium valproate has increased the levels of ethosuximide by about 50%. Sedation occurred and ethosuximide dose reductions were necessary. However, other studies have described no changes or even reduced ethosuximide levels when valproate was also given. Ethosuximide may also lower valproate levels.

> Monitor the effects of concurrent use for adverse effects such as sedation, and efficacy, adjusting the ethosuximide dose and increasing the valproate dose accordingly. Valproate levels may be helpful.

Etoposide

Etoposide + Phenobarbital ⚠

Etoposide clearance appears to be increased by almost 80% by phenobarbital, and this may result in reduced efficacy. Note that primidone is metabolised to phenobarbital and therefore may interact similarly.

> Monitor the outcome of concurrent use and be alert for the possible need to give larger doses of etoposide.

Etoposide + Phenytoin ⚠

Etoposide clearance appears to be increased by almost 80% by phenytoin, and this may result in reduced efficacy. Fosphenytoin, a prodrug of phenytoin, may interact similarly.

> Monitor the outcome of concurrent use and be alert for the possible need to give larger doses of etoposide.

Etoposide + Warfarin and other oral anticoagulants ❓

Etoposide, as part of several different antineoplastic regimens, has been seen to increase the INR of patients taking warfarin.

> These are isolated cases, and no specific drug interaction is established. Nevertheless, other factors due to the disease or patient might alter the response to anticoagulants. Therefore, the anticoagulant doses may need adjustment. Note that, from a disease perspective, when treating venous thromboembolic disease in patients with cancer, warfarin is generally inferior (higher risk of major bleeds and recurrent thrombosis) to low-molecular-weight heparins.

Exemestane

Exemestane + Herbal medicines or Dietary supplements ⚠

Rifampicin reduces the AUC and maximum levels of exemestane by 54% and 41%, respectively. St John's wort (*Hypericum perforatum*) is predicted to interact similarly.

> Monitor concurrent use for reduced exemestane efficacy. The US manufacturer recommends doubling the dose of exemestane to 50 mg daily in patients taking phenytoin or rifampicin. Similar dose adjustments may be necessary with St John's wort.

Exemestane + HRT

HRT would be expected to oppose the effects of anti-oestrogens such as exemestane.

> HRT and other oestrogens are often considered contraindicated in women taking anti-oestrogens. Some information suggests that there need not be a complete restriction on their concurrent use, but this needs confirmation.

Exemestane + Phenobarbital ⚠

Rifampicin reduces the AUC and maximum levels of exemestane by 54% and 41%, respectively. Phenobarbital (and therefore probably primidone) is predicted to interact similarly.

> Monitor concurrent use for reduced exemestane efficacy. The US manufacturer recommends doubling the dose of exemestane to 50 mg daily in patients taking phenytoin or rifampicin. Similar dose adjustments may be necessary with phenobarbital and primidone.

Exemestane + Phenytoin ⚠

Rifampicin reduces the AUC and maximum levels of exemestane by 54% and 41%, respectively. Phenytoin (and therefore probably fosphenytoin) is predicted to interact similarly.

> Monitor concurrent use for reduced exemestane efficacy. The US manufacturers suggest doubling the exemestane dose to 50 mg daily.

Exemestane + Rifampicin (Rifampin) ⚠

Rifampicin reduces the AUC and maximum levels of exemestane by 54% and 41%, respectively.

> It would seem prudent to monitor concurrent use for reduced exemestane efficacy. The manufacturers suggest doubling the exemestane dose to 50 mg daily.

Ezetimibe

Ezetimibe + Fibrates

Fenofibrate and gemfibrozil may modestly increase ezetimibe levels, whereas ezetimibe does not alter fenofibrate or gemfibrozil pharmacokinetics. However, both fibrates and ezetimibe increase the secretion of cholesterol into the bile, which increases the risk of gallstone formation.

> The pharmacokinetic changes are unlikely to be clinically relevant. The manufacturers of ezetimibe state that the safety of concurrent use with fibrates is not yet established and in the US, concurrent use is not recommended, except fenofibrate,

E

where longer-term safety studies have been undertaken. If gallstones or gall bladder disease is suspected in a patient receiving ezetimibe and fenofibrate then the combination should be discontinued.

Ezetimibe + Rifampicin (Rifampin)

Multiple doses of rifampicin decrease ezetimibe levels and almost totally abolish its effects.

It would be prudent to monitor concurrent use to ensure that ezetimibe is effective.

Ezetimibe + Statins

No pharmacokinetic interaction appears to occur between ezetimibe and the statins, but the incidence of rhabdomyolysis may be increased on concurrent use.

E

Patients taking statins should be counselled regarding myopathy (e.g. report any unexplained muscle pain, tenderness or weakness). This should be reinforced if they are also given ezetimibe. Note that the use of ezetimibe and a statin results in additive lipid-lowering effects, and combination preparations are available.

Ezetimibe + Warfarin and other oral anticoagulants

No clinically significant interaction occurred between ezetimibe and warfarin in one study. However, the manufacturers have received post-marketing reports of raised INRs in patients taking warfarin or fluindione after they were also given ezetimibe.

An interaction is not established. The manufacturers advise monitoring the prothrombin time in any patients taking a coumarin or indanedione and adjusting the dose as necessary.

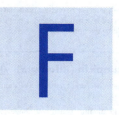

Famciclovir

Famciclovir + Probenecid [?]

The renal excretion of drugs similar to famciclovir is reduced by probenecid. Therefore the manufacturers of famciclovir suggest that probenecid may increase levels of penciclovir, the active metabolite of famciclovir, possibly resulting in increased adverse effects.

> As yet there seems to be no experimental or clinical evidence to show that this interaction occurs or that it is likely to be clinically important.

Felbamate

Felbamate + Gabapentin [?]

There is some evidence to suggest that the half-life of felbamate may be prolonged by gabapentin.

> The clinical importance of this interaction is unknown, but be alert for the need to reduce the felbamate dose.

Felbamate + Phenobarbital [!]

Felbamate normally causes a moderate increase of about 25 to 30% in phenobarbital levels (derived from phenobarbital or primidone). Phenobarbital toxicity has occurred in one patient when felbamate was added.

> Warn the patient to monitor for indicators of phenobarbital toxicity (drowsiness, ataxia or dysarthria), and take levels if necessary.

Felbamate + Phenytoin

Felbamate causes a moderate increase in phenytoin levels. Felbamate levels are reduced by phenytoin but the importance of this is uncertain. It seems possible that fosphenytoin, which is a prodrug of phenytoin, will interact similarly.

Warn the patient to monitor for indicators of phenytoin toxicity (blurred vision, nystagmus, ataxia or drowsiness). Take phenytoin levels and adjust the dose as necessary. The phenytoin dose may need to be reduced by up to 40%.

Felbamate + Valproate

Felbamate can raise valproate levels (by about 50% with a 2.4 g dose of felbamate), which may cause toxicity. Valproate may slightly decrease the clearance of felbamate.

Monitor valproate levels if toxicity is suspected (indicators of valproate toxicity include nausea, vomiting and dizziness); some have suggested a 30 to 50% dose reduction may be needed. Be aware that the felbamate dose may need to be decreased.

Fesoterodine

Fesoterodine + Macrolides

Ketoconazole increases fesoterodine levels up to about 2.5-fold by inhibiting CYP3A4. The macrolides inhibit CYP3A4 to varying extents (see macrolides, page 361), and therefore some may be expected to interact similarly.

The manufacturers state that the dose of fesoterodine should be restricted to 4 mg daily with potent CYP3A4 inhibitors; however note that they contraindicate the concurrent use of potent CYP3A4 inhibitors in those with moderate to severe hepatic or renal impairment. With other CYP3A4 inhibitors it may be prudent to monitor for an increase in fesoterodine adverse effects (e.g. dry mouth, dizziness, insomnia), and consider reducing the fesoterodine dose if these become troublesome.

Fesoterodine + Protease inhibitors

Ketoconazole increases fesoterodine levels up to about 2.5-fold by inhibiting CYP3A4. The protease inhibitors inhibit CYP3A4 to varying extents, but are generally considered to be potent CYP3A4 inhibitors, and therefore they may be expected to interact similarly.

The manufacturers state that the dose of fesoterodine should be restricted to 4 mg daily with potent CYP3A4 inhibitors; however note that they contraindicate the concurrent use of potent CYP3A4 inhibitors in those with moderate to severe hepatic or renal impairment. Monitor for an increase in fesoterodine adverse effects (e.g. dry mouth, dizziness, insomnia), and consider reducing the fesoterodine dose if these become troublesome.

Fibrates

Fibrates + Statins

Because of the increased risks of muscle toxicity (e.g. myopathy or rhabdomyolysis) it is generally accepted that use of a statin in conjunction with a fibrate should only be undertaken if the benefits outweigh the risks. The plasma levels of lovastatin, simvastatin, atorvastatin, and pravastatin are increased by gemfibrozil, the levels of fluvastatin are increased by bezafibrate, and the levels of pravastatin are increased by fenofibrate, which may increase the risks of myopathy.

In general, the concurrent use of a statin and a fibrate should only be undertaken if the benefits of treatment outweigh the risks, with the lowest necessary doses of each drug given. Patients taking statins should be counselled regarding myopathy (e.g. report any unexplained muscle pain, tenderness or weakness). This should be reinforced if they are also given a fibrate. The concurrent use of lovastatin with gemfibrozil should be avoided in patients with compromised liver or renal function. The maximum generally recommended dose for lovastatin is 20 mg and for simvastatin is 10 mg in patients taking a fibrate; the exception being fenofibrate with simvastatin, where no dose restrictions are deemed necessary. An atorvastatin starting dose of 10 mg is suggested for patients taking a fibrate. The US manufacturer suggests a maximum dose of 10 mg of rosuvastatin in patients taking gemfibrozil. The UK manufacturer recommends starting with a 5-mg dose of rosuvastatin, and contraindicates the 40-mg dose, in any patient taking a fibrate. The manufacturer of bezafibrate contraindicates the use of any statin if a number of conditions considered to be risk factors for myopathy (such as renal impairment and hypothyroidism) are present.

Fibrates + Ursodeoxycholic acid (Ursodiol)

The concurrent use of fibrates is predicted to decrease the efficacy of ursodeoxycholic acid by increasing cholesterol elimination in the bile and thus encourage gallstone formation.

The manufacturers do not recommend concurrent use.

Fibrates + Warfarin and other oral anticoagulants

The fibrates increase the effects of the coumarins and fatalities have resulted from this interaction. Most data is with the coumarins, although case reports suggest the indanediones may interact similarly. Gemfibrozil did not interact in a controlled study, although two cases of an interaction have been reported.

Evidence is not available for all combinations of fibrates and coumarins or indanediones, but it would seem prudent to expect them all to interact, to a greater or lesser extent. Coumarin and indanedione dose reductions may be needed to avoid the risk of bleeding. Monitor the INR and adjust the dose accordingly.

Flecainide

Flecainide + H$_2$-receptor antagonists

Cimetidine can increase flecainide plasma levels by about 30%.

> The clinical importance of this interaction does not appear to have been assessed, but be alert for the need to reduce the flecainide dose if cimetidine is added. The interaction is expected to be enhanced in the presence of renal impairment.

Flecainide + Lumefantrine ✕

The manufacturer of a preparation containing artemether and lumefantrine notes that *in vitro* lumefantrine significantly inhibits CYP2D6. They therefore contraindicate any drug that is metabolised by CYP2D6, and specifically name flecainide.

> These contraindications seem unnecessarily restrictive, especially as flecainide is not contraindicated with other established inhibitors of CYP2D6. Until more is known, it would be prudent to closely monitor the effects of any CYP2D6 substrate in patients given lumefantrine.

Flecainide + NSAIDs

Because valdecoxib (the metabolite of parecoxib) increases *dextromethorphan* levels about 3-fold and celecoxib increases *dextromethorphan* levels about 2.4-fold, the manufacturers predict that the levels of flecainide (which is similarly metabolised) will also be raised by these coxibs.

> The general importance of this interaction is unclear. Monitor concurrent use for adverse effects, and consider reducing the dose of the antiarrhythmic if these become troublesome.

Flecainide + Protease inhibitors ✕

Ritonavir increases plasma levels of flecainide. This increases the risk of arrhythmias and other adverse effects. Ritonavir-boosted protease inhibitors are expected to interact similarly.

> Concurrent use is generally contraindicated. If concurrent use is necessary, monitor carefully for flecainide adverse effects (abdominal pain, dizziness and cardiovascular effects) and adjust the flecainide dose if required.

Flecainide + Ranolazine

Ranolazine increases the levels of *metoprolol* by about 80% (by inhibiting CYP2D6). The manufacturers predict that flecainide will be similarly affected.

> Be aware of a possible interaction if flecainide adverse effects (such as abdominal pain, dizziness, hypotension, bradycardia) occur. The manufacturer of ranolazine suggests a dose reduction of flecainide may be needed.

F

Flecainide + SSRIs ⚠️

Fluoxetine and paroxetine are known moderate inhibitors of CYP2D6, the isoenzyme involved in flecainide metabolism. Concurrent use is therefore expected to raise flecainide levels and one case report with paroxetine supports this suggestion. The manufacturers of escitalopram predict that it may also interact in this way (although any effect is likely to be modest).

> There appear to be no reported interactions, but, given that fluoxetine interacts this way with other CYP2D6 substrates (such as propafenone, page 434), it would seem prudent to be alert for an increase in flecainide adverse effects (such as dizziness, nausea, and tremor) and consider a flecainide dose reduction if necessary.

Flecainide + Terbinafine ⚠️

In vitro studies suggest that terbinafine is an inhibitor of CYP2D6. It may therefore be expected to increase the plasma levels of drugs that are substrates of this enzyme, such as flecainide.

> Until more is known it would seem wise to be aware of the possibility of an increase in adverse effects if flecainide is given with terbinafine and consider a dose reduction if necessary.

F

Flutamide

Flutamide + Theophylline ❓

The manufacturer of flutamide notes that cases of increased theophylline plasma levels have been reported in patients taking these two drugs together.

> The manufacturers suggest the reason for this is that flutamide and theophylline are both metabolised by the cytochrome P450 isoenzyme CYP1A2; however, note that interactions by this mechanism are rarely clinically relevant.

Flutamide + Warfarin and other oral anticoagulants ⚠️

Case reports suggest that in some patients flutamide may increase the effects of warfarin. The interaction developed over 2 months in some cases but developed within 4 days in another.

> An interaction is not established. Nevertheless, the manufacturer of flutamide recommends that the prothrombin time be carefully monitored when these drugs are given with coumarins, adjusting the dose when necessary.

Folates

Folates + **Methotrexate**

Folic acid or folinic acid are sometimes added if low-dose methotrexate is given for rheumatoid arthritis or psoriasis to reduce adverse effects. Folinic acid is frequently used to minimise toxicity with high-dose methotrexate.

Patients taking methotrexate should avoid the inadvertent use of folates in multivitamin preparations.

Folates + **Phenobarbital**

If folic acid supplements are given to treat folate deficiency, which can be caused by the use of phenobarbital or primidone, the antiepileptic levels may fall, leading to decreased seizure control in some patients.

Monitor phenobarbital levels and adjust the dose of phenobarbital or primidone accordingly.

F

Folates + **Phenytoin**

If folic acid supplements are given to treat folate deficiency, which can be caused by the use of phenytoin, phenytoin levels may fall, leading to decreased seizure control in some patients. Reductions in phenytoin levels of 16 to 50% have been described with folic acid doses between 5 mg and 15 mg; doses as low as folic acid 1 mg may interact.

Monitor phenytoin levels and adjust the dose accordingly. Fosphenytoin is a prodrug of phenytoin. Although it does not appear to have been studied, it may interact similarly.

Folates + **Sulfasalazine**

Sulfasalazine can reduce the absorption of folic acid by about 30%.

The clinical significance of this interaction is unclear. Note that sulfasalazine is itself associated with blood dyscrasias due to folate deficiency, and this may be treated with folic acid or folinic acid.

Food

Food + **Furazolidone** ⊗

After 5 to 10 days of use furazolidone has MAO-inhibitory activity about equivalent to that of the antidepressant MAOIs. It may therefore be expected to interact with tyramine-rich foods.

It would seem prudent to warn patients given furazolidone not to take any of the foods or drinks that are prohibited with non-selective MAOIs. See MAOIs, page 301.

Food + Griseofulvin ❓

The rate and probably extent of griseofulvin absorption is increased by food, especially high-fat meals.

Griseofulvin should be taken with or after food to ensure adequate absorption.

Food + Isoniazid ⚠

The absorption of isoniazid is reduced by food. Patients taking isoniazid who eat some foods, particularly fish from the scombroid family (e.g. tuna, mackerel, salmon) that are not fresh, may experience an exaggerated histamine poisoning reaction e.g. chills, diarrhoea, flushing and itching of the skin, headache, tachycardia, vomiting, wheeze. Cheese has also been implicated in this reaction, but the adverse effects may be due to the weak MAOI effects of isoniazid rather than histamine poisoning.

For maximal absorption isoniazid should be taken without food, hence the manufacturer's guidance to take it at least 30 minutes before or 2 hours after food. There is no need to introduce general dietary restrictions, but if any of these reactions is experienced, examine the patient's diet and advise the avoidance of any probable offending foodstuffs.

Food + Isotretinoin ❓

The absorption of isotretinoin is approximately doubled by food.

Isotretinoin should be taken with food to maximise absorption.

Food + Levodopa ❓

The timing of meals and the type of diet, particularly high-protein diets, may affect the absorption of levodopa possibly leading to fluctuations in disease control.

If problems occur, a change in the pattern of drug and food administration on a trial-and-error basis may be helpful. Multiple small doses of levodopa and spreading out the intake of proteins may also diminish the effects of these interactions. Taking levodopa with food may help to minimise adverse effects such as anorexia, nausea, vomiting, and diarrhoea.

Food + Linezolid ⚠

Linezolid has some MAOI activity and therefore has the potential to cause potentially life-threatening hypertensive crisis when taken with tyramine-rich food (e.g. cheeses,

F

salami, yeast extracts, pickled herrings). A severe hypertensive reaction crisis of the proportions possible with the antidepressant MAOIs seems unlikely as linezolid only modestly increases the blood pressure in response to tyramine.

> Patients taking linezolid should not consume excessive amounts of tyramine-rich foods and drinks (100 mg of tyramine per meal is recommended by the manufacturers).

Food + Lumefantrine ❓

Food, especially high-fat food (including soya milk), markedly increases the absorption of lumefantrine.

> As soon as patients can tolerate food, lumefantrine should be taken with food to increase absorption. Patients who remain averse to food during treatment should be closely monitored since they may be at greater risk of recrudescence (reappearance of the disease after a period of inactivity).

Food + Macrolides

Food reduces the absorption of azithromycin from capsules but does not affect the AUC of azithromycin from tablets or suspension.

> Azithromycin capsules should be taken at least one hour before or 2 hours after a meal. Azithromycin suspension and tablets may be taken without regard to food.

F

Food + MAOIs ✖

A potentially life-threatening hypertensive crisis can develop in patients taking non-selective MAOIs who eat tyramine-rich food (e.g. cheeses, salami, yeast extracts, pickled herrings) and drinks (e.g. some beers and wines) or young broad bean pods, which contain dopa. Fatalities have occurred.

> As little as 20 mg of tyramine can raise the blood pressure by 30 mmHg in patients taking tranylcypromine. However, because tyramine levels vary so much it is impossible to guess the amount of tyramine present in any food or drink. Fermented or aged foods, such as cheeses (particularly over-ripe or strong smelling cheeses), sausages and beer, or smoked meats tend to be the most common tyramine-rich foods. There is no guarantee that patients who have uneventfully eaten these hazardous foodstuffs on many occasions may not eventually experience a full-scale hypertensive crisis, if all the possible variables conspire together. Therefore tyramine-rich foods should be avoided. In addition, avoidance of the prohibited foods should be continued for 2 to 3 weeks after stopping the MAOI to allow full recovery of the enzymes.

Food + Moclobemide

Tyramine 150 mg has been found to cause a 30 mmHg rise in systolic blood pressure when given with moclobemide. No reports of the potentially life-threatening hypertensive reactions seen with non-selective MAOIs appear to have been published for moclobemide.

Note that 150 mg of tyramine is equivalent to that found in about 200 g of Stilton cheese or 300 g of Gorgonzola cheese, which are really excessive amounts of cheese to be eaten in a few minutes. Most patients therefore do not need to follow the special dietary restrictions required with the non-selective MAOIs, but, to be on the safe side, the manufacturers of moclobemide advise all patients to avoid large amounts of tyramine-rich foods, because a few individuals may be particularly sensitive to its effects.

Food + NRTIs

Food decreases the absorption of didanosine by up to 50%.

Buffered didanosine should be taken at least 30 minutes before or 2 hours after food. Enteric coated didanosine should be taken 2 hours before or after food.

Food + NSAIDs

Food reduces the rate of absorption but has little or no clinically relevant effect on the extent of absorption of most NSAIDs.

The small changes seen will have no clinical relevance if these drugs are being used regularly to treat chronic pain and inflammation. However, if they are being used for the treatment of acute pain, administration on an empty stomach would be preferable in terms of onset of effect. However, it is usually recommended that NSAIDs are given with or after food, in an attempt to minimise their gastrointestinal adverse effects.

Food + Penicillamine

Food can reduce the absorption of penicillamine by about 50%.

If maximal effects are required penicillamine should be taken at least 30 minutes before food.

Food + Penicillins

Food can reduce the absorption of ampicillin by about 30%, and the peak levels and AUC of phenoxymethylpenicillin by about 50%. Limited evidence suggests that food has no significant effect on the bioavailability of flucloxacillin.

Ampicillin and phenoxymethylpenicillin should be taken one hour before food or on an empty stomach. Despite the apparent lack of interaction with flucloxacillin, it is recommended that it should be taken one hour before food or on an empty stomach to optimise absorption.

Food + **Protease inhibitors**

Food increases the bioavailability of atazanavir, ritonavir-boosted darunavir, ritonavir-boosted lopinavir soft capsules and solution, nelfinavir, saquinavir, and tipranavir, but decreases that of indinavir and fosamprenavir suspension. Food only minimally affects the bioavailability of amprenavir, fosamprenavir tablets and ritonavir.

Indinavir should be given one hour before or 2 hours after meals, or with light meals only, unless it is taken with ritonavir, when it may be taken without regard to food. Atazanavir, ritonavir-boosted darunavir, ritonavir-boosted lopinavir (capsules and oral solution), nelfinavir, and tipranavir should be taken with food to enhance bioavailability. Saquinavir (soft and hard capsules) should be taken with or up to 2 hours after a meal. The US manufacturers of amprenavir say that it should not be given with high-fat meals, but otherwise it may be given with or without food. Fosamprenavir suspension should be taken without food, although to improve tolerability and compliance, if necessary, children may take it with food. Fosamprenavir tablets may be taken without regard to food intake. Ritonavir capsules and solution should preferably be taken with food.

Food + **Proton pump inhibitors**

Food reduces the bioavailability of lansoprazole and esomeprazole by up to 70%.

It is recommended that lansoprazole should not be given with food. The manufacturers recommend that, to achieve optimal efficacy, lansoprazole should be given in the morning at least 30 minutes before food. Esomeprazole capsules and suspension should be taken one hour before meals.

Food + **Quinolones**

Dairy products reduce the bioavailability of ciprofloxacin (AUC reduced by about 30%) and norfloxacin (peak plasma levels reduced by about 50%).

The effect of these changes on the control of infection is uncertain but it would seem prudent to advise patients not to take these dairy products within one to 2 hours of either ciprofloxacin or norfloxacin. Enoxacin, lomefloxacin, and ofloxacin do not appear to interact significantly with food. They therefore may provide a useful alternative to the interacting quinolones. Consider also enteral feeds, page 286.

Food + **Rifampicin (Rifampin)**

Food delays and reduces the absorption of rifampicin.

Rifampicin should be taken on an empty stomach, 30 minutes before a meal, or 2 hours after a meal to ensure rapid and complete absorption.

Food + **Strontium**

The manufacturer notes that food, milk and dairy products reduce the bioavailability of strontium by about 60 to 70%, when compared with administration 3 hours after a meal.

> Strontium should not be taken within 2 hours of eating. The manufacturer recommends that it should be taken at bedtime, at least 2 hours after eating.

Food + Tetracyclines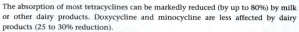

The absorption of most tetracyclines can be markedly reduced (by up to 80%) by milk or other dairy products. Doxycycline and minocycline are less affected by dairy products (25 to 30% reduction).

> It is usual to recommend that tetracyclines are taken one hour before food or 2 hours after food to avoid an interaction with all forms of dietary calcium. Note that lymecycline appears not to interact.

Food + Warfarin and other oral anticoagulants

Cranberry juice ❓

A number of case reports suggest that cranberry juice can increase the INR of patients taking warfarin, and one patient has died as a result of this interaction. Other patients have developed unstable INRs, or, in one isolated case, a reduced INR. However, in several controlled studies, cranberry juice did not alter the anticoagulant effect or the pharmacokinetics of warfarin, or had only very minor effects on the INR.

> An interaction is not established. It could also be that there is no specific interaction, and that the case reports just represent idiosyncratic reactions in which other unknown factors (e.g. altered diet) were more important. In 2004, on the basis of the then available case reports and lack of controlled studies, the CSM/MHRA in the UK advised that patients taking warfarin should avoid drinking cranberry juice unless the health benefits are considered to outweigh any risks. They recommended increased INR monitoring for any patient taking warfarin and who has a regular intake of cranberry juice (and cranberry capsules or concentrates). These might still be prudent precautions, although the controlled studies now available do provide some reassurance that, in otherwise healthy individuals, moderate amounts of cranberry juice are unlikely to have an important impact on anticoagulation.

Foods, general ❓

A number of foodstuffs have been implicated in interactions with warfarin. Some of these were not thought to be related to their vitamin K content. These include:

- antagonism of the effects of warfarin by ice cream, avocado, soybean protein, and soybean oil and other intravenous lipids
- an increase in prothrombin time with the use of aspartame or following the consumption of mango fruit

> These reactions seem unlikely to be of general importance, although bear them in mind in case of an unexpected response to oral anticoagulants.

Foods containing vitamin K ❓

The effects of warfarin can be reduced or abolished by vitamin K, including that found in health foods, food supplements, enteral feeds or exceptionally large amounts of some green vegetables or green tea.

Patients should be counselled about the effects of dietary supplements or dramatic dietary alterations when they start taking vitamin K antagonist anticoagulants (coumarins and indanediones).

Natto ❌

Natto, a Japanese food made from fermented soya bean, can reduce the effects of warfarin.

Patients should be advised to avoid natto until more is known about this interaction.

Pomegranate juice ❓

Case reports suggest that pomegranate juice increases the INR in response to warfarin. Other coumarins could potentially interact similarly.

There is currently insufficient evidence to suggest that patients taking warfarin should avoid pomegranate juice, but it may be prudent to consider pomegranate juice consumption in a patient with otherwise unexplained fluctuations in INR, or unexpectedly raised INRs.

F

Furazolidone

Furazolidone + Nasal decongestants ❌

After 5 to 10 days of use, furazolidone has MAO-inhibitory activity about equivalent to that of the non-selective MAOIs. Concurrent use with drugs such as phenylpropanolamine or ephedrine, may be expected to result in a potentially serious rise in blood pressure.

Although reports of hypertensive crises with furazolidone appear lacking it would still seem prudent to warn patients to avoid any of the nasal decongestants with indirect sympathomimetic activity (e.g. ephedrine, pseudoephedrine, phenylpropanolamine).

Fusidic acid

Fusidic acid + Protease inhibitors ⚠

A patient taking fusidic acid with saquinavir and ritonavir developed elevated fusidic acid levels with toxicity, and elevated saquinavir and ritonavir levels (roughly 4-fold increases).

> The clinical significance of this case is unclear. It has been suggested that fusidic acid be avoided in patients on these protease inhibitors. However, if the combination is needed it would seem sensible to monitor concurrent use carefully so any elevation in levels is detected before they become problematic.

Fusidic acid + Statins ?

Isolated cases of rhabdomyolysis have been described in patients given atorvastatin or simvastatin with fusidic acid.

> The general significance of this interaction is unclear. Patients given statins should be counselled regarding myopathy (e.g. report any unexplained muscle pain, tenderness or weakness). Reinforce this if fusidic acid is given to a patient taking atorvastatin or simvastatin.

F

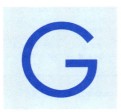

Galantamine

Galantamine + Quinidine

Paroxetine increases the risk of galantamine adverse effects (in particular nausea and vomiting) probably by inhibiting the metabolism of galantamine by CYP2D6. The manufacturers therefore predict that other CYP2D6 inhibitors (such as quinidine) will interact similarly.

> If the adverse effects of galantamine (e.g. nausea and vomiting) develop or worsen, consider reducing its dose.

Galantamine + SSRIs ⚠

Paroxetine increases the risk of galantamine adverse effects probably by inhibiting the metabolism of galantamine by CYP2D6. The manufacturers therefore predict that other CYP2D6 inhibitors (such as fluoxetine) will interact similarly. They also name fluvoxamine but note that fluvoxamine is usually considered to be a *weak* inhibitor of this isoenzyme.

> If the adverse effects of galantamine (e.g. nausea and vomiting) develop or worsen, consider reducing its dose.

Ganciclovir

Valganciclovir is a prodrug of ganciclovir and therefore has the potential to interact similarly.

Ganciclovir + Imipenem

The manufacturer notes that generalised seizures have been reported in patients who received ganciclovir and imipenem with cilastatin. Note that both ganciclovir and imipenem alone may cause seizures. Valganciclovir is a prodrug of ganciclovir and would therefore be expected to interact similarly.

> The manufacturer recommends that ganciclovir and its prodrug valganciclovir should not be used with imipenem unless the benefits outweigh the risks.

Ganciclovir + Mycophenolate ❓

No clinically significant pharmacokinetic interaction appears to occur between ganciclovir and mycophenolate. However, the manufacturers state that in renal impairment there may be competition for tubular secretion and increased concentrations of both drugs may occur. There are reports of neutropenia in patients taking mycophenolate with ganciclovir, and the risks of myelotoxicity appear to be increased if mycophenolate is given with valganciclovir (especially in high dose).

> No action is needed, but increased monitoring may be prudent in patients with reduced renal function. Both mycophenolate mofetil and ganciclovir and its prodrug, valganciclovir, have the potential to cause neutropenia and leucopenia, therefore patients should be closely monitored for additive toxicity.

Ganciclovir + NRTIs

Didanosine ⚠️

In several studies ganciclovir has been found to raise the maximum levels and AUC of didanosine by about 50% and 80%, respectively, even when the drugs are given 2 hours apart. Other studies have suggested that the efficacy of ganciclovir may be reduced by didanosine. Valganciclovir is a prodrug of ganciclovir and would therefore be expected to interact similarly.

> The clinical significance of these pharmacokinetic changes is unclear. Until more is known it would seem prudent to monitor concurrent use for didanosine toxicity and ganciclovir efficacy.

Tenofovir ⚠️

The manufacturers state that the concurrent use of tenofovir (which may cause renal impairment) and other nephrotoxic drugs such as ganciclovir (and therefore probably valganciclovir) has not been evaluated.

> If both drugs are given the manufacturers advise that renal function should be monitored at least weekly.

Zidovudine ⚠️

Anaemia, neutropenia, leucopenia and gastrointestinal disturbances were seen when zidovudine and ganciclovir were used concurrently. The dose of zidovudine had to be reduced to 300 mg daily in many patients. Valganciclovir is a prodrug of ganciclovir and would therefore be expected to interact similarly.

> The clinical significance of the pharmacokinetic changes is unclear. Until more is known, patients should be closely monitored for zidovudine toxicity (such as neutropenia) on concurrent use.

G

Ganciclovir + **Probenecid**

Probenecid reduces the renal excretion of ganciclovir and increases its AUC by about 50%.

> The clinical importance of this interaction is uncertain. Be alert for increased ganciclovir adverse effects (such as diarrhoea, nausea, neutropenia and thrombocytopenia) if probenecid is given with ganciclovir or its prodrug, valganciclovir. Ganciclovir eye drops are unlikely to interact.

Gestrinone

Gestrinone + **Phenobarbital**

The manufacturers state that phenobarbital (and therefore probably primidone, which is metabolised to phenobarbital) may increase the metabolism of gestrinone and thereby reduce its effects.

> Be aware that gestrinone may not be as effective if phenobarbital or primidone are given concurrently.

Gestrinone + **Phenytoin**

The manufacturers state that phenytoin (and therefore probably fosphenytoin, a prodrug of phenytoin) may increase the metabolism of gestrinone and thereby reduce its effects.

> Be aware that gestrinone may not be as effective if phenytoin or fosphenytoin are given concurrently.

Gestrinone + **Rifampicin (Rifampin)**

The manufacturers state that rifampicin may increase the metabolism of gestrinone and thereby reduce its effects.

> Be aware that gestrinone may not be as effective if rifampicin is also given.

G

Glucagon

Glucagon + **Warfarin and other oral anticoagulants**

The anticoagulant effects of warfarin are rapidly and markedly increased by glucagon in large doses (total dose exceeding 50 mg over 2 days), and bleeding can occur. This interaction did not occur in patients given, in total, less than 30 mg of glucagon over 1 to 2 days.

> It has been suggested that if glucagon 25 mg per day or more is given for two or more days, the dose of warfarin should be reduced in anticipation of the interaction, and prothrombin times closely monitored. Information about other anticoagulants is lacking, but it would be prudent to assume that all coumarins will interact similarly.

Gold

Gold + Leflunomide

The manufacturers state that the concurrent use of leflunomide and gold has not yet been studied but it would be expected to increase the risk of serious adverse reactions (haematological toxicity or hepatotoxicity).

> The manufacturers advise avoiding concurrent use. As the active metabolite of leflunomide has a long half-life of 1 to 4 weeks a washout with colestyramine or activated charcoal may decrease the risks of toxicity if patients are to be switched to other DMARDs.

Gold + Penicillamine ⊗

Gold appears to increase the risk of penicillamine toxicity.

> Avoid concurrent use. Increased penicillamine monitoring should be considered in those with previous adverse effects to gold, as these patients are likely to experience increased adverse effects to penicillamine.

Grapefruit juice

In general, grapefruit juice inhibits intestinal CYP3A4, and only slightly affects hepatic CYP3A4. This is demonstrated by the fact that intravenous preparations of drugs that are metabolised by CYP3A4 are not much affected, whereas oral preparations of the same drugs are, and their levels are increased by grapefruit juice. Some drugs that are not metabolised by CYP3A4 show decreased levels with grapefruit juice. This is probably because grapefruit juice is an inhibitor of some drug transporters. The active constituent of grapefruit juice is uncertain. However, grapefruit contains naringin, which degrades during processing to naringenin, a substance known to inhibit CYP3A4. Because of this, it has been assumed that whole grapefruit will not interact, but that processed grapefruit juice will. However, subsequently some reports have implicated the whole fruit. Other possible active constituents in the whole fruit include bergamottin and dihydroxybergamottin.

G

Grapefruit juice + **Phosphodiesterase type-5 inhibitors**

Grapefruit juice slightly increases the AUC of sildenafil. Tadalafil and vardenafil are predicted to interact similarly.

It has been suggested that although the pharmacokinetic changes are unlikely to be clinically significant, the combination is best avoided because concurrent use results in an increased variability in sildenafil pharmacokinetics. However, this seems over-cautious, as reduced doses of sildenafil can be given with more potent CYP3A4 inhibitors. The manufacturers of tadalafil and vardenafil advise caution and avoidance, respectively, in those who drink grapefruit juice.

Grapefruit juice + **Ranolazine**

Ketoconazole increases ranolazine levels, which increases the risk of QT prolongation and potentially life-threatening arrhythmias. Although not specifically studied grapefruit juice would be expected to interact similarly.

The manufacturer contraindicates concurrent use.

Grapefruit juice + **Sirolimus**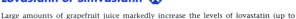

The manufacturers predict that grapefruit juice may raise sirolimus levels, probably because *ketoconazole* has been shown to do so (both ketoconazole and grapefruit juice can inhibit CYP3A4 by which sirolimus is metabolised).

G

The extent of any change in sirolimus levels is uncertain. The manufacturers suggest that concurrent use should be avoided.

Grapefruit juice + **Statins**

Lovastatin or Simvastatin

Large amounts of grapefruit juice markedly increase the levels of lovastatin (up to 12-fold) and simvastatin (up to 9-fold).

Large increases in the levels of lovastatin and simvastatin are potentially hazardous because elevated statin levels carry the risk of toxicity (muscle damage and the possible development of rhabdomyolysis). As even small quantities of grapefruit juice can significantly affect simvastatin levels the UK manufacturer says that concurrent use should be avoided, whereas the US manufacturers recommend restricting intake to less than 1 litre daily.

Atorvastatin

Grapefruit juice increases atorvastatin levels by about 50% (a modest increase).

In general, the occasional glass of grapefruit juice would not appear to be a problem; the UK manufacturer suggests that large quantities (unspecified) should be avoided. Remember, any patient on a statin should be told to report any unexplained muscle pain, tenderness or weakness.

Grapefruit juice + **Tacrolimus**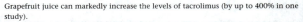

Grapefruit juice can markedly increase the levels of tacrolimus (by up to 400% in one study).

> The manufacturers of tacrolimus advise avoiding concurrent use. This would appear prudent. Patients should be informed of the potential risk of this interaction.

Griseofulvin

Griseofulvin + **Phenobarbital**

The antifungal effects of griseofulvin can be reduced (levels reduced by about one-third) or even abolished by the concurrent use of phenobarbital. Note that primidone is metabolised to phenobarbital and may therefore interact similarly.

> Concurrent use should be well monitored to confirm that griseofulvin is effective. If appropriate, a non-interacting antiepileptic such as valproate may be considered.

Griseofulvin + **Warfarin and other oral anticoagulants**

The anticoagulant effects of warfarin can be reduced by griseofulvin in some patients. In one patient a 41% increase in the dose of warfarin was needed. Other coumarins may interact similarly.

> Monitor the anticoagulant effect if griseofulvin is added or withdrawn in patients taking a coumarin, and adjust the dose as necessary. Note that in one patient the interaction took 12 weeks to develop.

Guanethidine

Guanethidine + **Inotropes and Vasopressors**

The pressor effects of noradrenaline (norepinephrine), phenylephrine, metaraminol and other related drugs can be increased in the presence of guanethidine. In addition the incidence and severity of cardiac arrhythmias is increased. Dopamine would be expected to interact similarly. Some of these drugs can also be used as eye drops, and in this situation their mydriatic effects are similarly enhanced and prolonged by guanethidine.

> The doses of these inotropes or vasopressors should be reduced appropriately in

patients taking guanethidine; monitor the outcome of concurrent use carefully. Consider also the possibility of an arrhythmogenic effect.

Guanethidine + Methylphenidate

The antihypertensive effects of guanethidine can be reduced or abolished by methylphenidate. The blood pressure may even rise higher than before treatment with the antihypertensive.

The concurrent use of guanethidine and methylphenidate should be avoided.

Guanethidine + Nasal decongestants

The antihypertensive effects of guanethidine can be reduced or abolished by ephedrine. The blood pressure may even rise higher than before treatment with the antihypertensive. Other related drugs, such as pseudoephedrine and phenylpropanolamine, that are used as cough and cold remedies, may also interact in this way.

Concurrent use should be avoided. Warn patients about the use of non-prescription nasal decongestants containing any of these drugs to relieve the nasal stuffiness commonly associated with the use of guanethidine and related drugs.

Guanethidine + Tricyclics ⚠

The antihypertensive effects of guanethidine are reduced or abolished by amitriptyline, desipramine, imipramine, nortriptyline and protriptyline. Doxepin in doses of 300 mg or more daily interacts similarly, but in smaller doses it may not interact, although one case is reported with doxepin 100 mg daily.

Not every combination of guanethidine and a tricyclic antidepressant has been studied but all are expected to interact similarly. Concurrent use should be avoided unless the effects are very closely monitored and the interaction balanced by raising the dose of the antihypertensive.

G

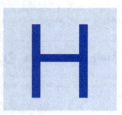

H₂-receptor antagonists

Cimetidine is a non-specific enzyme inhibitor and therefore interacts with a number of cytochrome P450 substrates. Other H$_2$-receptor antagonists do not have enzyme-inhibitory effects and therefore do not interact in this way. They may therefore provide useful alternatives to cimetidine. However, note that if an interaction occurs due to an alteration in gastric pH, all H$_2$-receptor antagonists would be expected to interact similarly.

H₂-receptor antagonists + Lidocaine

Cimetidine modestly reduces the clearance of intravenous lidocaine and raises its levels (by about 30% within 6 hours in one study). Lidocaine toxicity may occur if the dose is not reduced. However, not all patients are affected.

> Monitor all patients closely for evidence of toxicity (e.g. bradycardia, hypotension, pins and needles) and, if possible, consider checking lidocaine levels regularly. A reduced infusion rate may be needed. Ranitidine does not interact and so would appear to be a suitable alternative to cimetidine.

H₂-receptor antagonists + Macrolides

Cimetidine can almost double the levels of erythromycin, although this has only been seen in a single dose study. A single case report describes reversible deafness attributed to this interaction.

> Evidence for this interaction is very limited and its general importance is uncertain. If deafness occurs, stop the erythromycin. Ranitidine is a possible non-interacting alternative, as are azithromycin and clarithromycin.

H₂-receptor antagonists + Mirtazapine

Cimetidine increases the AUC and peak levels of mirtazapine by 54% and 22%, respectively. Mirtazapine does not appear to affect the pharmacokinetics of cimetidine.

> The manufacturers advise that the mirtazapine dose may need to be reduced during concurrent use and increased if cimetidine is stopped. Monitor for an increase in adverse effects (e.g. oedema, drowsiness, headache) when starting cimetidine.

H₂-receptor antagonists + **Moclobemide**

Cimetidine increases the levels of moclobemide by almost 40%.

> Some consider no dose adjustment to be necessary. One manufacturer recommends that moclobemide should be started at the lowest therapeutic dose in patients taking cimetidine, with the dose of moclobemide titrated as required. If cimetidine is given to a patient taking stable doses of moclobemide, the dose of the moclobemide should initially be reduced by 50% and later adjusted as necessary.

H₂-receptor antagonists + **NNRTIs**

Antacids roughly halve the AUC of delavirdine, and H₂-receptor antagonists would be expected to interact similarly.

> Long-term concurrent use of H₂-receptor antagonists with delavirdine is not recommended.

H

H₂-receptor antagonists + **Opioids**

Cimetidine increases the levels of alfentanil, and some preliminary observations suggest that cimetidine may increase the half-life of fentanyl. Isolated reports describe adverse reactions in patients taking methadone, morphine, or mixed opium alkaloids when cimetidine was also given, or morphine when ranitidine was also given.

> The clinical relevance of these effects on alfentanil and fentanyl are unknown. However, the UK manufacturer of alfentanil warns that cimetidine could increase the risk of respiratory depression, and that it may be necessary to lower the dose of alfentanil; monitor concurrent use carefully, or consider using ranitidine, which does not appear to interact. The case reports are not expected to be of general significance, although some manufacturers advise caution on concurrent use.

H₂-receptor antagonists + **Pentoxifylline**

Cimetidine moderately increases pentoxifylline levels and adverse effects, such as headache and nausea, are more common.

> Be aware that the adverse effects of pentoxifylline may be increased, and if necessary decrease its dose.

H₂-receptor antagonists + **Phenytoin**

Phenytoin levels are raised by cimetidine (maximum rise of 280% over 3 weeks). Very rarely bone marrow depression develops on concurrent use. Limited evidence suggests that low (non-prescription) doses of cimetidine may not interact. Fosphenytoin, a prodrug of phenytoin, may interact similarly.

> Monitor phenytoin levels and adjust the dose accordingly. Alternatively other H₂-receptor antagonists (ranitidine, famotidine, nizatidine) do not usually interact, although isolated cases have been reported. Be alert for signs of phenytoin toxicity (e.g. blurred vision, nystagmus, ataxia or drowsiness) when these H₂-receptor antagonists are first given.

H₂-receptor antagonists + **Phosphodiesterase type-5 inhibitors**

Cimetidine increases the AUC of sildenafil by 56%.

> Both increased efficacy and adverse effects may occur. For erectile dysfunction, the UK manufacturer of sildenafil suggests that a low starting dose of 25 mg should be used if cimetidine is given, although the modest increase in levels seems unlikely to cause particular problems. For pulmonary hypertension, no dose adjustment of sildenafil is necessary. The US manufacturers do not recommend any additional precautions.

H₂-receptor antagonists + **Procainamide**

Cimetidine can increase procainamide levels by more than 50%, which may lead to procainamide toxicity.

> Patients, particularly the elderly and those with renal impairment, should be closely monitored for signs of procainamide toxicity, and a dose reduction should be considered. Ranitidine and famotidine appear to interact only minimally or not at all.

H₂-receptor antagonists + **Propafenone**

Cimetidine raised the mean peak and steady-state plasma propafenone levels by 24% and 22%, respectively, but these did not reach statistical significance.

> No action is thought to be needed.

H₂-receptor antagonists + **Protease inhibitors**

Atazanavir and fosamprenavir levels are reduced by H₂-receptor antagonists such as ranitidine, probably by affecting gastric acidity. Amprenavir is predicted to be similarly affected. Not all H₂-receptor antagonists have been studied, but they would be expected to interact similarly. Saquinavir levels may be increased (more than doubled) by cimetidine.

> The manufacturers suggest that ritonavir-boosted atazanavir should be given once

daily with food, at the same time or at least 10 hours after famotidine 20 mg twice daily (or the comparable dose of another H$_2$-receptor antagonist). In the US, famotidine up to 40 mg twice daily may be given to treatment-naive patients, with the same dose and dose interval as the lower famotidine dose. In the UK, if famotidine 40 mg twice daily or more is required, then the manufacturers suggest considering increasing the dose of ritonavir-boosted atazanavir to 100/400 mg. For unboosted atazanavir in treatment-naive patients, the US manufacturer recommends a dose of 400 mg should be given once daily with food, 2 hours before and at least 10 hours after the dose of the H$_2$-receptor antagonist; the maximum dose of famotidine should not exceed 20 mg as a single dose or 40 mg daily. The UK manufacturer suggests that no fosamprenavir dose adjustment is needed with ranitidine or other H$_2$-receptor antagonists; however, the US manufacturer says the combination should be used with caution because fosamprenavir may become less effective. Increased monitoring should be considered to check for saquinavir adverse effects if cimetidine is given.

H$_2$-receptor antagonists + Quinidine ⚠

Cimetidine can raise quinidine levels and toxicity may develop in some patients.

Be alert for changes in the response to quinidine if cimetidine is started or stopped. Ideally quinidine levels should be monitored and the dose reduced as necessary. Reductions of 25% (oral) to 35% (intravenous) have been suggested.

H$_2$-receptor antagonists + Quinine ⚠

The clearance of quinine is reduced by cimetidine, resulting in a 42% increase in the AUC of quinine.

The clinical importance of this is uncertain, but be particularly alert for any evidence of quinine adverse effects during concurrent use. Note that ranitidine appears not to interact.

H$_2$-receptor antagonists + Sirolimus ⚠

The manufacturers of sirolimus predict that its levels will be increased by cimetidine.

Sirolimus levels and/or effects (e.g. on renal function) should be monitored as a matter of routine, but it may be prudent to increase monitoring if cimetidine is started or stopped.

H$_2$-receptor antagonists + SSRIs ❓

Citalopram, escitalopram, paroxetine and sertraline levels are moderately increased by cimetidine. Some individual patients had greater increases in SSRI levels.

Initial dose reductions are not needed, but be aware that some patients may have an increase in SSRI adverse effects (dry mouth, nausea, diarrhoea, dyspepsia, tremor, ejaculatory delay, sweating), in which case dose reductions may be appropriate.

H₂-receptor antagonists + Tacrine

Cimetidine increases the levels of tacrine by up to about 50%, possibly increasing tacrine beneficial and adverse effects.

Monitor concurrent use for an increase in tacrine adverse effects (nausea, vomiting, diarrhoea).

H₂-receptor antagonists + Theophylline

Cimetidine raises theophylline levels (by about one-third) and toxicity has been seen. The interaction is unlikely to be clinically relevant in most patients with low-dose (non-prescription) cimetidine.

Monitor theophylline levels if cimetidine is added or withdrawn: initial theophylline dose reductions of 30 to 50% have been suggested. The peak effect appears to occur after 3 days. Alternatively, use ranitidine or famotidine, which appear not to interact.

H₂-receptor antagonists + Tricyclics

The concurrent use of cimetidine can raise the levels of amitriptyline, desipramine, doxepin, imipramine and nortriptyline. Severe adverse effects have occurred in a few patients. Other tricyclic antidepressants are expected to interact similarly.

Patients taking tricyclics and cimetidine should be monitored for evidence of increased toxicity (dry mouth, urinary retention, blurred vision, constipation, tachycardia, postural hypotension). Reduce the tricyclic dose if necessary. Ranitidine does not appear to interact.

H₂-receptor antagonists + Triptans

Cimetidine raises the AUC of zolmitriptan by almost 50%.

The UK manufacturer recommends a zolmitriptan dose reduction to a maximum of 5 mg in 24 hours if patients are also taking cimetidine. The US manufacturer does not suggest a dose adjustment.

H₂-receptor antagonists + Warfarin and other oral anticoagulants

The anticoagulant effects of warfarin can be increased by cimetidine. Severe bleeding has occurred in a few patients but some show no interaction at all. Acenocoumarol and phenindione seem to interact similarly.

Monitor the INR if cimetidine is added or withdrawn. The interaction is rapid and may occur within days and even as early as after 24 hours. Famotidine, nizatidine and ranitidine usually appear to be non-interacting alternatives, although isolated cases of bleeding have been seen.

Heparin

Heparin + Nitrates

Some studies claim that the effects of heparin are reduced by the concurrent infusion of nitrates, but others have not confirmed this interaction.

> On balance it appears that a clinically relevant interaction is generally unlikely to be seen. Furthermore, given that heparin is routinely monitored, it is likely that if an interaction did occur, it would be rapidly detected.

Heparin + NSAIDs

Ketorolac

The risk of bleeding is said to be particularly high if ketorolac is used with anticoagulants including heparin. However, one study found no increase in bleeding time when ketorolac was given with heparin.

> The CSM in the UK and the manufacturer of ketorolac state that the concurrent use of anticoagulants is contraindicated, and they include low doses of heparin. Conversely, the US manufacturers of ketorolac advise that physicians should carefully weigh the benefits against the risks and use heparin with ketorolac only extremely cautiously.

NSAIDs, general ⚠

An increased risk of bleeding occurs when NSAIDs (that have antiplatelet actions) are given with heparin. Anticoagulants can exacerbate gastrointestinal bleeding caused by NSAIDs. Cases of spinal haematomas after epidural anaesthesia have been reported with the concurrent use of heparin and NSAIDs.

> Concurrent use is not uncommon, but prescribers should be aware that there is an increased risk of bleeding and monitor appropriately. Extreme caution is needed if concurrent use is considered appropriate in patients undergoing epidural anaesthesia.

Heparin + Prasugrel ❓

No significant interaction was reported between prasugrel and a single intravenous bolus of heparin; however, the manufacturers advise that there is a possible increased risk of bleeding on concurrent use. The use of prasugrel and heparin may contribute to the development of epidural or spinal haematoma after epidural anaesthesia.

> Concurrent use need not be avoided, but be aware of the potential for this interaction if bleeding occurs. Extreme caution is needed if concurrent use is considered appropriate in patients undergoing epidural anaesthesia.

H

Heparin + **Ticlopidine**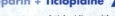

Concurrent use of ticlopidine with heparin increases haemorrhagic risk, and may contribute to the development of epidural or spinal haematoma after epidural anaesthesia.

If concurrent use is undertaken, there should be close clinical and laboratory monitoring. Extreme caution is needed if concurrent use is considered appropriate in patients undergoing epidural anaesthesia.

Herbal medicines or Dietary supplements

There seem to be few clinical reports of interactions between herbal medicines (with the exception of St John's wort) or dietary supplements and so recommendations regarding the interactions are often difficult to make. An additional problem in interpreting these interactions, is that the interacting constituent of the herb is usually not known and is therefore not standardised for. It could vary widely between different products, and batches of the same product. Bear this in mind.

Herbal medicines or Dietary supplements + **HRT**

The hormones in HRT are similar to those used in hormonal contraceptives, and so may be affected by enzyme-inducing drugs, such as St John's wort (*Hypericum perforatum*), in the same way as contraceptives, page 236. Reduced effects are therefore possible.

Any interaction would be most likely to be noticed where HRT is prescribed for menopausal vasomotor symptoms, but might be difficult to detect where the indication is osteoporosis. Further study is needed to confirm the importance of this possible interaction. The interaction is not relevant to HRT applied locally for menopausal vaginitis.

Herbal medicines or Dietary supplements + **Imatinib**

St John's wort (*Hypericum perforatum*) slightly reduces the levels of imatinib.

The manufacturers suggest that concurrent use should be avoided. If this is not possible, monitor the outcome of concurrent use and adjust the dose of imatinib as necessary.

Herbal medicines or Dietary supplements + Lithium

Herbal diuretic

A woman developed lithium toxicity after taking a herbal diuretic containing corn silk, *Equisetum hyemale*, juniper, ovate buchu, parsley and bearberry.

> This interaction is similar to that seen with prescription diuretics, page 269. Concurrent use needs monitoring, and patients should be encouraged to seek advice before self-medicating.

St John's wort (Hypericum perforatum)

A case report describes mania in a patient taking St John's wort and lithium.

> The general importance of this interaction is unclear. Bear it in mind in case of an unexpected response to treatment.

Herbal medicines or Dietary supplements + MAOIs

Two patients developed headache, insomnia, and in one case hallucinations, when they took phenelzine with ginseng.

> The general importance of these poorly documented early cases is unclear. Nevertheless, consider the possibility of an interaction in case of an unexpected response to treatment with phenelzine (or potentially any MAOI) in a patient taking any type of ginseng.

Herbal medicines or Dietary supplements + NNRTIs

There is evidence to suggest that St John's wort (*Hypericum perforatum*) may decrease the levels of nevirapine (clearance increased by 35%). Delavirdine, efavirenz and etravirine would be expected to interact similarly.

> The available evidence supports the advice issued by the CSM in the UK, that St John's wort may decrease the levels of the NNRTIs with possible loss of HIV suppression. Concurrent use should be avoided.

Herbal medicines or Dietary supplements + NSAIDs

Ginkgo biloba

Case reports describe fatal intracerebral bleeding in a patient taking *Ginkgo biloba* with ibuprofen, and prolonged bleeding and subdural haematomas in a patient taking *Ginkgo biloba* with rofecoxib. Studies with diclofenac and flurbiprofen showed that *Ginkgo biloba* had no effect on the pharmacokinetics of these drugs.

> The evidence from these reports is too slim to advise patients against taking NSAIDs and *Ginkgo biloba* concurrently, but some do recommend caution. Medical professionals should be aware of the possibility of increased bleeding tendency with *Ginkgo biloba* and monitor patients appropriately.

H

Tamarindus indica

Tamarindus indica (tamarind) fruit extract caused a 2-fold increase in the AUC of ibuprofen.

The clinical relevance of this interaction is unknown, but large rises in the ibuprofen levels may result in toxicity.

Herbal medicines or Dietary supplements + Opioids ✖

St John's wort (*Hypericum perforatum*) decreased methadone levels by up to 60% in one study, and withdrawal symptoms have been reported.

Advise patients taking methadone to avoid St John's wort. It may be prudent to follow the same advice for other opioids that are mainly metabolised by CYP3A4, such as buprenorphine, fentanyl or alfentanil.

Herbal medicines or Dietary supplements + Penicillins ⚠

Chewing khat reduces the absorption of ampicillin, and to a lesser extent amoxicillin, but the effects are minimal 2 hours after khat chewing stops.

The authors of one of the studies concluded that both ampicillin and amoxicillin should be taken 2 hours after khat chewing to ensure that maximum absorption occurs.

Herbal medicines or Dietary supplements + Phenobarbital ✖

St John's wort (*Hypericum perforatum*) is predicted to reduce the levels of phenobarbital (and therefore possibly primidone-derived phenobarbital).

Until more is known, it would probably be prudent to avoid concurrent use. The CSM in the UK advise that St John's wort should be stopped and that the phenobarbital dose should be adjusted.

Herbal medicines or Dietary supplements + Phenytoin

Ayurvedic medicines ✖

A case report, and an *animal* study, indicate that an antiepileptic Ayurvedic herbal preparation, SRC (*Shankhapushpi*), can markedly reduce phenytoin levels, leading to an increased seizure frequency. SRC is a syrup prepared from *Convolvulus pluricaulis* leaves, *Nardostachys jatamansi* rhizomes, *Onosma bracteatum* leaves and flowers, and the whole plant of *Centella asiatica*, *Nepeta hindostana* and *Nepeta elliptica*.

Shankhapushpi (SRC) is given because it has some antiepileptic activity but there is little point in combining it with phenytoin if the outcome is a fall in phenytoin levels, accompanied by an increase in seizure frequency. For this reason concurrent use should be avoided. It would seem prudent to be similarly cautious with the use of fosphenytoin, a prodrug of phenytoin.

St John's wort (Hypericum perforatum)

St John's wort is predicted to reduce the levels of phenytoin. Fosphenytoin, a prodrug of phenytoin, may interact similarly.

Until more is known, it would probably be prudent to avoid concurrent use in patients taking phenytoin, especially as phenytoin is a substrate of CYP2C19, which St John's wort appears to induce. The CSM in the UK advise that St John's wort should be stopped and that the phenytoin dose should be adjusted.

Herbal medicines or Dietary supplements + Phosphodiesterase type-5 inhibitors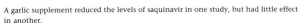

St John's wort is predicted to reduce the levels of phosphodiesterase type-5 inhibitors, because other inducers of CYP3A4 have been shown to do so. For example, the AUC of sildenafil is reduced by about 70% by *bosentan* and the AUC of tadalafil is reduced by 88% by *rifampicin*. Vardenafil is also metabolised by CYP3A4, and therefore its levels may possibly be lowered by St John's wort.

If these phosphodiesterase type-5 inhibitors are not effective in patients taking St John's wort, consider reviewing the need for concurrent use. If concurrent use is necessary, a dose increase in the phosphodiesterase type-5 inhibitor may be required.

Herbal medicines or Dietary supplements + Protease inhibitors

Garlic ✗

A garlic supplement reduced the levels of saquinavir in one study, but had little effect in another.

All garlic supplements should probably be avoided if saquinavir is ever given as the sole protease inhibitor (not recommended). The clinical relevance of this interaction with ritonavir-boosted saquinavir is unclear, but note that no significant interaction appears to occur with ritonavir.

St John's wort (Hypericum perforatum) ✗

St John's wort causes a marked reduction in the levels of indinavir, which may result in HIV treatment failure. Other protease inhibitors, whether used alone or ritonavir-boosted, are predicted to interact similarly.

The advice of the CSM in the UK is that patients taking protease inhibitors should avoid St John's wort, and that anyone already taking both should stop the St John's wort and have their HIV RNA viral load measured. The manufacturers also note that protease inhibitor levels may increase on stopping St John's wort, and the dose may need adjusting. They note that the inducing effect may persist for up to 2 weeks after stopping treatment with St John's wort.

Herbal medicines or Dietary supplements + **Proton pump inhibitors**

Both *Gingko biloba* and St John's wort (*Hypericum perforatum*) induce the metabolism of omeprazole, and this might result in reduced efficacy. Other proton pump inhibitors are likely to be similarly affected.

> There is insufficient evidence to suggest that these herbs should be avoided in patients taking proton pump inhibitors. However, the potential reduction in their efficacy should be borne in mind, particular where the consequences may be serious, such as in patients with healing ulcers.

Herbal medicines or Dietary supplements + **Ranolazine**

Rifampicin (*rifampin*) reduces ranolazine levels by 95%, and loss of efficacy is expected. St John's wort is predicted to interact in the same way as rifampicin.

> The manufacturers recommend avoiding concurrent use. In the absence of any information on the magnitude of the effect of St John's wort on ranolazine levels, this seems prudent.

Herbal medicines or Dietary supplements + **Sirolimus**

The manufacturers predict that St John's wort (*Hypericum perforatum*) may lower sirolimus levels, probably because *rifampicin* (*rifampin*), another CYP3A4 inducer, has been shown to do so.

> The extent of any change in sirolimus levels is uncertain, but if concurrent use cannot be avoided it would seem prudent to increase the frequency of monitoring of sirolimus levels.

Herbal medicines or Dietary supplements + **SSRIs**

Ayahuasca

A man taking fluoxetine experienced symptoms of serotonin syndrome after drinking the psychoactive beverage ayahuasca (also known as caapi, daime, hoasca, natema, yage), which is characteristically derived from the vine *Banisteriopsis caapi*.

> This appears to be the only report of an interaction. However, as ayahuasca contains monoamine oxidase-inhibiting harmala alkaloids concurrent use with any SSRIs may potentially cause serotonin syndrome, page 454.

St John's wort (Hypericum perforatum)

Cases of severe sedation, mania and serotonin syndrome, page 454, have been reported in patients taking St John's wort with SSRIs.

> The incidence of an interaction is probably small, but because of the potential

severity of the reaction some suggest avoiding the concurrent use of any SSRI and St John's wort. The CSM in the UK advise that St John's wort should be stopped if patients are taking an SSRI.

Herbal medicines or Dietary supplements + **Statins**

St John's wort (*Hypericum perforatum*) appears to modestly reduce the levels of atorvastatin and simvastatin.

The significance of this interaction is unclear but it may be prudent to consider an interaction if lipid-lowering targets are not met, and advise the patient to stop taking St John's wort or adjust the dose of atorvastatin or simvastatin if needed. Pravastatin does not appear to interact.

Herbal medicines or Dietary supplements + Tacrolimus

St John's wort (*Hypericum perforatum*) has been found, on average, to decrease tacrolimus maximum levels by 65% and its AUC by 32%. However, the decrease in AUC ranged from 15% to 64%, with one patient having a 31% *increase* in AUC.

Given the unpredictability of the interaction (and the variability in content of St John's wort products) it would seem prudent to avoid St John's wort in transplant patients, and possibly patients taking tacrolimus for other indications. If St John's wort is withdrawn monitor tacrolimus levels and adjust the dose accordingly.

Herbal medicines or Dietary supplements + Ticlopidine

Ginkgo biloba has been associated with platelet, bleeding and clotting disorders and there are isolated reports of serious adverse reactions after its concurrent use with antiplatelet drugs including ticlopidine.

The evidence is too slim to advise patients against taking ticlopidine with *Ginkgo biloba*. However, caution should be exercised if *Ginkgo biloba* is used with any drug that affects platelet aggregation as bleeding has been seen with the use of *Ginkgo biloba* alone. Patients should be told to seek professional advice if any bleeding problems arise.

Herbal medicines or Dietary supplements + Trazodone

Coma developed in an elderly patient with Alzheimer's disease after she took trazodone with *Ginkgo biloba*. She later recovered.

This appears to be an isolated case, from which no general conclusions can be drawn.

H

Herbal medicines or Dietary supplements + Tricyclics ✔

The levels of amitriptyline and its metabolite nortriptyline are modestly reduced by St John's wort (*Hypericum perforatum*). Other tricyclics would be expected to interact similarly.

> The clinical significance of this interaction is unknown, although it is likely to be small. However, bear it in mind should an unexpected reduction in tricyclic efficacy occur. Both the tricyclics and St John's wort are antidepressants, but whether concurrent use is beneficial or safe is not known. Further study is needed.

Herbal medicines or Dietary supplements + Triptans ✖

Serotonin syndrome has been reported in a patient taking eletriptan and St John's wort (*Hypericum perforatum*). This reaction is possible with any triptan and St John's wort.

> The CSM suggest that patients taking triptans should not take St John's wort; however, most manufacturers generally advise caution, which seems prudent, see serotonin syndrome, page 454.

Herbal medicines or Dietary supplements + Venlafaxine

Jujube ❓

An isolated report describes an acute serotonin reaction when venlafaxine was given with a Chinese herbal remedy, jujube (sour date nut; suanzaoren; *Ziziphus jujuba*).

> Patients should be asked about the use of herbal remedies and advised to discontinue them before prescribing antidepressant drugs if there is any possibility of an interaction.

St John's wort (Hypericum perforatum) ⚠

A possible case of serotonin syndrome has been reported in a patient taking venlafaxine and St John's wort.

> Caution is advised if venlafaxine is given with other drugs that affect the serotonergic neurotransmitter systems, such as St John's wort. See serotonin syndrome, page 454, for further monitoring advice.

Herbal medicines or Dietary supplements + Warfarin and other oral anticoagulants

Boldo ❓

A report describes a woman on warfarin whose INR rose modestly when she began to take boldo and fenugreek. She was eventually restabilised with a 15% dose reduction.

> Evidence is limited to one isolated case. Because of the many other factors

influencing anticoagulant control, it is not possible to reliably ascribe a change in INR specifically to a drug interaction in a single case report without other supporting evidence. Advise patients to discuss the use of any herbal products they wish to try, and to increase monitoring if this is thought advisable.

Chamomile

A single case describes a woman taking warfarin who developed a marked increase in her INR with bleeding complications 5 days after she started drinking chamomile tea (an infusion of *Matricaria chamomilla* (German chamomile)) and using a chamomile-based skin lotion.

Note that there appear to be no reports of German chamomile alone causing anticoagulation, which might suggest that the risk of an additive effect is small. Because of the many other factors influencing anticoagulant control, it is not possible to reliably ascribe a change in INR specifically to a drug interaction in a single case report without other supporting evidence. Advise patients to discuss the use of any herbal products they wish to try, and to increase monitoring if this is thought advisable.

Chinese angelica (Angelica sinensis) ⊗

Two case reports describe a very marked increase in the anticoagulant effects of warfarin when Chinese angelica was added.

Patients taking warfarin and related anticoagulants should be warned of the potential risks of also taking Chinese angelica. Until more information is available, Chinese angelica should be avoided unless the effects on anticoagulation can be monitored.

Cucurbita

The INR of a patient taking warfarin increased from 2.4 to 3.5 after he took curbicin, which contains saw palmetto (*Serenoa repens*) and *Cucurbita pepo*.

Evidence is limited to one isolated case. Because of the many other factors influencing anticoagulant control, it is not possible to reliably ascribe a change in INR specifically to a drug interaction in a single case report without other supporting evidence. Advise patients to discuss the use of any herbal products they wish to try, and to increase monitoring if this is thought advisable.

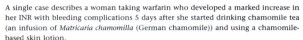

Danshen ⊗

Several case reports indicate that danshen (the root of *Salvia miltiorrhiza*), a Chinese herbal remedy, can increase the effects of warfarin resulting in bleeding. There seems to be no evidence about other related anticoagulants, but it seems possible that they may be similarly affected.

Avoid concurrent use where possible. However, if concurrent use is felt desirable it would seem sensible to warn patients to be alert for any signs of bruising or bleeding, and report these immediately, should they occur.

Fenugreek

A report describes a woman taking warfarin whose INR rose modestly when she began to take boldo and fenugreek. She was eventually restabilised with a 15% dose reduction.

Evidence is limited to one isolated case. Because of the many other factors influencing anticoagulant control, it is not possible to reliably ascribe a change in INR specifically to a drug interaction in a single case report without other supporting evidence. Advise patients to discuss the use of any herbal products they wish to try, and to increase monitoring if this is thought advisable.

Fish oils ▲

The use of warfarin with fish oils did not alter warfarin efficacy in two studies, nor the incidence of bleeding episodes in another. However, in one of the studies, fish oil significantly prolonged bleeding time. There are a couple of reports of an increased INR in patients taking warfarin and fish oils.

This interaction is not established. Based on the possible moderate increase in bleeding times with high-dose fish oils, the manufacturers of one product say that patients receiving anticoagulants should be monitored (e.g. for bruising or bleeding), and the dose of anticoagulant adjusted as necessary. Note that monitoring the INR would not pick up this pharmacodynamic interaction.

Garlic ❓

Two patients taking warfarin and one taking fluindione developed increased INRs after the addition of garlic capsules. One patient developed haematuria. However, a controlled study with warfarin suggests no interaction occurs.

This interaction seems rare, but bear it in mind in case of unexpected bleeding. It is worth noting that there have been cases of spontaneous bleeding attributed to garlic alone. In addition, garlic may have some antiplatelet effects, and although there appear to be no clinical reports of an adverse interaction, it may be prudent to consider the potential for an increase in the severity of bleeding if garlic is given with anticoagulants.

Ginkgo biloba ❓

Evidence from studies suggests that *Ginkgo biloba* does not interact with warfarin. However, an isolated report describes intracerebral haemorrhage associated with the use of *Ginkgo biloba* and warfarin

There is insufficient evidence to justify telling patients taking warfarin to avoid *Ginkgo biloba* but, because bleeding has been reported with *Ginkgo biloba* alone, they should be told to monitor for early signs of bruising or bleeding and seek informed professional advice if any bleeding problems arise.

Ginseng ▲

One pharmacological study found that *Panax quinquefolius* (American ginseng) modestly decreased the effect of warfarin, whereas another study found that *Panax ginseng* (Asian ginseng) did not alter the effect of warfarin. Two case reports describe decreased warfarin effects, one with thrombosis, attributed to the use of ginseng (probably *Panax ginseng*). Note that there have been reports of spontaneous bleeding with ginseng alone, and *Panax ginseng* has been found to contain antiplatelet components.

Be alert for a possible decrease in the effects of warfarin and related drugs in patients using ginseng, particularly *Panax quinquefolius*. Patients should be warned to monitor for early signs of bruising or bleeding and seek informed professional advice if any bleeding problems arise.

Glucosamine +/- Chondroitin

A couple of reports suggest that glucosamine with or without chondroitin may increase the INR in patients taking warfarin. In contrast, one case of a *decreased* INR has been reported when glucosamine was taken with acenocoumarol.

An interaction would seem to be rare, and there do not appear to have been any controlled studies of this interaction. The cases described suggest it would be prudent to monitor the INR more closely if glucosamine is started. If a patient shows an unexpected change in INR, bear in mind the possibility of self-medication with supplements such as glucosamine.

Lycium barbarum

One patient developed a raised INR after taking a tea made from the fruits of *Lycium barbarum* L. (also known as Chinese wolfberry, gou qi zi, Fructus Lycii Chinensis, or *Lycium chinense*).

Evidence is limited to one isolated case. Because of the many other factors influencing anticoagulant control, it is not possible to reliably ascribe a change in INR specifically to a drug interaction in a single case report without other supporting evidence. Advise patients to discuss the use of any herbal products they wish to try, and to increase monitoring if this is thought advisable.

Quilinggao ❓

A single case report describes a man taking warfarin who had a marked increase in his INR with bleeding complications, 9 days after he switched the brand of quilinggao (a Chinese herbal product made from a mixture of herbs) he was using.

The general importance of this isolated case report is unknown, but bear it in mind in case of an increased response to anticoagulant treatment.

Saw palmetto ❓

The INR of a patient taking warfarin increased from 2.4 to 3.5 after he took curbicin, which contains saw palmetto and cucurbita. Excessive bleeding during surgery has been reported in another patient who had been taking saw palmetto.

Because of the many other factors influencing anticoagulant control, it is not possible to reliably ascribe a change in INR specifically to a drug interaction in a single case report without other supporting evidence. Advise patients to discuss the use of any herbal products they wish to try, and to increase monitoring if this is thought advisable.

St John's wort (Hypericum perforatum) ✕

St John's wort can cause a moderate reduction in the anticoagulant effects of phenprocoumon and warfarin.

It would be prudent to monitor the INRs of patients taking any coumarin if they start taking St John's wort, being alert for the need to slightly raise the anticoagulant dosage. However, note that the CSM in the UK advise against the concurrent use of St Johnãs wort with warfarin: if St John's wort is being taken by patients also taking anticoagulants the herb should be stopped and the anticoagulant dose adjusted as necessary.

Ubidecarenone (Coenzyme Q10)

Coenzyme Q10 did not alter the INR or required warfarin dose in a controlled study in patients stabilised on warfarin. However, cases of either reduced, or transiently increased anticoagulant effects have been reported in patients taking warfarin and ubidecarenone.

The general importance of this interaction is unknown. Until more is known it would seem prudent to increase the frequency of INR monitoring in patients taking warfarin if coenzyme Q10 is started.

HRT

As HRT contains many of the same hormones as the contraceptives, studies with contraceptives, page 233, may be applicable to HRT and *vice versa*, although the relative doses should be borne in mind.

HRT + Letrozole ✖

HRT would be expected to diminish the effects of letrozole (which has anti-oestrogenic effects).

Some information suggests that there need not be a complete restriction on their concurrent use, but this needs confirmation. Until then, concurrent use should be avoided: the manufacturers contraindicate concurrent use.

HRT + Levothyroxine ⚠

Oral oestrogens appear to increase the requirement for levothyroxine in some patients.

It would be prudent to monitor thyroid function several months after starting or stopping oral oestrogens to check levothyroxine requirements. Transdermal HRT would not be expected to interact, but this needs confirmation.

HRT + MAO-B inhibitors ✖

In a controlled study, the AUC of selegiline was modestly increased by estradiol-containing HRT (60%), but this was not considered to be clinically significant.

One UK manufacturer of selegiline advises that the concurrent use of HRT should be avoided. If concurrent use is necessary, monitor for increased selegiline adverse effects (such as nausea, constipation, hypotension and diarrhoea).

HRT + Modafinil ?

The hormones in HRT are similar to those used in oral hormonal contraceptives, and so may be affected by enzyme-inducing drugs in the same way as contraceptives, page 238. Reduced effects are therefore possible if modafinil is also given.

Any interaction would be most likely to be noticed where HRT is prescribed for menopausal vasomotor symptoms. Further study is needed to confirm the importance of this possible interaction. The interaction is not relevant to HRT applied locally.

HRT + NNRTIs ?

The hormones in HRT are similar to those used in oral hormonal contraceptives, and so may be affected by enzyme-inducing drugs, such as nevirapine and efavirenz, in the same way as contraceptives, page 238. Reduced effects are therefore possible if either of these drugs is also given.

Any interaction would be most likely to be noticed where HRT is prescribed for menopausal vasomotor symptoms. Further study is needed to confirm the importance of this possible interaction. The interaction is not relevant to HRT applied locally.

HRT + Phenobarbital ?

The hormones in HRT are similar to those used in oral hormonal contraceptives, and so may be affected by enzyme-inducing drugs in the same way as contraceptives, page 240. Reduced effects are therefore possible if phenobarbital or primidone is also given.

Any interaction would be most likely to be noticed where HRT is prescribed for menopausal vasomotor symptoms. Further study is needed to confirm the importance of this possible interaction. The interaction is not relevant to HRT applied locally.

HRT + Phenytoin ?

The hormones in HRT are similar to those used in oral hormonal contraceptives, and so may be affected by enzyme-inducing drugs in the same way as contraceptives, page 240. Reduced effects are therefore possible if phenytoin or fosphenytoin is also given.

Any interaction would be most likely to be noticed where HRT is prescribed for menopausal vasomotor symptoms. Further study is needed to confirm the importance of this possible interaction. The interaction is not relevant to HRT applied locally.

HRT + Protease inhibitors ?

The hormones in HRT are similar to those used in oral hormonal contraceptives, and so may be affected by enzyme-inducing drugs in the same way as contraceptives,

H

page 240. Reduced effects are therefore theoretically possible if a protease inhibitor is also given; however, note that some protease inhibitors have actually *increased* hormone levels.

Any interaction resulting in reduced effect would be most likely to be noticed where HRT is prescribed for menopausal vasomotor symptoms. Further study is needed to confirm the importance of this possible interaction but it may be prudent to use the lowest possible dose of HRT and gradually titrate to effect. The interaction is not relevant to HRT applied locally.

HRT + Rifabutin ❓

The hormones in HRT are similar to those used in oral hormonal contraceptives, and so may be affected by enzyme-inducing drugs in the same way as contraceptives, page 241. Reduced effects are therefore possible if rifabutin is also given.

Any interaction would be most likely to be noticed where HRT is prescribed for menopausal vasomotor symptoms. Further study is needed to confirm the importance of this possible interaction. The interaction is not relevant to HRT applied locally.

HRT + Rifampicin (Rifampin) ❓

The hormones in HRT are similar to those used in oral hormonal contraceptives, and so may be affected by enzyme-inducing drugs in the same way as contraceptives, page 241. Reduced effects are therefore possible if rifampicin is also given.

Any interaction would be most likely to be noticed where HRT is prescribed for menopausal vasomotor symptoms. Further study is needed to confirm the importance of this possible interaction. The interaction is not relevant to HRT applied locally.

HRT + Tacrine ❓

HRT (conjugated oestrogens, estradiol or estrone sulfate) increases the AUC of tacrine by 60% (and even up to 3-fold in one individual) and reduces its clearance by about 30%.

The importance of this interaction is unclear. Increased tacrine levels may increase both the efficacy and adverse effects of tacrine. Monitor patients for signs of tacrine toxicity and consider a tacrine dose reduction if indicated.

HRT + Tamoxifen ❌

HRT would be expected to diminish the effects of tamoxifen and other anti-oestrogens.

Some information suggests that there need not be a complete restriction on their concurrent use, but this needs confirmation. Until then, concurrent use should be avoided: the manufacturers contraindicate concurrent use.

HRT + **Topiramate**

The hormones in HRT are similar to those used in oral hormonal contraceptives, and so may be affected by enzyme-inducing drugs in the same way as contraceptives, page 242. Reduced effects are therefore possible if topiramate is also given.

Any interaction would be most likely to be noticed where HRT is prescribed for menopausal vasomotor symptoms. Further study is needed to confirm the importance of this possible interaction. The interaction is not relevant to HRT applied locally.

HRT + **Toremifene**

HRT would be expected to diminish the effects of toremifene (which has anti-oestrogenic effects).

Some information suggests that there need not be a complete restriction on their concurrent use, but this needs confirmation. Until then, concurrent use should be avoided: the manufacturers contraindicate concurrent use.

HRT + **Ursodeoxycholic acid (Ursodiol)**

Ursodeoxycholic acid does not affect the bioavailability of ethinylestradiol. However, oestrogens may decrease the effectiveness of ursodeoxycholic acid by increasing the elimination of cholesterol in bile.

The manufacturers suggest that concurrent use should be avoided.

HRT + **Warfarin and other oral anticoagulants**

There is conflicting data on whether or not the use of HRT (oral or topical) affects warfarin or phenindione dosing. In one case, the acenocoumarol dose was increased by 75% when oral conjugated oestrogens were changed to transdermal estradiol. Tibolone may increase the INR in some patients taking warfarin or phenindione.

Direct information is limited. Note that, because of the increased risk of developing venous thromboembolism with HRT, the use of HRT in women already receiving an anticoagulant requires careful consideration of the risks and benefits. If the combination is used be aware that the anticoagulant response may be affected. Increased INR monitoring is advised when starting tibolone in patients stabilised on warfarin, other coumarins, or indanediones.

H

5-HT₃-receptor antagonists

5-HT₃-receptor antagonists + **Opioids** ⚠

Ondansetron reduces the analgesic efficacy of tramadol and at least double the dose was required in one clinical study. This resulted in more vomiting despite the ondansetron. Although not tested, other 5-HT₃-receptor antagonists would be expected to interact similarly.

> It would seem prudent to use alternative analgesics if ondansetron is required.

5-HT₃-receptor antagonists + SSRIs

Symptoms similar to serotonin syndrome have been reported in two patients receiving paroxetine and ondansetron or sertraline and dolasetron.

> It has been suggested that a variant of serotonin syndrome, page 454, may rarely be seen when 5-HT₃-receptor antagonists and SSRIs are given together, and clinicians should consider this possibility if both drugs are given.

Hydralazine

Hydralazine + NSAIDs

Indometacin abolished the hypotensive effects of intravenous hydralazine in one study, but did not affect it in another.

> Although information is limited, various NSAIDs have been reported to reduce the efficacy of other antihypertensive drug classes. It would be prudent to monitor the concurrent use of hydralazine and NSAIDs.

H

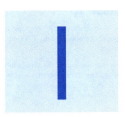

Imatinib

Imatinib + Levothyroxine

Patients taking levothyroxine who have previously undergone a total thyroidectomy may develop markedly elevated TSH levels and become clinically hypothyroid after taking imatinib.

TSH levels should be closely monitored in thyroidectomy patients taking levothyroxine if they are given imatinib, anticipating the need to increase the levothyroxine dose. It has been suggested that the dose of levothyroxine should be doubled before starting imatinib.

Imatinib + Macrolides

Ketoconazole increases the AUC of imatinib by 40%. Macrolides such as erythromycin, clarithromycin and telithromycin are, like ketoconazole, inhibitors of CYP3A4. The manufacturers of imatinib therefore predict that some macrolides will raise imatinib levels.

An interaction is not established and the outcome of concurrent use with the macrolides is uncertain. It may be prudent to be alert for increased imatinib adverse effects (such as bone marrow suppression and diarrhoea) if these macrolides are given. Other macrolides may also interact, although it seems unlikely that they all will, see macrolides, page 361.

Imatinib + Phenobarbital

Rifampicin decreases the AUC of imatinib by 74%. The manufacturers suggest that phenobarbital (and therefore probably primidone) will interact similarly.

The manufacturers suggest that concurrent use should be avoided. However, if this is not possible it would be prudent to monitor the outcome of concurrent use, and increase the imatinib dose as necessary: an increase of at least 50% has been suggested by the US manufacturer.

Imatinib + **Phenytoin** ⚠

Rifampicin decreases the AUC of imatinib by 74%. The manufacturers suggest that phenytoin (and therefore possibly fosphenytoin) will interact similarly: there is some data to support this prediction.

> The manufacturers suggest that concurrent use should be avoided. However, if this is not possible it would be prudent to monitor the outcome of concurrent use, and increase the imatinib dose as necessary: an increase of at least 50% has been suggested by the US manufacturer.

Imatinib + **Protease inhibitors** ❓

Single-dose *ketoconazole* (a potent CYP3A4 inhibitor) modestly raised the AUC of a single-dose of imatinib by about 40%. Other potent CYP3A4 inhibitors are predicted to interact similarly. The manufacturers name atazanavir, indinavir, nelfinavir, ritonavir, and saquinavir.

> The manufacturers advise caution, although the clinical relevance of the modest increase is as yet unclear. Bear the possibility of an interaction in mind should an increase in imatinib adverse effects (such as bone marrow suppression and diarrhoea) occur.

Imatinib + **Rifampicin (Rifampin)** ⚠

Rifampicin decreases the AUC of imatinib by 74%.

> The manufacturers suggest that concurrent use should be avoided. However, if this is not possible it would be prudent to monitor the outcome of concurrent use, and increase the imatinib dose as necessary: an increase of at least 50% has been suggested by the US manufacturer.

Imatinib + **Statins** ⚠

Imatinib increased the maximum levels of simvastatin 2-fold and the AUC 3-fold in one study. Lovastatin, and possibly atorvastatin, may interact similarly.

> These rises increase the risk of simvastatin toxicity (most notably myopathy and rhabdomyolysis), for which reason the simvastatin dose should be reduced appropriately. Patients given any of these statins and imatinib should be counselled regarding myopathy (e.g. report any unexplained muscle pain, tenderness or weakness).

Imatinib + **Warfarin and other oral anticoagulants** ⚠

The manufacturers suggest that imatinib may inhibit the metabolism of warfarin. This suggestion seems to be based on an observation in one patient, and *in vitro* studies that show that imatinib can inhibit CYP2C9, which is involved in the metabolism of warfarin.

> The manufacturers say that patients needing anticoagulation should be given

heparin or a low-molecular-weight heparin. If warfarin is given, it may be prudent to increase the frequency of INR monitoring.

Imipenem

Imipenem + Valproate

Case reports describe reduced valproate levels after imipenem was given. This has led to seizures.

Although evidence is limited this is in line with the way other carbapenems interact. It would be prudent to monitor valproate levels in any patient given carbapenems. The valproate dose may need to be increased. Consider using another antibacterial, or an alternative to valproate; limited evidence suggests that carbamazepine and phenytoin are not affected. Note that imipenem should be used with caution in patients with a history of seizures.

Inotropes and Vasopressors

Inotropes and Vasopressors + Linezolid

Because of its weak MAO-inhibitory properties, the manufacturers of linezolid suggest that it may interact with adrenaline (epinephrine), dopamine, dobutamine, and noradrenaline (norepinephrine) in the same way as the non-selective MAOIs. However, the evidence available suggests that blood pressure rises are only very moderate and certainly unlikely to be of the hypertensive crisis proportions seen with the non-selective MAOIs.

The manufacturers contraindicate the use of sympathomimetics with linezolid unless there are facilities available for close observation of the patient and monitoring of blood pressure.

Inotropes and Vasopressors + MAO-B inhibitors

A case report describes a hypertensive reaction attributed to the concurrent use of dopamine and selegiline.

The manufacturers of selegiline recommend that dopamine should be used cautiously, if at all, in patients who are receiving selegiline long-term or who have received selegiline in the 2 weeks before needing dopamine.

Inotropes and Vasopressors + **MAOIs**

Dopamine, Dopexamine, Metaraminol or Phenylephrine

Metaraminol and phenylephrine are vasopressors with both direct and indirect sympathomimetic actions. This means that it may cause serious and potentially fatal hypertensive reactions in patients taking MAOIs. Dopamine and dopexamine may possibly interact similarly.

Avoid the use of these vasopressors in patients who are either taking MAOIs or who have stopped taking them in the previous 2 weeks. One UK manufacturer of dopamine suggests that patients who have been taking an MAOI should be given a starting dose of dopamine that is one-tenth of the usual dose.

Other inotropes and vasopressors

The pressor effects of inotropes and vasopressors with indirect sympathomimetic actions, such as adrenaline (epinephrine), isoprenaline (isoproterenol), noradrenaline (norepinephrine) and methoxamine may be unchanged or only moderately increased in patients taking MAOIs. The increase may be somewhat greater in those who show a significant hypotensive response to the MAOI. Dobutamine would be expected to interact similarly.

Although this interaction is unlikely to be important in most patients, some may experience greater effects. The manufacturers of the MAOIs contraindicate concurrent use, although some consider this overly cautious.

Inotropes and Vasopressors + **Phenytoin**

There is some limited evidence that patients needing dopamine to support their blood pressure can become severely hypotensive if phenytoin is added to their treatment.

Blood pressure is doubtless being monitored in patients receiving dopamine, and should be measured when phenytoin is given intravenously. However, more frequent monitoring may be necessary as this interaction appears to develop rapidly.

Inotropes and Vasopressors + **Tricyclics**

Patients taking tricyclic antidepressants show a grossly exaggerated response (hypertension, cardiac arrhythmias, etc.) to parenteral noradrenaline (norepinephrine), adrenaline (epinephrine), and to a lesser extent, to phenylephrine.

The parenteral use of these inotropes should, where possible, be avoided in patients taking tricyclic antidepressants. If they must be used, the rate and amount injected must be very much reduced. The risk is probably lower when drugs such as adrenaline (epinephrine) are used with a local anaesthetic for surface or infiltration anaesthesia, or nerve block and anecdotal evidence suggests that concurrent use is common; however, it would still seem advisable to be aware of the potential for interaction. The effects of phenylephrine given orally or as nasal drops does not appear to have been studied. Nevertheless, one manufacturer of an eye drop preparation contraindicates concurrent use.

Iron

Iron + Levodopa

The absorption of levodopa can be reduced by 30 to 50% by ferrous sulfate due to levodopa chelation. Therefore all iron compounds are expected to act similarly. Carbidopa levels are also reduced by iron. There is some evidence that this interaction causes a decrease in symptom control.

Be alert for any signs of reduced levodopa efficacy. If this occurs, separating the administration of the iron as much as possible seems likely to be an effective way of managing this interaction.

Iron + Levothyroxine

Ferrous sulfate (and therefore probably other iron compounds) causes a reduction in the effects of levothyroxine.

Be alert for this effect if both drugs are given, and monitor thyroid hormone levels if an interaction is suspected: adjust the levothyroxine dose accordingly.

Iron + Methyldopa

The antihypertensive effects of methyldopa can be reduced by ferrous sulfate or ferrous gluconate. Most other iron compounds are expected to interact similarly.

Monitor the effects of concurrent use and increase the methyldopa dose as necessary. Separating the dosages by up to 2 hours apparently only partially reduces the effects of this interaction.

Iron + Mycophenolate

One study found that oral iron compounds markedly reduced the absorption of mycophenolate. However, four subsequent studies, including one of identical design to the first study, found that oral iron compounds had no significant effect on the absorption of mycophenolate.

On balance, it would appear that oral iron compounds do not alter the pharmacokinetics of mycophenolate, and that no special precautions are required on concurrent use.

Iron + Penicillamine

The absorption of penicillamine can be reduced as much as two-thirds by oral iron.

For maximal absorption give the iron at least 2 hours after the penicillamine. Do not stop iron suddenly in a patient stabilised on penicillamine as the marked increase in absorption that follows may precipitate penicillamine toxicity.

Iron + **Proton pump inhibitors**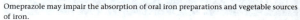

Omeprazole may impair the absorption of oral iron preparations and vegetable sources of iron.

> Many factors and disease states can affect oral iron absorption. However bear these reports in mind should a patient taking any proton pump inhibitor fail to respond to treatment with oral iron.

Iron + **Quinolones**

Iron compounds reduce the absorption of many of the quinolones. In descending order the extent of the interaction appears to be: norfloxacin, levofloxacin, ciprofloxacin, moxifloxacin, gatifloxacin, ofloxacin/sparfloxacin. Serum levels of the antibacterial may become subtherapeutic as a result.

> Most quinolones should not be taken at the same time as iron. As the quinolones are rapidly absorbed, taking them 2 hours before the iron should largely avoid this interaction. The exceptions are fleroxacin, which appears not to interact, and lomefloxacin, which seems to interact only minimally.

Iron + **Tetracyclines**

The absorption of the tetracyclines is markedly reduced by concurrent use. Tetracycline levels are reduced by 30 to 90% and their therapeutic effectiveness may be reduced or even abolished. The absorption of iron may also be reduced.

> The extent of the reductions depends on a number of factors.

- the particular tetracycline used: tetracycline and oxytetracycline were affected the least in one study.
- the time interval between the administration of the two drugs: giving the iron 3 hours before or 2 to 3 hours after the antibacterial is satisfactory with tetracycline, but one study found that even 11 hours was inadequate for doxycycline.
- the particular iron compound used: the reduction in tetracycline levels with ferrous sulfate was 80 to 90%; with ferrous fumarate, succinate and gluconate, 70 to 80%; with ferrous tartrate, 50%; and with ferrous sodium edetate, 30%. This was with doses containing equivalent amounts of elemental iron.

The interaction can therefore be accommodated by separating the doses as much as possible. It would also seem logical to choose one of the iron preparations causing minimal interference, but it seems unlikely that there will be a clinically significant difference between those that are commonly available (i.e. sulfate, fumarate and gluconate).

Isoniazid

Isoniazid + Levodopa

Levodopa-induced dyskinesias are improved by isoniazid, but the control of Parkinson's disease is worsened. This may take several weeks to develop.

The combination need not be avoided, but be aware that an adjustment in treatment may be needed if parkinsonism deteriorates.

Isoniazid + Paracetamol (Acetaminophen)

Hepatotoxicity has been seen with the combination of isoniazid and paracetamol, usually in patients who have taken more than 4 g of paracetamol daily, but occasionally in those taking normal doses.

A cautious approach would be to limit paracetamol intake, but information is very limited and more study is needed to confirm any interaction.

Isoniazid + Phenytoin

Phenytoin levels can be raised by isoniazid and some patients may develop toxicity. If both rifampicin (rifampin) and isoniazid are given, phenytoin levels may fall in patients who are fast acetylators of isoniazid, but may occasionally rise in those who are slow acetylators (said to be about 50% of the population).

It is unlikely that the acetylator status of the patient will be known. Therefore monitor phenytoin adverse effects (e.g. blurred vision, nystagmus, ataxia or drowsiness) and phenytoin levels and adjust the dose accordingly. In some patients the interaction has taken several weeks to develop.

Isoniazid + Theophylline

Two short-term studies found that theophylline levels were slightly increased by isoniazid and a case of theophylline toxicity supports this finding. However, another short-term study found that isoniazid slightly increased theophylline clearance.

The outcome of concurrent use is uncertain but it would be prudent to be alert for any evidence of increased theophylline levels and toxicity if isoniazid is given. It may take 3 to 4 weeks for this interaction to develop.

Isotretinoin

Isotretinoin + Tetracyclines ✗

The development of 'pseudotumour cerebri' (benign intracranial hypertension) has been associated with the concurrent use of isotretinoin and tetracyclines.

> The manufacturers of isotretinoin contraindicate its use with tetracyclines.

Isotretinoin + Vitamin A ⚠

A condition similar to vitamin A (retinol) overdose may occur if isotretinoin and vitamin A are given concurrently.

> The manufacturers of isotretinoin state that high doses of vitamin A (more than 4000 to 5000 units daily, the recommended daily allowance) should be avoided.

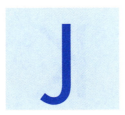

No interactions have been included for drugs beginning with the letter J.

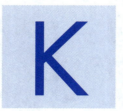

Kaolin

Kaolin + Quinidine

Limited evidence from single-dose studies suggests that kaolin-pectin may reduce the absorption of quinidine and lower its levels (salivary concentration reduced by about 50%; which correlates with serum levels).

Be alert for the need to increase the quinidine dose if kaolin-pectin is used concurrently.

Kaolin + Tetracyclines

Kaolin-pectin reduces the absorption of tetracycline by about 50%.

If these two drugs are given together, consider separating the doses by at least 2 hours to minimise admixture in the gut. Information about other tetracyclines is lacking, but be alert for them to interact similarly.

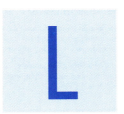

Lamotrigine

Lamotrigine + **Oxcarbazepine**

Oxcarbazepine appears to lower lamotrigine levels by about 15 to 75%. Lamotrigine appears to increase the levels of the active metabolite of oxcarbazepine. Not all studies have found these effects.

> The clinical relevance of any interaction is uncertain, but it seems possible that some patients will have significantly reduced lamotrigine levels. Monitor concurrent use carefully, being aware that dose adjustments may be necessary. The importance of the increase in oxcarbazepine metabolite levels is less clear.

Lamotrigine + **Phenobarbital**

Phenobarbital has been associated with reduced lamotrigine levels (reduction of about 50% in one study). Lamotrigine does not appear to affect phenobarbital or primidone levels.

> Phenobarbital induces the metabolism of lamotrigine, and the recommended starting dose and long-term maintenance dose of lamotrigine in patients already taking phenobarbital or primidone is twice that of patients receiving lamotrigine monotherapy. However, note that if they are also taking valproate in addition to phenobarbital, the lamotrigine dose should be reduced.

Lamotrigine + **Phenytoin**

Phenytoin has been associated with reduced lamotrigine levels (reduction of almost two-thirds in one study). Lamotrigine has no effect on phenytoin levels.

> Phenytoin (and therefore probably fosphenytoin) induces the metabolism of lamotrigine, and the recommended starting dose and long-term maintenance dose of lamotrigine in patients already taking phenytoin is twice that of patients receiving lamotrigine monotherapy. However, note that if they are also taking valproate in addition to phenytoin, the lamotrigine dose should be reduced.

Lamotrigine + **Protease inhibitors**

Ritonavir-boosted atazanavir, lopinavir and saquinavir moderately reduce lamotrigine levels, whereas the protease inhibitor levels did not appear to be altered. Reduced lamotrigine levels should be anticipated with any ritonavir-boosted regimen.

> Lamotrigine efficacy should be monitored in patients taking any ritonavir-boosted regimen (seizures have occurred as a result of this interaction). Anticipate the need to increase the lamotrigine dose.

Lamotrigine + **Rifampicin (Rifampin)**

Rifampicin increases the clearance of lamotrigine and reduces its AUC by 97% and 44%, respectively. A lamotrigine dose increase was required in one case report.

> Information is limited but rifampicin could reduce the efficacy of lamotrigine. Monitor the patient and increase the lamotrigine dose if required.

Lamotrigine + **Valproate**

The levels of lamotrigine can be increased by sodium valproate. Small increases, decreases or no changes in sodium valproate levels have been seen with lamotrigine. Concurrent use has been associated with skin rashes and other toxic reactions.

> Monitor the outcome of concurrent use. The lamotrigine dose should be reduced by about half when valproate is added to avoid possible toxicity (sedation, tremor, ataxia, fatigue, rash). In patients already taking valproate, the manufacturer of lamotrigine recommends a lamotrigine starting dose that is half that of lamotrigine monotherapy, irrespective of whether they are also receiving enzyme-inducing antiepileptics, and a very gradual dose titration. The development of rashes should be investigated promptly.

Lanthanum

Lanthanum + **Levothyroxine**

Lanthanum carbonate decreases levothyroxine absorption and the reduced thyroxine levels that result seem likely to be of clinical importance.

> Other absorption interactions of lanthanum can be minimised by separating the doses by 2 hours. Even so, the outcome should be monitored so that any necessary thyroid hormone dose adjustments can be made.

Lanthanum + **Tetracyclines**

The bioavailability of tetracyclines is expected to be reduced by lanthanum, as

L

concurrent use may result in the formation of insoluble chelates (as with other polyvalent cations).

It is recommended that tetracycline are not taken within 2 hours of a dose of lanthanum.

Leflunomide

Leflunomide + Methotrexate

Although no pharmacokinetic interaction appears to occur between methotrexate and leflunomide, elevated liver enzyme levels have been seen.

The UK manufacturers state that concurrent use is not advisable. The US manufacturers state that if concurrent use is undertaken, monitoring should be increased to monthly intervals. Close liver enzyme monitoring is also recommended if switching between these drugs, and colestyramine or activated charcoal washout recommended as it may reduce the risk of toxicity when switching from leflunomide to methotrexate.

Leflunomide + Penicillamine

The manufacturers state that the concurrent use of leflunomide and penicillamine has not yet been studied but it would be expected to increase the risk of serious adverse reactions (haematological toxicity or hepatotoxicity).

The manufacturers advise avoiding concurrent use. As the active metabolite of leflunomide has a long half-life of 1 to 4 weeks, a washout of colestyramine or activated charcoal is recommended if patients are to be switched to other DMARDs as this may reduce the risk of toxicity.

Leflunomide + Phenytoin

In vitro studies have found that the active metabolite of leflunomide is an inhibitor of CYP2C9, the isoenzyme concerned with the metabolism of phenytoin and fosphenytoin.

Although no cases of phenytoin toxicity appear to have been reported as a result of this interaction, caution is advisable, especially as leflunomide has, in practice, been seen to inhibit the metabolism of other CYP2C9 substrates. Monitor for phenytoin toxicity (e.g. blurred vision, nystagmus, ataxia or drowsiness) and take levels as necessary. Adjust the phenytoin dose accordingly.

Leflunomide + Rifampicin (Rifampin)

Rifampicin increases the levels of the active metabolite of leflunomide by 40%.

There would seem to be no reason for avoiding concurrent use, but the

L

manufacturers advise caution as levels may build up over time. It may be prudent to increase the frequency of leflunomide monitoring if these two drugs are used together.

Leflunomide + Vaccines ❌

The body's immune response is suppressed by leflunomide. The antibody response to vaccines may be reduced and the use of live attenuated vaccines may result in generalised infection.

For many inactivated vaccines even the reduced response seen is considered clinically useful and, in the case of renal transplant patients, influenza vaccination is actively recommended. If a vaccine is given, it may be prudent to monitor the response, so that alternative prophylactic measures can be considered where the response is inadequate. Note that even where effective antibody titres are produced, these may not persist as long as in healthy subjects, and more frequent booster doses may be required. The use of live vaccines is generally considered to be contraindicated. Ideally vaccines should take place before immunosuppressive treatment is started, and live vaccines should not be given for up to 6 months after treatment has stopped.

Leflunomide + Warfarin and other oral anticoagulants ⚠

Leflunomide appears to raise the INR of patients taking warfarin. Case reports describe bleeding, and INRs as high as 6 and 11. Other coumarins may be similarly affected.

It would seem prudent to closely monitor the INR of any patient taking a coumarin who starts taking leflunomide.

Levodopa

Levodopa + MAOIs ❌

A rapid, serious and potentially life-threatening hypertensive reaction can occur in patients taking MAOIs if they are also given levodopa.

An interaction with levodopa given with carbidopa or benserazide is unlikely. Even so, the manufacturers continue to list the MAOIs among their contraindications and say that patients should not be given levodopa during treatment with MAOIs, nor for 14 days after an MAOI has been stopped.

Levodopa + Methyldopa ⚠

Methyldopa can increase the effects of levodopa. This has allowed a dose reduction of about 30 to 70% in some patients taking levodopa alone, but the benefit may only be temporary and dyskinesias may be worsened in some patients. A small increase in the hypotensive actions of methyldopa may also occur, see also Antihypertensives, page 89.

> This interaction is expected to be minimised in the presence of carbidopa or benserazide and so it seems unlikely that a dose reduction of levodopa would usually be required. The increased hypotensive effects seem to be small, but be aware they are possible.

Levodopa + Metoclopramide

Metoclopramide is a centrally-acting dopamine antagonist, which can oppose the effects of levodopa and worsen Parkinson's disease. It also stimulates gastric emptying and this may lead to a small increase in the bioavailability of levodopa.

> Concurrent use should generally be avoided. However if concurrent use of metoclopramide is essential, monitor the outcome closely. Note that domperidone is the antiemetic of choice in Parkinson's disease.

Levodopa + Penicillamine

Penicillamine can raise levodopa levels in some patients. This may improve the control of the parkinsonism but the adverse effects of levodopa may also be increased.

> Concurrent use need not be avoided, but monitor for an increase in the adverse effects of levodopa.

Levodopa + Phenytoin

The therapeutic effects of levodopa can be reduced or abolished by phenytoin.

> Evidence is limited (effects in 5 patients only). If concurrent use is necessary, it would seem prudent to monitor concurrent use for any evidence of reduced levodopa efficacy. It seems possible that fosphenytoin, a prodrug of phenytoin, could have similar effects.

Levodopa + Pyridoxine ❓

The effects of levodopa are reduced or abolished by pyridoxine, but this interaction does not occur when levodopa is given with the dopa-decarboxylase inhibitors carbidopa or benserazide, as is usual clinical practice.

> In the rare cases that levodopa is used alone, pyridoxine in doses as low as 5 mg daily can reduce the effects of levodopa and should therefore be avoided. Warn patients about proprietary pyridoxine-containing preparations such as multi-vitamins and supplements. There is no evidence to suggest that a low-pyridoxine diet is desirable.

L

Levodopa + SSRIs

The use of an SSRI is often beneficial in patients with Parkinson's disease taking levodopa. However, sometimes parkinsonian symptoms are worsened.

> In some cases parkinsonism can, rarely, be worsened by SSRIs. Concurrent use is valuable and need not be avoided, but monitor the outcome and withdraw the SSRI if necessary.

Levothyroxine

Levothyroxine + Orlistat

Orlistat may decrease the absorption of levothyroxine. This resulted in hypothyroidism in one patient.

> One manufacturer of levothyroxine recommends that the administration of levothyroxine and orlistat should be separated by 4 hours. It may be prudent to monitor the response to concurrent use, to ensure that this is effective.

Levothyroxine + Phenobarbital

An isolated report describes a reduction in the response to levothyroxine in a patient given secobarbital with amobarbital. It seems possible that all barbiturates may interact in this way. Note that phenobarbital has been shown to reduce the levels of endogenous thyroid hormones in some studies.

> The general importance of this interaction is almost certainly small, but be alert for any evidence of changes in thyroid status if barbiturates are added or withdrawn from patients taking levothyroxine. Monitor thyroid hormones levels if an interaction is suspected, and adjust the levothyroxine dose accordingly.

Levothyroxine + Phenytoin

An isolated report describes a patient, previously well maintained on levothyroxine, who developed clinical hypothyroidism when also given phenytoin. Phenytoin can reduce endogenous thyroid hormone levels, but clinical hypothyroidism caused by an interaction seems to be rare.

> The general importance of this interaction seems small, but be alert for any evidence of changes in thyroid status if phenytoin is added or withdrawn from patients taking levothyroxine. Monitor thyroid hormones levels if an interaction is suspected and adjust the levothyroxine dose accordingly.

Levothyroxine + Protease inhibitors

Isolated case reports describe increased levothyroxine dose requirements in patients given ritonavir-boosted lopinavir, ritonavir-boosted saquinavir, nelfinavir and possibly indinavir, but one report describes decreased levothyroxine requirements in a patient given indinavir.

> Direct information is limited and the presence of an interaction seems to depend on the individual protease inhibitor, how it affects glucuronidation, and how much remaining thyroid function a patient has. Until more is known about this interaction it would seem prudent to monitor thyroid function more closely if a protease inhibitor is given to a patient with pre-existing thyroid dysfunction.

Levothyroxine + Raloxifene

Two patients developed increased levothyroxine requirements after taking raloxifene for a number of months.

> Consider monitor TSH levels if both drugs are given, especially if symptoms of hypothyroidism develop. If TSH levels are raised, try separating administration by 12 hours before increasing the levothyroxine dose.

Levothyroxine + Rifampicin (Rifampin)

Two case reports suggest that rifampicin might possibly reduce the effects of thyroid hormones.

> The evidence for this interaction is by no means conclusive. Bear this interaction in mind if rifampicin is given to a patient taking levothyroxine. If symptoms of hypothyroidism develop, monitor thyroid hormone levels, and adjust the dose of levothyroxine accordingly.

Levothyroxine + Sevelamer

Sevelamer decreases levothyroxine absorption and appears to increase levothyroxine requirements.

> It would be prudent to monitor levothyroxine requirements in patients requiring sevelamer. Whether separation of administration would minimise any interaction remains to be demonstrated, but, where absorption is a problem, the manufacturers generally recommend avoiding giving other drugs at least 1 hour before or 3 hours after sevelamer.

Levothyroxine + SSRIs

The concurrent use of sertraline may oppose the effects of levothyroxine (TSH levels elevated) in some patients.

> These cases draw attention to the need to monitor the effects of giving sertraline to

L

patients taking thyroid hormones, the dose of which may need to be increased. However, note that this interaction seems relatively rare.

Levothyroxine + Sucralfate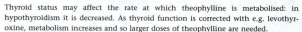

Sucralfate may reduce levothyroxine absorption, but not all studies have found this effect.

An interaction is not established; however, it might be prudent to avoid taking sucralfate until a few hours after levothyroxine. Patients should be advised accordingly and the response well monitored.

Levothyroxine + Theophylline

Thyroid status may affect the rate at which theophylline is metabolised: in hypothyroidism it is decreased. As thyroid function is corrected with e.g. levothyroxine, metabolism increases and so larger doses of theophylline are needed.

Monitor the outcome of resolving hypothyroidism, checking that the effects of theophylline are adequate. Monitor theophylline levels as necessary and adjust the theophylline dose as necessary.

Levothyroxine + Tricyclics

The antidepressant response to imipramine, amitriptyline and possibly other tricyclics can be accelerated by the use of thyroid hormones. Isolated cases of paroxysmal atrial tachycardia, thyrotoxicosis and hypothyroidism have been attributed to concurrent use.

These apparent interactions remain unexplained and concurrent use seems generally advantageous. Unless problems arise there would seem to be no good reason for avoiding concurrent use.

Levothyroxine + Warfarin and other oral anticoagulants

The anticoagulant effects of acenocoumarol, phenindione, and warfarin are increased by thyroid hormones and bleeding has been seen. This is largely due to alteration of thyroid function, rather than a direct drug-drug interaction.

Hypothyroid patients taking an anticoagulant who are subsequently given thyroid hormones as replacement therapy will need a downward adjustment of the anticoagulant dose as treatment proceeds. Monitor the INR (weekly has been suggested) until patients are euthyroid, and adjust the coumarin or indanedione dose as necessary.

L

Lidocaine

Lidocaine + Phenobarbital

Lidocaine levels, following slow intravenous injection, may be up to about 30% lower in patients who are taking phenobarbital. It seems likely that other barbiturates will interact similarly.

> It may be necessary to increase the dose of lidocaine to achieve the desired therapeutic response in patients taking phenobarbital or other barbiturates.

Lidocaine + Phenytoin

The incidence of central adverse effects may be increased following the concurrent use of lidocaine and phenytoin. Sinoatrial arrest has been reported in one patient receiving the combination. Lidocaine levels may be reduced by phenytoin. Fosphenytoin, a prodrug of phenytoin, may interact similarly.

> The clinical significance of this interaction is most likely to be small. However, the sinoatrial arrest emphasises the need to exercise caution when giving two drugs that have cardiodepressant actions.

Lidocaine + Protease inhibitors

Ritonavir may increase levels of lidocaine more than 3-fold, which would be expected to increase the risk of lidocaine adverse effects, including arrhythmias. Other protease inhibitors may interact similarly.

> The manufacturers of darunavir, indinavir, nelfinavir and tipranavir contraindicate the concurrent use either of lidocaine, or of drugs with a narrow therapeutic range that are metabolised by CYP3A4, which could reasonably be expected to include lidocaine. If concurrent use cannot be avoided, it would seem prudent to monitor closely for lidocaine adverse effects (e.g. light-headedness, paraesthesia), monitoring lidocaine levels if possible. Reduce the lidocaine dose as necessary.

Linezolid

L

Linezolid is a non-selective, reversible inhibitor of MAO, and it therefore shares some of the interactions of the MAOIs. However, its effects are weak, and serious adverse interactions of the magnitude seen with the MAOIs do not seem to occur. However, some caution is prudent if linezolid is given with drugs that interact with MAOIs.

Linezolid + MAO-B inhibitors ❌

The manufacturers of linezolid state that its effects are likely to be additive with any other drug that inhibits MAO-B.

The use of linezolid is contraindicated with and with 2 weeks of the use of any drug with MAO-inhibitory effects.

Linezolid + MAOIs ❌

The manufacturers of linezolid state that its effects are likely to be additive with any other drug that inhibits either MAO-A or MAO-B, because their MAO-inhibitory activities are predicted to be additive.

The use of linezolid is contraindicated with and with 2 weeks of the use of any drug with MAO-inhibitory effects.

Linezolid + Mirtazapine ❌

In theory the use of mirtazapine and linezolid may result in serotonin syndrome. One patient developed symptoms similar to serotonin syndrome, page 454 while taking these drugs.

The UK manufacturer of linezolid contraindicates the concurrent use of serotonergic drugs unless it is essential. If concurrent use is necessary, patients should have their blood pressure monitored and be closely observed.

Linezolid + Moclobemide ❌

The manufacturers of linezolid state that its effects are likely to be additive with any other drug that inhibits MAO-A, because their MAO-inhibitory activities are predicted to be additive.

The use of linezolid is contraindicated with and within 2 weeks of the use of any drug with MAO-inhibitory effects.

Linezolid + Nasal decongestants ❌

Because of its weak MAO-inhibitory properties, the manufacturers of linezolid predict its use with drugs such as phenylpropanolamine and pseudoephedrine will result in raised blood pressure. However, the evidence available suggests that blood pressure rises are only very moderate and certainly unlikely to be of the hypertensive crisis proportions seen with the antidepressant MAOIs.

The manufacturers contraindicate the use of pseudoephedrine and phenylpropanolamine with linezolid unless there are facilities available for close observation of the patient and monitoring of blood pressure. In addition, they advise careful dose titration. Patients should be warned about cough and cold remedies containing these and related drugs.

L

Linezolid + Opioids

The use of pethidine (meperidine) with MAOIs has resulted in a potentially life-threatening reaction in a few patients. Excitement, muscle rigidity, hyperpyrexia, flushing, sweating and unconsciousness occur very rapidly. Respiratory depression and hypotension have also been seen. Because linezolid has weak MAOI properties the manufacturers predict it may interact similarly. A case report supports this prediction.

> Avoid concurrent use unless facilities are available for close observation and monitoring of blood pressure.

Linezolid + SSRIs

Several case reports describe the development of serotonin syndrome in patients given linezolid with SSRIs (citalopram, escitalopram, fluoxetine, paroxetine and sertraline are implicated).

> The interaction is probably rare. The manufacturers of linezolid contraindicate concurrent use unless patients are closely observed for serotonin syndrome and have their blood pressure monitored. See serotonin syndrome, page 454 for more information.

Linezolid + Tricyclics

Serotonin syndrome, page 454, is predicted to occur when linezolid is used with tricyclics.

> The UK manufacturer contraindicates concurrent use unless patients are closely observed for serotonin syndrome and have their blood pressure monitored.

Linezolid + Venlafaxine ⊗

In theory the use of venlafaxine and linezolid may result in serotonin syndrome, page 454. Case reports describe a number of patients who developed symptoms similar to serotonin syndrome while taking these drugs.

> The interaction is probably rare. The UK manufacturer contraindicates concurrent use unless patients are closely observed for signs and symptoms of serotonin syndrome, and have their blood pressure monitored.

Lithium

Lithium is given under close supervision with regular monitoring of serum concentrations because there is a narrow margin between therapeutic concentrations and those that are toxic. The dose of lithium is adjusted to give levels of 0.4 to 1 mmol/L, although it should be noted that this is the range used in the UK, and other ranges have been quoted. Initially weekly monitoring is advised, dropping to every 3 months for those on stable regimens. It is usual to take lithium samples about 10 to 12 hours after the last oral dose. Adverse effects that are not usually considered serious include nausea, weakness, fine tremor, mild polydipsia and polyuria. If levels rise into the 1.5 to 2 mmol/L range, toxicity usually occurs, and may present as lethargy, drowsiness, coarse hand tremor, lack of coordination, muscular weakness, increased nausea and vomiting, or diarrhoea. Higher levels result in neurotoxicity, which manifests as ataxia, giddiness, tinnitus, confusion, dysarthria, muscle twitching, nystagmus, and even coma or seizures. Cardiovascular symptoms may also develop and include ECG changes and circulatory problems, and there may be a worsening of polyuria. Virtually all of the reports are concerned with the carbonate, but sometimes lithium is given as other compounds. There is no reason to believe that these lithium compounds will interact any differently to lithium carbonate.

Lithium + Maprotiline

The concurrent use of *tricyclic antidepressants* and lithium has been successful but some patients may develop adverse effects. Serotonin syndrome, page 454, and neuroleptic malignant syndrome have been reported. One study suggests that maprotiline interacts similarly.

> If both drugs are used monitor for any evidence of neurotoxicity.

Lithium + Methyldopa

Symptoms of lithium toxicity, not always associated with raised lithium levels, have been described in patients and healthy subjects when they were also given methyldopa.

> If both drugs are given, the effects should be closely monitored (see lithium, page 355). Monitoring lithium levels may be unreliable because symptoms of toxicity can occur even though the levels remain within the normally accepted therapeutic range.

Lithium + Metronidazole

The lithium levels of 3 patients were raised following the use of metronidazole. However, 2 of these patients had evidence of renal impairment, and one other report describes safe concurrent use.

> Some have recommended that a reduction in the lithium dose should be considered, especially in patients maintained at relatively high lithium levels. Patients taking lithium should be aware of the symptoms of lithium toxicity (see lithium, page 355) and told to report them immediately should they occur. This should be reinforced when they are given metronidazole.

Lithium + NSAIDs

NSAIDs may increase lithium levels leading to toxicity, but there is great variability between different NSAIDs and also between individuals taking the same NSAID. For example, studies have found that celecoxib causes a modest 17% increase in lithium levels, yet case reports describe increases of up to about 350%. Similar effects occur with other NSAIDs, and it seems likely that all NSAIDs will interact similarly. However, note that sulindac seems unique in that it is the only NSAID that has been reported to also cause a *decrease* in lithium levels.

> NSAIDs should be avoided, especially if other risk factors for lithium toxicity (such as advanced age, impaired renal function, decreased sodium intake, volume depletion, renal artery stenosis, and heart failure) are present, unless lithium levels can be very well monitored (initially every few days) and the lithium dose reduced appropriately. Patients taking lithium should be aware of the symptoms of lithium toxicity (see lithium, page 355) and told to report them immediately should they occur. This should be reinforced when they are given an NSAID.

Lithium + Phenytoin

Lithium toxicity has been seen in patients also taking phenytoin.

> The interaction is not well established. Patients taking lithium should be aware of the symptoms of lithium toxicity (see lithium, page 355) and told to immediately report them should they occur. This should be reinforced when they are given phenytoin. Increased lithium monitoring does not appear to be of value in this situation as the interaction occurred in patients with lithium levels within the normally accepted range.

Lithium + Sibutramine

There are no reports of adverse reactions between sibutramine and lithium but the US manufacturers have warned that concurrent use may theoretically lead to the potentially fatal serotonin syndrome.

> Serotonin syndrome appears to occur rarely with other serotonergic drugs and lithium. If concurrent use is considered necessary, monitor closely for symptoms of serotonin syndrome, page 454. If these symptoms occur treatment should be withdrawn.

Lithium + SSRIs

The concurrent use of lithium and SSRIs can be advantageous and uneventful, but various kinds of neurotoxicities have occurred. Isolated reports describe the development of symptoms similar to those of serotonin syndrome in patients taking lithium with fluoxetine, fluvoxamine, paroxetine and possibly citalopram. In addition, fluoxetine appears to have caused increases and decreases in lithium levels.

> If lithium is used with an SSRI be alert for any evidence of toxicity (see serotonin syndrome, page 454). If these symptoms occur treatment should be withdrawn.

Lithium + Theophylline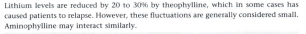

Lithium levels are reduced by 20 to 30% by theophylline, which in some cases has caused patients to relapse. However, these fluctuations are generally considered small. Aminophylline may interact similarly.

> Monitor lithium levels if theophylline or aminophylline is also given, and adjust the lithium dose if necessary. Note that, in rare cases lithium has been associated

L

with QT prolongation. In theory, this may be exacerbated by hypokalaemia caused by the xanthines. For more information, see Drugs that prolong the QT interval, page 277.

Lithium + Tricyclics ⚠

The concurrent use of a tricyclic antidepressant and lithium can be beneficial in some patients. However, some patients may rarely develop adverse effects, a few of them severe. Cases of neurotoxicity, serotonin syndrome and neuroleptic malignant syndrome have been reported.

If both drugs are used be alert for any evidence of neurotoxicity (see under serotonin syndrome, page 454).

Lithium + Triptans ❓

Case reports describe the development of serotonin syndrome in patients taking sumatriptan and lithium. This is in line with the known effects of lithium and the triptans.

If lithium is used with any triptan be alert for any evidence of toxicity (see serotonin syndrome, page 454). If these symptoms occur treatment should be withdrawn.

Lithium + Venlafaxine ⚠

Studies suggest that no clinical pharmacokinetic interaction appears to occur if venlafaxine is given with lithium. However, serotonin syndrome has been reported in some patients on concurrent use.

If both drugs are used, monitor for any evidence of neurotoxicity (see under serotonin syndrome, page 454).

Loperamide

Loperamide + Protease inhibitors ❓

Loperamide reduces the bioavailability of saquinavir by about 50%. Ritonavir increases the levels of loperamide without increasing its CNS adverse effects, and saquinavir similarly increases the bioavailability of loperamide by about 40%. Conversely, tipranavir alone, and in combination with ritonavir, *reduces* the bioavailability and levels of loperamide and its metabolites.

Monitor patients to ensure that saquinavir remains effective. The increase in loperamide bioavailability is not expected to be clinically significant in the case of saquinavir and ritonavir. The clinical relevance of the decrease in loperamide bioavailability with tipranavir alone or ritonavir-boosted tipranavir is unknown,

L

but may not be important as loperamide is thought to have a local action in the gut.

Loperamide + Quinidine

Quinidine increases absorption of loperamide into the brain resulting in respiratory depression.

Be alert for the CNS adverse effects of loperamide (such as drowsiness) if quinidine is given. If adverse effects are troublesome consider reducing the dose of loperamide.

Low-molecular-weight heparins

Low-molecular-weight heparins + NSAIDs

Ketorolac

The effects of low-molecular-weight-heparins can be increased by other drugs that affect anticoagulation, platelet function or increase the risks of bleeding, such as NSAIDs. Cases of severe bleeding and prolonged bleeding times have been reported with ketorolac. Concurrent use is considered to be a contributing factor in the development of spinal or epidural haematoma occurring after lumbar puncture.

The CSM in the UK and the UK manufacturers say that ketorolac is contraindicated with anticoagulants. Conversely, the US manufacturers of ketorolac advise that physicians should carefully weigh the benefits against the risks and use heparins with ketorolac only extremely cautiously. Extreme caution is needed if concurrent use is considered appropriate in patients undergoing epidural anaesthesia.

Other NSAIDs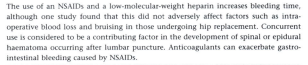

The use of an NSAIDs and a low-molecular-weight heparin increases bleeding time, although one study found that this did not adversely affect factors such as intra-operative blood loss and bruising in those undergoing hip replacement. Concurrent use is considered to be a contributing factor in the development of spinal or epidural haematoma occurring after lumbar puncture. Anticoagulants can exacerbate gastro-intestinal bleeding caused by NSAIDs.

Concurrent use is not uncommon, but prescribers should be aware that there is an increased risk of bleeding and monitor appropriately. Extreme caution is needed if concurrent use is considered appropriate in patients undergoing epidural anaes-thesia.

L

Low-molecular-weight heparins + Prasugrel

In phase III studies, no clinically significant interaction was reported when low-molecular-weight heparins were given with prasugrel. Nevertheless, due to the actions of both drugs there is a possible increased risk of bleeding on concurrent use. Furthermore, the use of prasugrel and heparin may contribute to the development of epidural or spinal haematoma after epidural anaesthesia.

> Be aware of the potential for this interaction if bleeding occurs. Extreme caution is needed if concurrent use is considered appropriate in patients undergoing epidural anaesthesia.

Low-molecular-weight heparins + Ticlopidine

Concurrent use of ticlopidine with a low-molecular-weight heparin increases haemorrhagic risk. The risk of epidural or spinal haematomas with a low-molecular-weight heparin may be increased if they are used concurrently with other drugs affecting haemostasis, such as antiplatelet drugs.

> If concurrent use is undertaken, there should be close clinical and laboratory monitoring. Extreme caution is needed if concurrent use is considered appropriate in patients undergoing epidural or spinal anaesthesia.

Lumefantrine

Lumefantrine + Tricyclics

The manufacturer of a preparation containing artemether with lumefantrine notes that *in vitro* data indicate that lumefantrine significantly inhibits CYP2D6. As a consequence, they contraindicate the use of artemether with lumefantrine in patients taking any drug that is metabolised by CYP2D6 (they include imipramine, amitriptyline, and clomipramine as examples).

> These contraindications seem unnecessarily restrictive, especially as the tricyclics are not contraindicated with other established inhibitors of CYP2D6. Until more is known, it would be prudent to closely monitor the effects of any CYP2D6 substrate in patients given lumefantrine. However, more seriously, note that additive QT-prolonging effects are possible with some tricyclics and the artemether component, see drugs that prolong the QT interval, page 277.

L

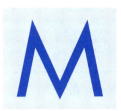

Macrolides

The macrolides are generally considered to be inhibitors of CYP3A4; however, it should be noted that they vary in the strength of their effect. Macrolides that are more potent inhibitors of CYP3A4 are likely to have greater effects on substrates of this isoenzyme, and therefore their use seems more likely to be associated with greater clinical consequences. Clinically, clarithromycin, erythromycin and telithromycin have the greatest effects, and are considered moderate CYP3A4 inhibitors (although note that some consider clarithromycin and telithromycin to be a potent inhibitor); josamycin, midecamycin and roxithromycin have more modest effects, while azithromycin, dirithromycin and spiramycin only inhibit CYP3A4 to a small or clinically irrelevant extent. Note that clarithromycin is often predicted to have a more potent effect on CYP3A4 than erythromycin, but in many clinical studies this has not been shown to be the case, for example, see under phosphodiesterase type-5 inhibitors, page 362.

Macrolides + Mirtazapine

The macrolides are predicted to inhibit the metabolism of mirtazapine by CYP3A4. Other CYP3A4 inhibitors (such as some azoles) have been shown to have this effect.

> The manufacturers advise caution on concurrent use. Monitor for adverse effects (e.g. sedation, fatigue, headache). Note that the macrolides differ in their ability to inhibit CYP3A4, see macrolides, above.

Macrolides + NNRTIs

Delavirdine may increase clarithromycin exposure (AUC doubled), whereas efavirenz, etravirine and nevirapine may reduce clarithromycin exposure (by about 30 to 40%) and increase the levels of the active hydroxy metabolite of clarithromycin. The levels of etravirine are modestly increased by clarithromycin.

> The manufacturer of delavirdine recommends that the dose of clarithromycin need only be reduced in patients with renal impairment. The clinical significance of the reduction in clarithromycin levels with efavirenz, etravirine and nevirapine is unknown and further experience of the use of these NNRTIs with clarithromycin

is needed. Until then, caution is warranted. Alternatives to clarithromycin should be considered, in particular for the treatment of *Mycobacterium avium* complex (MAC) infection. The UK manufacturer advises monitoring liver function tests if nevirapine is given with clarithromycin. The increase in etravirine levels by clarithromycin is not expected to be clinically relevant.

Macrolides + Opioids

Telithromycin inhibits the metabolism of oxycodone (by CYP3A4), leading to an increase in oxycodone levels and effects. Macrolides are predicted to increase the levels of buprenorphine by inhibiting CYP3A4. Other CYP3A4 inhibitors, such as the azoles, page 137 have been shown to interact in this way.

Monitor for an increase in oxycodone adverse effects. An oxycodone dose decrease of 25 to 50% may be necessary, with further titration according to response. There seems to be no information about other macrolides, but several (particularly clarithromycin and erythromycin) are known to inhibit CYP3A4 and may therefore be expected to interact similarly. It has been suggested that the macrolides that are potent CYP3A4 inhibitors (see macrolides, page 361) should be avoided when buprenorphine is used parenterally or sublingually as an analgesic. If concurrent use is essential in opioid addiction the manufacturers suggest that the buprenorphine dose should be halved. Note that additive QT-prolonging effects may occur in predisposed individuals taking macrolides and high-dose methadone, see drugs that prolong the QT interval, page 277.

Macrolides + Phenytoin

Clarithromycin ❓

Limited evidence suggests that clarithromycin may raise phenytoin levels. Fosphenytoin, a prodrug of phenytoin, may interact similarly.

The clinical importance of this interaction is unknown, but bear it in mind in case of an unexpected response to treatment. Indicators of phenytoin toxicity include blurred vision, nystagmus, ataxia or drowsiness. Note that erythromycin does not appear to interact.

Telithromycin ❌

As *rifampicin (rifampin)* reduces telithromycin levels by about 80%, and reduces its efficacy, the manufacturers predict that phenytoin (and therefore probably fosphenytoin, a prodrug of phenytoin) will interact similarly.

The manufacturers state that telithromycin should be avoided during and for up to 2 weeks after phenytoin has been taken. Note that erythromycin does not appear to interact.

Macrolides + Phosphodiesterase type-5 inhibitors

Sildenafil or Vardenafil ⚠

Erythromycin and clarithromycin increase the AUC of sildenafil 2- to 3-fold. It seems

M

likely that telithromycin will interact similarly. Erythromycin increases the AUC of vardenafil 4-fold; it seems likely that clarithromycin and telithromycin will interact similarly.

> Dosing guidance is given as follows:
> Sildenafil for erectile dysfunction – consider a starting dose of 25 mg.
> Sildenafil for pulmonary hypertension – with erythromycin consider reducing the oral sildenafil dose to 20 mg twice daily and the intravenous sildenafil dose to 10 mg twice daily; with clarithromycin or telithromycin 20 mg once daily and the intravenous sildenafil dose to 10 mg daily. However, note that erythromycin had a greater effect than clarithromycin in the studies.
> Vardenafil – the dose of vardenafil should not exceed 5 mg in 24 hours with erythromycin. The dose of vardenafil should not exceed 5 mg in 24 hours (UK) or 2.5 mg in 24 hours with clarithromycin (US). It would seem prudent to follow this advice for telithromycin.

Tadalafil

Erythromycin, clarithromycin, and therefore probably telithromycin, are expected to raise tadalafil levels by inhibiting its metabolism by CYP3A4. This effect has been seen with other inhibitors of CYP3A4 (up to 4-fold rise with ketoconazole). Other macrolides have less effect on CYP3A4, see macrolides, page 361, and therefore seem less likely to interact.

> The adverse effects of tadalafil may be increased in some patients. The manufacturers advise caution.

Macrolides + Protease inhibitors

Azithromycin with Nelfinavir ⚠

The pharmacokinetics of nelfinavir are minimally affected by azithromycin, but the AUC and maximum levels of azithromycin are roughly doubled by nelfinavir.

> The clinical significance of this interaction has not been established. Monitor for increased azithromycin adverse effects.

Clarithromycin with Protease inhibitors ⚠

Atazanavir almost doubled the AUC of clarithromycin, and reduced the AUC of its active metabolite by 70%. Similar, changes have been seen with darunavir, ritonavir-boosted tipranavir and ritonavir, but with these protease inhibitors the levels of the active metabolite of clarithromycin were almost totally abolished. Other ritonavir-boosted protease inhibitors would be expected to interact similarly. Clarithromycin appears to have relatively minor effects on the pharmacokinetics of atazanavir and ritonavir, but almost doubles the minimum levels of tipranavir (given as ritonavir-boosted tipranavir).

> As the levels of 14-hydroxyclarithromycin are significantly reduced it is generally advised that for most infections an alternative to clarithromycin should be considered with the exception of *Mycobacterium avium* complex infections, where this metabolite is inactive. If concurrent use is undertaken, some dose adjustments of the clarithromycin may be needed. Patients with renal impairment: the manufacturers of ritonavir and clarithromycin recommend a 50% reduction in the dose of clarithromycin for those with a creatinine clearance of 30 to 60 mL/minute

and a 75% reduction for clearances of less than 30 mL/minute. Some advise avoiding clarithromycin in doses exceeding 1 g daily. Similar clarithromycin dose reductions in renal impairment are recommended for a number of the ritonavir-boosted protease inhibitors. Patients with normal renal function: although most manufacturers suggest that no dose adjustment is necessary the UK manufacturer of tipranavir advises monitoring clarithromycin adverse effects in those taking a dose of clarithromycin of more than 500 mg twice daily and the US manufacturer of atazanavir suggests that the clarithromycin dose should be reduced by 50%. Note that clarithromycin has been associated with QT prolongation, and rises in its levels may increase this risk.

Erythromycin with Protease inhibitors

The concurrent use of fosamprenavir or amprenavir with erythromycin is predicted to increase the levels of both the protease inhibitor and erythromycin. The manufacturers predict that ritonavir (including ritonavir used to boost the levels of other protease inhibitors) will greatly elevate erythromycin levels. Ritonavir-boosted saquinavir is associated with a high risk of prolonging the QT interval; erythromycin (particularly intravenous erythromycin) may also prolong the QT interval. The manufacturers suggest that a serious prolongation is possible if they are used together.

Carefully monitor the outcome of giving erythromycin with amprenavir or fosamprenavir. Advise patients to be alert for erythromycin and amprenavir or fosamprenavir adverse effects (e.g. gastrointestinal effects, tremors). The concurrent use of erythromycin and ritonavir should not be undertaken unless the benefits outweigh the risks. Monitor for erythromycin adverse effects (e.g. gastrointestinal effects). Note that high levels of erythromycin can cause temporary hearing loss. Because of the potential risks of QT prolongation, one UK manufacturer contraindicates the concurrent use of erythromycin and saquinavir.

Telithromycin with Protease inhibitors

Ketoconazole increases the AUC of telithromycin 2-fold. Therefore the manufacturers predict that the exposure to telithromycin may be greater than 2-fold in the presence of ritonavir. Other protease inhibitors may interact similarly.

The manufacturers advise caution on concurrent use. Monitor for telithromycin adverse effects (such as diarrhoea, dizziness and headache). Note that concurrent use is contraindicated in severe hepatic or renal impairment.

Macrolides + Proton pump inhibitors

Clarithromycin almost doubles the levels of esomeprazole, lansoprazole and omeprazole. A small rise in the levels of clarithromycin also occurs, which may be therapeutically useful. Some very limited evidence indicates that erythromycin raises omeprazole levels, without altering its gastric acid lowering effect.

Given the wide use of *Helicobacter pylori* eradication regimens containing these drugs it seems unlikely that this interaction is detrimental.

Macrolides + Ranolazine

Ketoconazole increases the AUC, peak and trough levels, and half-life of ranolazine

2.5- to 4.5-fold. The dose-related adverse effects of ranolazine such as nausea and dizziness were increased by *ketoconazole*. Further, increases in plasma levels of ranolazine may cause significant QT prolongation and increase the risk of arrhythmias. Clarithromycin and telithromycin are expected to interact in the same way as ketoconazole, and erythromycin may also interact, but to a lesser extent.

The manufacturers of ranolazine contraindicate the concurrent use of clarithromycin, and the UK manufacturer also contraindicates telithromycin. The US manufacturer recommends that the dose of ranolazine should be limited to 500 mg twice daily when given to patients taking erythromycin, whereas the UK manufacturer recommends careful dose titration of ranolazine in patients taking erythromycin. Note that additive QT-prolonging effects may occur in some individuals taking macrolides and ranolazine, see Drugs that prolong the QT interval, page 277.

Macrolides + Reboxetine

The manufacturers predict that macrolides will decrease the clearance of reboxetine by inhibiting CYP3A4. Other CYP3A4 inhibitors have been shown to have this effect.

The manufacturers recommend that macrolides (they specifically name erythromycin) should not be given with reboxetine. Note that the macrolides differ in their ability to inhibit CYP3A4, see macrolides, page 361.

Macrolides + Rifabutin

Azithromycin

The concurrent use of rifabutin and azithromycin does not appear to alter the levels of either drug, but in one study a very high incidence of neutropenia and leucopenia was seen.

Until more information is available it would seem wise to monitor white cell counts during concurrent use.

Clarithromycin

Rifabutin markedly reduces clarithromycin levels, and clarithromycin increases rifabutin levels. There is an increased risk of uveitis and neutropenia with the combination.

Monitor the outcome of concurrent use to ensure treatment with the macrolide is effective. Because of the increased risk of uveitis the CSM in the UK says that consideration should be given to reducing the dose of rifabutin to 300 mg daily. If uveitis occurs the CSM recommends that rifabutin should be stopped and the patient should be referred to an ophthalmologist. Full blood counts should also be monitored with concurrent use.

M

Macrolides + Rifampicin (Rifampin)

Clarithromycin ⚠️

Limited evidence suggests that rifampicin markedly reduces the clarithromycin levels (90% in one study).

> Monitor the outcome of concurrent use to ensure clarithromycin treatment is effective.

Telithromycin ❌

Rifampicin reduces the AUC and maximum levels of telithromycin by 86% and 79% respectively.

> The UK manufacturers recommend that telithromycin should not be given during and for 2 weeks after the use of rifampicin.

Macrolides + Salbutamol (Albuterol) and related bronchodilators ❌

Ketoconazole increases the AUC of inhaled salmeterol 16-fold, which may result in systemic adverse effects adverse effects of salmeterol. Although, clinically significant effects were not seen on blood pressure, heart rate, blood glucose and blood potassium levels, this increase in the exposure to salmeterol increases the risk of QT prolongation. The manufacturers of salmeterol predict that clarithromycin and telithromycin will interact in the same way as *ketoconazole*.

> Avoid unless the benefits outweigh the risks. If clarithromycin or telithromycin and salmeterol are given be alert for salmeterol adverse effects such as hypokalaemia and tachycardia.

Macrolides + Sirolimus ❌

Erythromycin markedly increases sirolimus levels up to fivefold. A case of a marked increase in sirolimus levels and renal impairment has also been reported with clarithromycin.

> The US manufacturer advises avoiding concurrent use of sirolimus with erythromycin whereas the UK manufacturers advise monitoring sirolimus levels and decreasing the dose of both drugs as appropriate. They both state that concurrent use with clarithromycin or telithromycin should be avoided. If any macrolide is considered essential in a patient taking sirolimus, it would be prudent to closely monitor sirolimus levels and decrease the dose accordingly. Note that the macrolides differ in their ability to inhibit CYP3A4, see macrolides, page 361; other macrolides seem less likely to interact.

Macrolides + Solifenacin ⚠️

Ketoconazole increases solifenacin levels 2- to 3-fold by inhibiting CYP3A4. The macrolides inhibit CYP3A4 to varying extents (see macrolides, page 361), and therefore some may be expected to interact similarly.

It is recommended that the daily dose of solifenacin is limited to 5 mg daily in patients taking potent CYP3A4 inhibitors. The concurrent use of solifenacin is contraindicated in patients with severe renal impairment or moderate hepatic impairment who are taking potent CYP3A4 inhibitors. With other CYP3A4 inhibitors it may be prudent to monitor for an increase in fesoterodine adverse effects (e.g. dry mouth, dizziness, insomnia), and consider reducing the fesoterodine dose if these become troublesome.

Macrolides + Statins

Atorvastatin

Clarithromycin and erythromycin moderately raise the levels of atorvastatin. Note that the macrolides differ in their ability to inhibit CYP3A4, see macrolides, page 361; other macrolides may interact similarly but to varying extents.

Concurrent use of atorvastatin with clarithromycin or erythromycin should only be undertaken if the benefits outweigh the risks and lower doses of atorvastatin should be considered. The dose of atorvastatin should not exceed 20 mg daily with clarithromycin or alternatively (for short antibacterial courses) a temporary suspension of treatment with atorvastatin may be considered. Warn patients to be on the look out for symptoms of myopathy (e.g. muscle pain or weakness). Be especially cautious in patients also taking other drugs that interact with statins (e.g. fibrates and diltiazem). Note that the manufacturers of telithromycin contraindicate concurrent use.

Simvastatin or Lovastatin

The levels of simvastatin and lovastatin are increased by clarithromycin, erythromycin, telithromycin and other macrolides that inhibit CYP3A4 (see macrolides, page 361). Rhabdomyolysis has been seen.

Concurrent use is contraindicated and simvastatin and lovastatin should be temporarily withdrawn during short courses of clarithromycin, erythromycin or telithromycin .

Other statins

No interaction of note would be expected between fluvastatin, pravastatin or rosuvastatin and macrolides.

Although no interaction would generally be expected to occur note that there have been case reports of rhabdomyolysis in patients taking statin/macrolide combinations that have been predicted not to interact. Any patient taking a statin should be advised to look out for symptoms of myopathy (e.g. muscle pain or weakness). It may be prudent to reinforce this when macrolides are given.

Macrolides + Tacrolimus

Several patients have had marked increases in tacrolimus levels accompanied by evidence of renal toxicity when they also took erythromycin. The same interaction has been seen in patients given clarithromycin, and is predicted with josamycin. A case of raised tacrolimus levels has been reported with concurrent use of azithromycin.

> Tacrolimus levels and/or effects (e.g. on renal function) should be monitored as a matter of routine, but it may be prudent to increase monitoring if these macrolides are started or stopped. Note that the macrolides differ in their ability to inhibit CYP3A4, see macrolides, page 361.

Macrolides + Theophylline

Erythromycin ⚠

Theophylline levels can be increased by erythromycin and toxicity may develop. The onset may be delayed for 2 to 7 days. Erythromycin levels may be modestly reduced by theophylline.

> Monitor theophylline levels after 48 hours and adjust the dose accordingly. Monitor the effects of erythromycin to ensure that they are adequate. Intravenous erythromycin appears not to be affected.

Other macrolides ❓

Azithromycin, clarithromycin, dirithromycin, josamycin, midecamycin, spiramycin, and telithromycin normally only cause modest changes in theophylline levels or do not interact at all. However, there are unexplained and isolated case reports of theophylline toxicity with josamycin and clarithromycin. Roxithromycin usually has no relevant interaction but a significant increase in theophylline levels was seen in one study.

> The situation with roxithromycin is uncertain as only one study has suggested an interaction, but it would be prudent to be alert for the need to reduce the theophylline dose. It would also seem prudent to monitor the outcome of the use of the other macrolides because a few patients, especially those with theophylline levels at the high end of the therapeutic range, may need some small theophylline dose adjustments. In the case of azithromycin, care should be taken in adjusting the dose based on theophylline levels taken after about 5 days of concurrent use, as they may only be a reflection of a transient drop. In addition, acute infection *per se* may alter theophylline pharmacokinetics.

Macrolides + Tolterodine ⚠

The manufacturers of tolterodine warn that potent CYP3A4 inhibitors (they name clarithromycin and erythromycin) increase the risk of tolterodine toxicity. Other macrolides may also interact, see macrolides, page 361.

> Based on the interactions of other CYP3A4 inhibitors with tolterodine it may be prudent to monitor for adverse effects and to bear in mind the possibility of an interaction if antimuscarinic effects (dry mouth, constipation, drowsiness) are increased. However, note that the UK manufacturers advise avoiding concurrent use, whereas the US manufacturers suggest reducing the tolterodine dose to 1 mg twice daily.

M

Macrolides + **Toremifene**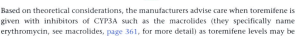

Based on theoretical considerations, the manufacturers advise care when toremifene is given with inhibitors of CYP3A such as the macrolides (they specifically name erythromycin, see macrolides, page 361, for more detail) as toremifene levels may be raised.

It would seem prudent to monitor for toremifene adverse effects (e.g. hot flushes, uterine bleeding, fatigue, nausea, dizziness) on concurrent use with the macrolides. Note that the manufacturers suggest that toremifene is associated with a high risk of QT prolongation and life-threatening arrhythmias. For general information on QT prolongation see drugs that prolong the QT interval, page 277.

Macrolides + **Trazodone**

Clarithromycin impaired the clearance of trazodone and enhanced its sedative effects in a study in healthy subjects.

The UK manufacturer of trazodone recommends that a lower dose of trazodone should be considered if it is given with a CYP3A4 inhibitor such as clarithromycin or erythromycin, but that concurrent use should be avoided where possible. Note that other macrolides may also interact, see macrolides, page 361.

Macrolides + **Triptans**

Erythromycin increased the maximum levels and AUC of eletriptan 2-fold and 3.6-fold, respectively, in one study.

The US manufacturer specifically recommends that eletriptan should not be given within 72 hours of potent CYP3A4 inhibitors, and they specifically name clarithromycin. The UK manufacturer suggests that concurrent use of erythromycin and other macrolide inhibitors of CYP3A4 (such as clarithromycin and telithromycin) should be avoided. Other macrolides seem less likely to interact, see macrolides, page 361.

Macrolides + **Warfarin and other oral anticoagulants**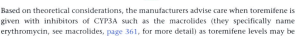

Most controlled studies suggest that macrolides do not cause clinically relevant changes in the pharmacokinetics or anticoagulant effects of warfarin. There is less information about other anticoagulants, but two retrospective studies of acenocoumarol and phenprocoumon have variously shown an increased risk (azithromycin, clarithromycin), a non-significant increased risk (erythromycin) or no increased risk of bleeding (clarithromycin, erythromycin, roxithromycin). Furthermore, a number of case reports describe marked increases in INRs and/or bleeding in patients taking coumarins and macrolides.

The available evidence suggests that, occasionally and unpredictably the effects of warfarin, acenocoumarol or phenprocoumon may be markedly increased by the macrolides. It would therefore be prudent to increase monitoring in all patients when they are first given any macrolide. There is some evidence that this may be particularly important in those who clear warfarin and other anticoagulants slowly

M

and who therefore only need low doses. The elderly in particular would seem to fall into this higher risk category.

Macrolides + Zafirlukast

Erythromycin reduces the mean plasma levels of zafirlukast by about 40%, which may reduce its anti-asthma effects.

If these drugs are given concurrently, be alert for a reduced response; however, note that the manufacturers do not suggest that an alteration in the zafirlukast dose is necessary.

MAO-B inhibitors

MAO-B inhibitors + MAOIs

Severe orthostatic hypotension has been seen in patients given selegiline with MAOIs.

Avoid concurrent use wherever possible. If both drugs are used, monitor initial doses very carefully so hypotension can be rapidly managed. Note that one of the manufacturers of selegiline contraindicates concurrent use and suggests that at least 14 days should elapse between stopping rasagiline and starting an MAOI. The manufacturers of rasagiline contraindicate concurrent use, presumably because of the way selegiline interacts. At least 14 days should elapse between stopping rasagiline and starting an MAOI.

MAO-B inhibitors + Moclobemide

The combination of an MAO-A inhibitor (moclobemide) with an MAO-B inhibitor (selegiline or rasagiline) causes MAO inhibition similar to that seen with the non-selective MAOIs.

Some manufacturers contraindicate concurrent use. If both drugs are given, patients should be given the same dietary restrictions for tyramine-rich foods and drinks (cheese, some wines and beers, etc.), which relate to the non-selective MAOIs. See food, page 301. It is suggested that if selegiline is replaced by moclobemide, the dietary restrictions can be relaxed after a wash-out period of about 2 weeks. If switching from moclobemide to selegiline, a wash-out period of 1 to 2 days is sufficient. Similar advice would seem prudent with rasagiline. Note that all of the interactions of the non-selective MAOIs, are likely to apply to patients taking this combination.

MAO-B inhibitors + Nasal decongestants

An isolated report describes a hypertensive crisis, which was attributed to an

M

interaction between selegiline, ephedrine, and maprotiline. Rasagiline is expected to interact like selegiline.

In general, if selegiline is used at recommended doses it is selective for MAO-B and no restrictions are required. Nevertheless, this report suggests that, rarely, interactions are still possible, and some consider that patients taking selegiline should try to avoid pseudoephedrine. The manufacturers of rasagiline recommend against concurrent use of nasal decongestants that are indirectly-acting sympathomimetics, such as ephedrine and pseudoephedrine, due to the risk of hypertensive crises.

MAO-B inhibitors + Opioids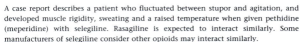

A case report describes a patient who fluctuated between stupor and agitation, and developed muscle rigidity, sweating and a raised temperature when given pethidine (meperidine) with selegiline. Rasagiline is expected to interact similarly. Some manufacturers of selegiline consider other opioids may interact similarly.

On the basis of this evidence the manufacturers of selegiline and rasagiline contraindicate pethidine (meperidine) and also suggest that pethidine should be avoided in the 14 days after rasagiline has been stopped. Some manufacturers of selegiline contraindicate concurrent use with all opioids, which is probably unnecessary, based on the evidence with non-selective MAOIs, page 374.

MAO-B inhibitors + Quinolones

Ciprofloxacin increases the AUC of rasagiline by 83%.

The clinical relevance of this pharmacokinetic interaction has not been assessed but it may be prudent to be alert for rasagiline adverse effects (e.g. headache, dyspepsia). Some other quinolones may also interact, see quinolones, page 444.

MAO-B inhibitors + SSRIs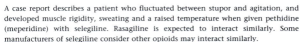

Although the safe concurrent use of selegiline and SSRIs has been reported in a number of patients, there are also documented cases of serotonin syndrome, page 454. Rasagiline is expected to interact similarly. Note that fluvoxamine would be expected to raise rasagiline levels and may therefore increase the risk of an interaction occurring.

The manufacturers of rasagiline recommend avoiding the concurrent use of fluoxetine and fluvoxamine. Rasagiline should not be started for 5 weeks after stopping fluoxetine or 2 weeks after starting fluvoxamine, and fluoxetine should not be started for 2 weeks after stopping rasagiline. Caution would also seem prudent with the other SSRIs. The manufacturers of selegiline contraindicate the concurrent use of SSRIs. In addition, selegiline should not be started for 5 weeks after stopping fluoxetine, 2 weeks after stopping sertraline, and one week after stopping other SSRIs. SSRIs should not be started for 2 weeks after stopping selegiline.

MAO-B inhibitors + Tricyclics

Rare cases of serotonin syndrome, page 454, and other CNS disturbances have been seen when selegiline is given with tricyclics. Rasagiline is expected to interact similarly.

If the combination is used the outcome should be well monitored, but the likelihood of problems seems to be small. Nevertheless, some manufacturers of selegiline advise avoiding the concurrent use of tricyclics. The manufacturers of rasagiline advise caution if it is given with antidepressants.

MAO-B inhibitors + Triptans ✖

One manufacturer of selegiline contraindicates the concurrent use of serotonin agonists (and name triptans as an example). This is presumably because of the theoretical risk of the serotonin syndrome, page 454.

Avoid concurrent use. The manufacturer states that at least 14 days should lapse between stopping selegiline and starting any potentially interacting drug.

MAO-B inhibitors + Venlafaxine ▲

Serotonin syndrome, page 454, has been reported when selegiline was given with venlafaxine. This is in line with the manufacturers' prediction and the way that other serotonergic drugs behave with selegiline. Rasagiline is expected to interact similarly.

The manufacturers of selegiline suggest that the concurrent use of venlafaxine should be avoided. A 2-week washout period would seem appropriate when switching from one of these drugs to the other. The manufacturers of rasagiline advise caution on the concurrent use of antidepressants.

MAOIs

This section covers the non-selective MAOIs. Other drugs with MAO-inhibitory properties, such as linezolid, moclobemide, and the MAO-B inhibitors, selegiline and rasagiline, are discussed in their own sections.

MAOIs + Maprotiline ✖

Toxic and sometimes fatal reactions (similar to or the same as serotonin syndrome, page 454) have very occasionally occurred in patients taking both MAOIs and *tricyclic antidepressants*. Maprotiline would be expected to interact similarly.

Avoid concurrent use. Maprotiline should not be started for 2 to 3 weeks after treatment with MAOIs has been stopped and an MAOI should not be started until at least 7 to 14 days after maprotiline has been stopped. If concurrent use is thought necessary it has been suggested that it should only be undertaken by specialists well aware of the problems and who can undertake adequate supervision.

M

MAOIs + Methyldopa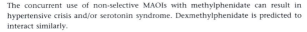

Theoretically hypertension may occur when non-selective MAOIs are taken with methyldopa, although additive blood-pressure lowering effects are also a possibility. The concurrent use of antidepressant MAOIs and methyldopa may not be desirable because methyldopa can sometimes cause depression.

It would seem prudent to avoid the combination wherever possible. Some manufacturers contraindicate concurrent use.

MAOIs + Methylphenidate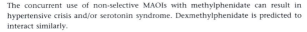

The concurrent use of non-selective MAOIs with methylphenidate can result in hypertensive crisis and/or serotonin syndrome. Dexmethylphenidate is predicted to interact similarly.

Methylphenidate and dexmethylphenidate should not be taken either with or within 14 days of an MAOI.

MAOIs + Mianserin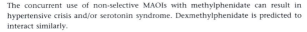

Toxic and sometimes fatal reactions (similar to or the same as serotonin syndrome, page 454) have very occasionally occurred in patients taking both MAOIs and *tricyclic antidepressants*. Case reports suggest that mianserin can interact similarly.

Avoid concurrent use. Mianserin should not be started for 2 to 3 weeks after treatment with MAOIs has been stopped and an MAOI should not be started until at least 7 to 14 days after mianserin has been stopped. If concurrent use is thought necessary it has been suggested that it should only be undertaken by specialists well aware of the problems and who can undertake adequate supervision.

MAOIs + Mirtazapine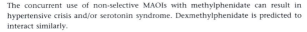

No data seem to be available about the concurrent use of mirtazapine with MAOIs.

The manufacturers say that the concurrent use of mirtazapine and the MAOIs should be avoided both during and within 2 weeks of stopping treatment. This is a general warning about the concurrent use of MAOIs that most of the manufacturers of antidepressants issue.

MAOIs + Nasal decongestants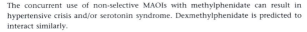

The concurrent use of a number of nasal decongestants with indirect sympathomimetic actions, such as ephedrine, phenylpropanolamine, and pseudoephedrine, and non-selective MAOIs can result in a potentially fatal hypertensive crisis.

Avoid concurrent use both during and for 2 weeks after stopping the MAOI. These drugs are found in many proprietary cough, cold and influenza preparations, or are used as appetite suppressants. Counsel patients accordingly.

MAOIs + Nefopam ❌

Nefopam has sympathomimetic activity, which theoretically may cause severe hypertension in those taking MAOIs.

> Concurrent use should be avoided. With other drugs that interact in the manner predicted it is usually advised that concurrent use should also be avoided for 2 weeks after the MAOI has been stopped.

MAOIs + Opioids ❌

The concurrent use of pethidine (meperidine) and an MAOI has resulted in a serious and potentially life-threatening reaction in several patients. Excitement, muscle rigidity, hyperpyrexia, flushing, sweating and unconsciousness can occur very rapidly. Respiratory depression and hypertension or hypotension have also been seen. Similar interactions have been seen if tramadol is taken with MAOIs. Isolated cases of adverse reactions (e.g. hypertension, hypotension, hyperthermia and tachycardia) have been reported after fentanyl or morphine were given to patients taking MAOIs.

> The interaction with pethidine (meperidine) is serious and potentially fatal, but the incidence is probably quite low. It may therefore be an idiosyncratic reaction. Nevertheless, it would be imprudent to give pethidine to any patient taking an MAOI. Bear in mind that the non-selective MAOIs are all essentially irreversible so that an interaction is possible for many days after their withdrawal (at least 2 weeks is the official advice). The manufacturers of tramadol contraindicate its use with MAOIs because of the risks of this reaction. Evidence for an interaction between other opioids and MAOIs is limited, and some of the cases appear to represent a different type of reaction to that seen with pethidine. Indeed, with some opioids there is evidence of safe concurrent use. Nevertheless, the manufacturers of many opioids contraindicate concurrent use both with and within 14 days of the use of an MAOI. These include alfentanil, buprenorphine, codeine, dextropropoxyphene (propoxyphene), diamorphine, dipipanone, fentanyl, hydromorphone, methadone, morphine and oxycodone.

MAOIs + Phenobarbital ❓

Although the MAOIs can enhance and prolong the activity of barbiturates in *animals*, only a few isolated cases of adverse responses (profound sedation) attributed to an interaction have been described.

> There is no well-documented evidence showing that concurrent use should be avoided, although some caution is clearly appropriate because of the case reports.

MAOIs + Reboxetine ❌

No data seem to be available about the concurrent use of reboxetine with MAOIs. However, the manufacturers predict that a hypertensive reaction is possible.

> Concurrent use should be avoided. With other drugs that interact in the manner predicted it is usually advised that concurrent use should also be avoided for 2 weeks after the MAOI has been stopped.

M

MAOIs + Salbutamol (Albuterol) and related bronchodilators

An isolated case of tachycardia and apprehension has been described after a patient with asthma taking phenelzine also took salbutamol (albuterol).

This appears to be an isolated case, and is probably not of general importance as the reaction is not in line with the expected pharmacological effects of concurrent use. Nevertheless, on the basis of interactions with other sympathomimetic drugs, one manufacturer of fenoterol (with ipratropium) advises caution if MAOIs are also given.

MAOIs + Sibutramine ✗

There are no reports of adverse reactions between sibutramine and the MAOIs but the manufacturers have suggested that, in theory, the potentially serious serotonin syndrome, page 454 could develop on concurrent use.

Concurrent use is contraindicated. The manufacturers state that 14 days should elapse between stopping either drug and starting the other.

MAOIs + SSRIs ✗

A number of case reports describe serotonin syndrome, page 454, in patients given SSRIs with MAOIs: some have been fatal.

Direct information about the interaction between MAOIs and SSRIs is limited, and given that concurrent use is contraindicated, further reports seem unlikely. The manufacturers say that the SSRIs should not be given within 14 days of discontinuing an irreversible MAOI. Moreover, the manufacturers of each SSRI give guidance on the appropriate intervals that should be left between stopping the SSRI and starting an MAOI; that is, 7 days for sertraline, citalopram, escitalopram, fluvoxamine or paroxetine (14 days in the US for citalopram, escitalopram, sertraline and paroxetine) and at least 5 weeks for fluoxetine, with an even longer interval if long-term or high-dose fluoxetine has been used.

MAOIs + Trazodone ✗

Toxic and sometimes fatal reactions (similar to or the same as serotonin syndrome, page 454) have very occasionally occurred in patients taking both MAOIs and *tricyclic antidepressants*. A case report suggests that trazodone may interact similarly; however, a small number of reports describe the successful use of low-dose trazodone with phenelzine for depression and insomnia.

Trazodone should not be started for 2 weeks after treatment with MAOIs has been stopped, and an MAOI should not be started until 1 week after trazodone has been stopped. If concurrent use is thought necessary it has been suggested that it should only be undertaken by specialists well aware of the problems and who can undertake adequate supervision.

M

MAOIs + Tricyclics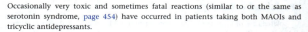

Occasionally very toxic and sometimes fatal reactions (similar to or the same as serotonin syndrome, page 454) have occurred in patients taking both MAOIs and tricyclic antidepressants.

> Concurrent use is contraindicated. Tricyclic antidepressants should not be started for 2 weeks after treatment with MAOIs has been stopped (3 weeks if starting clomipramine or imipramine), and an MAOI should not be started until at least 7 to 14 days after a tricyclic or related antidepressant has been stopped (3 weeks in the case of clomipramine or imipramine). If concurrent use is thought necessary it has been suggested that it should only be undertaken by specialists well aware of the problems and who can undertake adequate supervision.

MAOIs + Triptans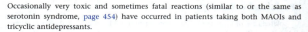

Some have suggested that there may be a pharmacodynamic interaction between MAOIs (both selective and non-selective) and triptans, which may result in serotonin syndrome.

> The manufacturers of rizatriptan and sumatriptan contraindicate the concurrent use of MAOIs. The US manufacturer contraindicates the use of zolmitriptan both during, and for 2 weeks after, the use of *moclobemide*, whereas the UK manufacturer restricts the dose of zolmitriptan to 5 mg in 24 hours. In the absence of any direct information it would seem prudent to apply these warnings to the use of non-selective MAOIs.

MAOIs + Tryptophan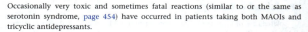

Although the concurrent use of MAOIs and tryptophan can be both safe and effective, a number of patients have developed severe behavioural and neurological signs of toxicity (some similar to serotonin syndrome, page 454) after taking MAOIs with tryptophan, and fatalities have occurred.

> It has been recommended that patients taking MAOIs should start treatment with a low dose of tryptophan (500 mg). This should be gradually increased while monitoring the patient for changes suggesting hypomania, and neurological changes, including ocular oscillations and upper motor neurone signs.

MAOIs + Venlafaxine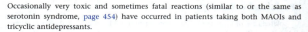

Serious and potentially life-threatening reactions (serotonin syndrome, page 454) can develop if venlafaxine and non-selective, irreversible MAOIs are given concurrently, or even sequentially if insufficient time is left in between.

> Concurrent use is contraindicated. The manufacturers of venlafaxine recommend that at least one week should elapse between stopping the venlafaxine and starting an MAOI, and 2 weeks between stopping an MAOI and starting venlafaxine.

Maprotiline

Maprotiline + Moclobemide

One study did not find a serious hypertensive reaction, like that seen with the tricyclics and the MAOIs, when maprotiline was given with moclobemide. Nevertheless, such a reaction is thought possible.

Concurrent use should be avoided. Moclobemide has a short duration of action so no treatment free period is required before starting a tricyclic or related antidepressant. However, some recommend waiting 24 hours. Moclobemide should not be started until at least one week after a tricyclic or related antidepressant has been stopped.

Mebendazole

Mebendazole + Phenobarbital

Carbamazepine and *phenytoin* lower mebendazole levels. Phenobarbital and primidone are expected to interact similarly.

When treating systemic worm infections it may be necessary to increase the mebendazole dose in patients taking phenobarbital or primidone. Monitor the outcome of concurrent use. This interaction is of no importance when mebendazole is used for intestinal worm infections where its action is a local effect on the worms in the gut.

Mebendazole + Phenytoin

Phenytoin lowers mebendazole levels. Fosphenytoin is expected to interact similarly.

When treating systemic worm infections it may be necessary to increase the mebendazole dose in patients taking phenytoin or fosphenytoin. Monitor the outcome of concurrent use. This interaction is of no importance when mebendazole is used for intestinal worm infections where its action is a local effect on the worms in the gut.

Medroxyprogesterone

For the interactions of medroxyprogesterone used as a progestogen-only contraceptive, consider contraceptives, page 233.

Medroxyprogesterone + **Warfarin and other oral anticoagulants**

High-dose medroxyprogesterone acetate (1 g daily) increases the half-life and reduces the clearance of warfarin by about 70% and 35%, respectively.

> Monitor the effect of concurrent use on the anticoagulant response and adjust the warfarin dose as necessary.

Mefloquine

Mefloquine + **Quinine**

Mefloquine levels may possibly be increased by quinine. In theory there is an increased risk of convulsions. The manufacturers advise avoidance of concurrent use because of the theoretical risk of QT prolongation. See Drugs that prolong the QT interval, page 277 for more information.

> It has been suggested that treatment with mefloquine should be delayed until 12 hours after the last dose of quinine.

Mefloquine + **Rifampicin (Rifampin)**

Rifampicin reduces the AUC of mefloquine by almost 70%.

> The clinical relevance of this is uncertain, but some suggest that simultaneous use should be avoided to prevent treatment failure and the risk of *Plasmodium falciparum* resistance to mefloquine. Until more is known, this would seem a sensible precaution.

Mefloquine + **Warfarin and other oral anticoagulants**

The effects of warfarin and an unnamed coumarin were increased in two patients who took mefloquine.

> Patients taking mefloquine should have their warfarin effects checked before travel to allow for monitoring of any changes in anticoagulant effects.

Melatonin

Melatonin + Quinolones

In a study, *fluvoxamine* raised melatonin levels 12-fold probably by inhibiting CYP1A2. All subjects reported marked drowsiness after melatonin intake that was even more pronounced when *fluvoxamine* was also given. The manufacturer predicts that the quinolones, page 444 will interact similarly, but note that they differ in their ability to inhibit this isoenzyme.

Be aware that excessive drowsiness and related adverse effects may occur on concurrent use.

Melatonin + SSRIs

In a study, fluvoxamine raised melatonin levels 12-fold. All subjects reported marked drowsiness after melatonin intake that was even more pronounced when fluvoxamine was also given.

The manufacturers advise avoiding concurrent use.

Melatonin + Warfarin and other oral anticoagulants

Case reports suggest that melatonin may raise or lower the INR in response to warfarin.

Until more is known, bear these cases in mind in the event of an unexpected change in coagulation status in patients also taking melatonin.

Meropenem

Meropenem + Probenecid

Probenecid increases the AUC of meropenem by about 50%.

The manufacturers say that because the potency and duration of meropenem are adequate without probenecid, they do not recommend concurrent use.

Meropenem + Valproate

Meropenem appears to dramatically and rapidly reduce valproate levels resulting, in some cases, in increased seizure frequency.

It would be prudent to monitor valproate levels in any patient given carbapenems.

M

The valproate dose may need to be increased. Consider using another antibacterial, or an alternative to valproate; limited evidence suggests that carbamazepine and phenytoin are not affected.

Methotrexate

Methotrexate + Neomycin ❓

The gastrointestinal absorption of methotrexate can be reduced by neomycin.

The significance of this interaction is unclear, but bear it in mind in case of an unexpected response to treatment.

Methotrexate + NSAIDs ⚠

Increased methotrexate toxicity, sometimes life-threatening, has been seen in a few patients also taking an NSAID, whereas other patients have taken NSAIDs with methotrexate uneventfully. The mechanism of this interaction suggests that all NSAIDs have the potential to interact similarly. The pharmacokinetics of methotrexate (reduced clearance) can also be changed by some NSAIDs.

Concurrent use need not be avoided but close monitoring is necessary. Tell patients to report symptoms such as sore throat, dyspnoea or cough. If high-dose methotrexate is given with an NSAID, monitor methotrexate levels and increase routine methotrexate monitoring (e.g. full blood count, liver function tests). The risk appears to be lowest in those taking low-dose methotrexate for psoriasis or rheumatoid arthritis, with normal renal function. Patients must be counselled regarding non-prescription NSAIDs.

Methotrexate + Penicillins ⚠

Reduced clearance and acute methotrexate toxicity has been attributed to the concurrent use of various penicillins (amoxicillin, benzylpenicillin, carbenicillin, dicloxacillin, flucloxacillin, mezlocillin, oxacillin, phenoxymethylpenicillin, piperacillin, and ticarcillin) in a small number of case reports.

Serious interactions between methotrexate and penicillins are uncommon. Risk factors are as yet unknown and even patients taking low doses of methotrexate have been affected. Given the current evidence monitoring is advisable. Full blood count should be routinely monitored with methotrexate alone: consider twice-weekly platelet and white cell counts for 2 weeks initially, with the measurement of methotrexate levels if toxicity is suspected.

Methotrexate + Probenecid ⚠

Probenecid markedly increases methotrexate levels (3- to 4-fold).

A marked increase in both the therapeutic and toxic effects of methotrexate can occur, apparently even with low doses if other risk factors are present (e.g. renal impairment, concurrent NSAIDs). Anticipate the need to reduce the dose of methotrexate and monitor the effects well if probenecid is also taken. If this is not possible, avoid the combination.

Methotrexate + Proton pump inhibitors

The excretion of methotrexate is reported to have been reduced in several patients given omeprazole and a few patients given lansoprazole. However, similar elevations in methotrexate levels in another patient taking omeprazole were independent of omeprazole use. One patient had myalgia and elevated 7-hydroxymethotrexate levels when treated with methotrexate and pantoprazole.

The general significance of this interaction is unclear but the risk seems greatest with high-dose methotrexate. Routine methotrexate monitoring should be adequate to detect any toxicity. If toxicity develops, consider the proton pump inhibitor as a possible cause.

Methotrexate + Quinolones

A report describes methotrexate toxicity in 2 patients also taking ciprofloxacin.

Full blood count should be monitored when methotrexate is used. If any abnormalities arise, consider this interaction as a possible cause.

Methotrexate + Tetracyclines

Two case reports describe the development of methotrexate toxicity in patients also taking tetracycline or doxycycline.

The general significance of this interaction is unclear, but bear it in mind in case of an unexpected response to treatment.

Methotrexate + Theophylline

In one study theophylline clearance was reduced by 19% after 6 weeks of treatment with intramuscular methotrexate 15 mg weekly. A few patients complained of nausea and the theophylline dose had to be reduced in one. It seems possible that aminophylline could be similarly affected.

The clinical importance of this change is unclear; however bear it in mind should increased theophylline adverse effects (such as nausea and vomiting) occur with concurrent use. Note that one UK manufacturer of low-dose methotrexate recommends monitoring theophylline levels.

Methotrexate + Trimethoprim

The concurrent use of low-dose methotrexate and trimethoprim or trimethoprim with sulfamethoxazole has resulted in several cases of severe bone marrow depression, some of which were fatal.

Full blood count should be monitored when methotrexate is used. If any abnormalities arise, consider this interaction as a possible cause. Note that trimethoprim (as co-trimoxazole) is commonly used in some cytotoxic regimens.

Methotrexate + Vaccines ❌

The immune response of the body is suppressed by cytotoxic antineoplastics. The effectiveness of vaccines may be poor and generalised infection may occur in patients immunised with live vaccines. In one study the antibody response to pneumococcal vaccination was reduced by 60% in patients receiving antineoplastics, and suboptimal responses to influenza and measles vaccines have been reported.

Live vaccines should not be given to patients who are receiving cytotoxics or other immunosuppressant antineoplastics. In the UK, it is recommended that live vaccines should not be given during or within at least 6 months of such treatment. Monitor the immune response to other types of vaccine. Consider whether vaccination can be carried out before or after methotrexate use.

Methylphenidate

Methylphenidate + Phenytoin ❓

Raised phenytoin levels and phenytoin toxicity have been seen in a few patients also given methylphenidate, but it is an uncommon reaction and two studies suggest that most patients do not experience an interaction. It seems possible that dexmethylphenidate, the d-isomer of methylphenidate, and fosphenytoin, a prodrug of phenytoin, could interact similarly.

This interaction is unlikely to be generally significant, but bear it in mind in case of an unexpected response to treatment. Indicators of phenytoin toxicity include blurred vision, nystagmus, ataxia or drowsiness.

Methylphenidate + SSRIs ❓

Isolated reports describe delirium in one patient and a seizure in another when methylphenidate was taken with sertraline.

The general significance of these cases is likely to be small, especially when set in the context of beneficial concurrent use with SSRIs (fluoxetine, paroxetine, sertraline). However, if adverse CNS effects become troublesome, it may be worth considering this interaction as a possible cause: in both cases the adverse effects resolved when one of the drugs was withdrawn.

M

Methylphenidate + **Tricyclics**

Several studies have reported an increase in imipramine or desipramine levels following the addition of methylphenidate, which can be of benefit but may also increase adverse effects. Isolated cases of behavioural problems have been seen, but a large review indicates the absence of a clinically significant interaction. Dexmethylphenidate, the d-isomer of methylphenidate, would be expected to interact similarly.

> The combination of methylphenidate and tricyclic antidepressants may be beneficial but may result in an increase in tricyclic adverse effects. If concurrent use is necessary it would seem prudent to monitor for adverse tricyclic effects (e.g. dry mouth, blurred vision, urinary retention) and adjust the dose of the tricyclic as necessary.

Metoclopramide

Metoclopramide + **Paracetamol (Acetaminophen)**

Metoclopramide increases the rate of absorption of paracetamol and raises its maximum plasma levels.

> As the total amount of paracetamol absorbed was unchanged this interaction is unlikely to be clinically significant, although a more rapid onset of action may be advantageous.

Metoclopramide + **SSRIs**

Case reports describe serotonin syndrome, page 454, in patients taking SSRIs with metoclopramide. Extrapyramidal symptoms have occurred in patients given fluoxetine, fluvoxamine or sertraline with metoclopramide.

> Information seems to be limited to these reports, but they highlight the fact that care should be taken if two drugs with the potential to cause the same adverse effects are used together. Some monitoring for increased adverse effects would be advisable if an SSRI is taken with metoclopramide.

Metronidazole

Metronidazole + **Phenobarbital**

Phenobarbital markedly increases the metabolism of metronidazole, and treatment failure as a result of this interaction has been reported in both adults and children. Primidone is metabolised to phenobarbital and would be expected to interact similarly. Other barbiturates are also expected to interact.

> Monitor the effects of concurrent use and anticipate the need to increase the metronidazole dose by 2- to 3-fold.

Metronidazole + Phenytoin

One study found that the half-life of intravenous phenytoin was modestly prolonged by metronidazole, whereas another found that metronidazole did not affect the pharmacokinetics of oral phenytoin. An anecdotal report describes a few patients who developed toxic phenytoin levels when given metronidazole. Fosphenytoin, a prodrug of phenytoin, may interact similarly.

> This interaction is unlikely to be generally significant, but bear it in mind in case of an unexpected response to treatment. Indicators of phenytoin toxicity include blurred vision, nystagmus, ataxia or drowsiness.

Metronidazole + Warfarin and other oral anticoagulants

The anticoagulant effects of warfarin can be markedly increased by metronidazole and bleeding has been seen. Tinidazole may interact similarly.

> Monitor the INR if either metronidazole or tinidazole is given with warfarin and adjust the warfarin dose accordingly. Nothing seems to be documented about other anticoagulants but it would be prudent to expect the coumarins to behave similarly.

Mexiletine

Mexiletine + Opioids

The absorption of mexiletine is reduced in patients following a myocardial infarction, and very markedly reduced and delayed if opioids (diamorphine or morphine) are given concurrently. Other opioids may interact similarly.

> The delay and reduction in the absorption would seem to limit the value of oral mexiletine during the first few hours after a myocardial infarction, particularly if opioid analgesics are used. The manufacturer suggests that a higher loading dose of oral mexiletine may be preferable in this situation. Alternatively, an intravenous dose of mexiletine may be given.

Mexiletine + Phenytoin

Phenytoin halves the AUC of mexiletine. Fosphenytoin, a prodrug of phenytoin, may interact similarly.

> It seems likely that the fall in mexiletine levels will be clinically important in at least some individuals. Monitor for mexiletine efficacy, and where possible monitor mexiletine levels. Raise the dose if necessary.

M

Mexiletine + **Protease inhibitors**

Ritonavir appears to increase the levels of mexiletine, probably by inhibiting CYP2D6. Tipranavir would be expected to interact similarly. The other protease inhibitors do not significantly affect CYP2D6 and would not be expected to increase mexiletine levels alone; however, they are usually given with low-dose ritonavir as a pharmacological booster.

> Until more is known, it would seem prudent to monitor any patient taking mexiletine with ritonavir, tipranavir or any ritonavir-boosted protease inhibitor for an increase in mexiletine adverse effects (such as nausea, tremor, hypotension), and titrate the mexiletine dose slowly, according to clinical response.

Mexiletine + **Rifampicin (Rifampin)**

The clearance of mexiletine is increased by rifampicin. The mexiletine AUC was reduced by about 40% in one study.

> It seems likely that the fall in mexiletine levels will be clinically important in some individuals. Monitor for mexiletine efficacy, and where possible monitor mexiletine levels. Raise the dose if necessary.

Mexiletine + **SSRIs**

Fluvoxamine increases the AUC of mexiletine by 55% by inhibiting its metabolism by CYP1A2. Fluoxetine and paroxetine might also be expected to interact, by inhibiting mexiletine metabolism by CYP2D6

> There appear to be no reported interactions with fluoxetine or paroxetine, but given the way they interact with other CYP2D6 substrates some interaction seems possible. However, note that other CYP2D6 inhibitors have only modest effects on mexiletine metabolism. Nevertheless, until more is known it may be prudent to be alert for mexiletine adverse effects (e.g. nausea, tremor, hypotension) in patients given fluoxetine or paroxetine. If they develop, consider an interaction as a possible cause. Similar caution seems warranted with fluvoxamine.

Mexiletine + **Terbinafine**

In vitro studies suggest that terbinafine is an inhibitor of CYP2D6. It may therefore be expected to increase the plasma levels of other drugs that are substrates of this enzyme, such as mexiletine.

> Until more is known it would seem wise to be aware of the possibility of an increase in adverse effects (e.g. nausea, tremor, hypotension) if mexiletine is given with terbinafine. Consider a dose reduction if necessary.

Mexiletine + **Theophylline**

Theophylline levels are increased by mexiletine and toxicity may occur.

> Monitor concurrent use and reduce the theophylline dose as necessary. It has been suggested that 50% dose reductions may be required.

Mexiletine + Tizanidine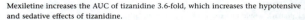

Mexiletine increases the AUC of tizanidine 3.6-fold, which increases the hypotensive and sedative effects of tizanidine.

> If concurrent use is necessary, consider reducing the dose of tizanidine or use the lowest possible starting dose (2 to 4 mg) titrated to effect. Monitor closely for adverse effects such as bradycardia, hypotension and drowsiness.

Mianserin

Mianserin + Moclobemide ✖

A number of studies suggest that no interaction, or only a moderate non-significant rise in *tricyclic antidepressant* levels occurs when they are given with moclobemide. However, several case reports describe serotonin syndrome, page 454, in patients receiving the combination. There is little evidence regarding mianserin, but it seems likely that it could interact similarly.

> Concurrent use should be avoided. Moclobemide has a short duration of action so no treatment free period is required before starting a tricyclic or related antidepressant. However, some recommend waiting 24 hours. Moclobemide should not be started until at least one week after a tricyclic or related antidepressant has been stopped.

Mianserin + Phenobarbital ⚠

Mianserin levels can be markedly reduced by phenobarbital. Note that primidone is metabolised to phenobarbital and therefore may interact similarly.

> Monitor the response to mianserin and increase the dose as necessary. Note that mianserin lowers the convulsive threshold and may therefore be inappropriate for patients with epilepsy.

Mianserin + Phenytoin ⚠

Mianserin levels can be markedly reduced by phenytoin. Fosphenytoin, a prodrug of phenytoin, may interact similarly.

> Monitor the response to mianserin and increase the dose as necessary. Note that mianserin lowers the convulsive threshold and may therefore be inappropriate for patients with epilepsy.

Mianserin + Warfarin and other oral anticoagulants ❓

Mianserin increased the response to warfarin in one patient. A case of decreased

M

acenocoumarol efficacy has also been reported with mianserin. However on the whole concurrent use seems uneventful.

The general significance of the case reports is unknown, but bear it in mind in case of an excessive response to anticoagulant treatment.

Mifepristone

Mifepristone + NSAIDs

Theoretically NSAIDs might reduce the efficacy of mifepristone, and combined use is often not recommended. However, evidence from two studies with naproxen and diclofenac suggests no reduction in mifepristone efficacy.

Because of theoretical concerns of antagonistic effects, NSAID analgesics have been avoided in protocols for medical abortion. However, the limited available evidence suggests that this might not be necessary. Nevertheless, some NSAID manufacturers continue to advise that NSAIDs should not be used for 8 to 12 days after mifepristone.

Mirtazapine

Mirtazapine + Phenobarbital

Phenytoin decreases the AUC and maximum levels of mirtazapine by 47% and 33%, respectively. Phenobarbital (and therefore primidone) would be expected to interact similarly.

The mirtazapine dose may need to be increased in the presence of phenobarbital or primidone. Monitor concurrent use to ensure mirtazapine is effective. Note that mirtazapine can lower the seizure threshold, and therefore its use should be carefully considered in patients given barbiturates for epilepsy.

Mirtazapine + Phenytoin

Phenytoin decreases the AUC and maximum levels of mirtazapine by 47% and 33%, respectively. Fosphenytoin, a prodrug of phenytoin, may interact similarly.

The mirtazapine dose may need to be increased in the presence of phenytoin or fosphenytoin. Monitor concurrent use to ensure mirtazapine is effective. Note that, mirtazapine can lower the seizure threshold, and therefore its use should be carefully considered in patients with epilepsy.

Mirtazapine + **Protease inhibitors**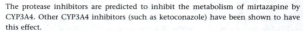

The protease inhibitors are predicted to inhibit the metabolism of mirtazapine by CYP3A4. Other CYP3A4 inhibitors (such as ketoconazole) have been shown to have this effect.

The manufacturers advise caution on concurrent use. Monitor for adverse effects (most commonly sedation, fatigue, headache).

Mirtazapine + **Rifampicin (Rifampin)**

Rifampicin is predicted to lower mirtazapine levels. Other enzyme inducers (e.g. phenytoin) have been shown to have this effect.

The mirtazapine dose may need to be increased during concurrent use. Monitor to ensure that mirtazapine is effective.

Mirtazapine + **SSRIs** ❓

There are a couple of isolated cases of possible serotonin syndrome, page 454, when mirtazapine was used with fluoxetine and fluvoxamine, and there is a report of hypomania associated with the concurrent use of sertraline. Restless legs syndrome occurred with fluoxetine and mirtazapine. Fluvoxamine markedly increased plasma levels of mirtazapine in two cases.

Caution is warranted on concurrent use. Monitor for adverse effects (most commonly sedation, fatigue, headache) and be aware that CNS excitation may occur. Extra caution might be appropriate with fluvoxamine, as the limited evidence suggests that this might markedly raise mirtazapine levels. However, this needs confirming.

Mirtazapine + **Warfarin and other oral anticoagulants** ❓

Mirtazapine may cause small, clinically insignificant increases in INR in patients taking warfarin.

No action needed. One UK manufacturer of mirtazapine very cautiously advises that the prothrombin time should be controlled if mirtazapine is given with warfarin; however, another manufacturer does not consider monitoring to be necessary.

Moclobemide

Moclobemide + **Nasal decongestants** ❌

The concurrent use of ephedrine and moclobemide raises blood pressure, and this has resulted in palpitations and headache. Other related drugs (e.g. pseudoephedrine) would be expected to interact with the MAOIs similarly.

> The manufacturers of moclobemide advise avoiding drugs such as ephedrine, pseudoephedrine and phenylpropanolamine. Patients taking MAOIs should be strongly warned not to take any of these drugs either with or for 2 weeks after stopping their MAOI.

Moclobemide + Opioids

Animal studies suggest that moclobemide may potentiate the effects of the opioids. A report of suspected serotonin syndrome in a patient given pethidine (meperidine) in addition to her usual treatment with moclobemide, nortriptyline and lithium, adds some weight to this suggestion. Similar predictions have been made for tramadol, and serotonin syndrome, page 454, has been seen in a patient given tramadol with moclobemide and clomipramine.

> Concurrent use should be avoided or undertaken with great caution. One manufacturer of moclobemide suggests that opioid dose adjustments may be needed. Note that the concurrent use of pethidine (meperidine) with moclobemide is contraindicated.

Moclobemide + SSRIs

Some studies suggest that moclobemide may not interact with the SSRIs, but there have been case reports of serotonin syndrome, page 454 in patients taking the combination.

> Concurrent use is contraindicated. Because the effects of moclobemide are readily reversible, only one day need elapse between stopping moclobemide and starting an SSRI. However, if stopping an SSRI and starting moclobemide the same intervals as for the irreversible MAOIs, page 375 are required.

Moclobemide + Trazodone

Isolated cases of serotonin syndrome, page 454 have been reported in patients receiving trazodone and moclobemide. A small number of reports describe the successful use of low-dose trazodone with moclobemide for depression and insomnia.

> The balance of the evidence suggests that concurrent use is favourable if the dose of trazodone is low (200 mg daily or less). No specific advice appears to have been given for moclobemide with higher doses, but, because of its half-life, a 24-hour washout is usually considered appropriate when starting potentially interacting drugs in patients who have been taking moclobemide.

Moclobemide + Tricyclics

A number of studies suggest that no interaction, or only a moderate non-significant rise in tricyclic antidepressant levels occurs when they are given with moclobemide.

However, several case reports describe serotonin syndrome, page 454 in patients receiving the combination.

> Concurrent use should be avoided. Moclobemide has a short duration of action so no treatment free period is required before starting a tricyclic antidepressant. However, some recommend waiting 24 hours. Moclobemide should not be started until at least one week after a tricyclic antidepressant has been stopped.

Moclobemide + Triptans

Moclobemide markedly inhibits the metabolism of rizatriptan, modestly inhibits the metabolism of zolmitriptan and approximately doubles the bioavailability of sumatriptan. Note that there is a potential risk of serotonin syndrome, page 454 if triptans are given with moclobemide.

> The manufacturers contraindicate the use of moclobemide with rizatriptan or sumatriptan. In the UK, a maximum intake of 5 mg of zolmitriptan in 24 hours is recommended by the manufacturers, whereas in the US the combination is contraindicated.

Moclobemide + Venlafaxine

The concurrent use of moclobemide and venlafaxine has led to the potentially fatal serotonin syndrome, page 454.

> Concurrent use is contraindicated. The UK manufacturer of venlafaxine states that a withdrawal period shorter than 14 days may be used before starting venlafaxine (with other similar interactions with moclobemide 24 to 48 hours has been said to be adequate). At least 7 days should elapse between stopping venlafaxine and starting moclobemide.

Modafinil

Modafinil + Phenytoin

Modafinil may inhibit the metabolism of phenytoin. The manufacturers predict that phenytoin may reduce the levels of modafinil. Fosphenytoin, a prodrug of phenytoin, may interact similarly.

> Monitor for evidence of increased phenytoin effects and toxicity (blurred vision, nystagmus, ataxia or drowsiness). An effect on modafinil seems unlikely as it has multiple routes of metabolism; nevertheless it may be prudent to monitor for modafinil efficacy.

M

Montelukast

Montelukast + **Phenobarbital**

Phenobarbital reduces the AUC and maximum levels of montelukast by 38% and 20%, respectively. Note that primidone is metabolised to phenobarbital and therefore may interact similarly.

The manufacturers advises caution on concurrent use, especially in children. Monitor for a reduction in montelukast efficacy but note that dose adjustments seem unlikely to be needed.

Montelukast + **Phenytoin**

Phenytoin (and therefore possibly fosphenytoin) is predicted to reduce montelukast levels.

The manufacturers advise caution on concurrent use, especially in children. Monitor for a reduction in montelukast efficacy but note that dose adjustments seem unlikely to be needed.

Montelukast + **Rifampicin (Rifampin)**

Rifampicin is predicted to reduce montelukast levels.

The manufacturers advise caution on concurrent use, especially in children. Monitor for a reduction in montelukast efficacy but note that dose adjustments seem unlikely to be needed.

Moxonidine

Moxonidine + **Tricyclics** ✕

Tricyclic antidepressants may antagonise the blood-pressure lowering effects of clonidine, page 225. As moxonidine is related to clonidine it is expected to interact similarly. Tricyclics can also cause postural hypotension, which could potentially be additive with the effects of moxonidine.

The manufacturers of moxonidine advise avoiding tricyclic antidepressants, because of the lack of clinical experience of concurrent use. If the combination is used, it would be prudent to carefully monitor blood pressure.

M

Mycophenolate

Mycophenolate + Rifampicin (Rifampin)

Rifampicin reduces the levels of mycophenolic acid (the active metabolite of mycophenolate) and increases the levels of the metabolite associated with mycophenolate adverse effects. An isolated case describes increased mycophenolate dose requirements in a patient taking rifampicin.

Mycophenolate should be closely monitored for both reduced efficacy and increased adverse effects if rifampicin is given, and the dose adjusted as required, both on starting and stopping rifampicin.

Mycophenolate + Sevelamer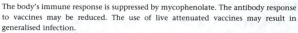

Sevelamer reduces the AUC of mycophenolate by 25%.

The clinical significance of this interaction is unclear, but it would seem prudent to monitor mycophenolate levels in any patient given sevelamer. One UK manufacturer of mycophenolate mofetil recommends that drugs for which a reduction in bioavailability could be clinically important should be taken at least 1 hour before or three 3 hours after taking sevelamer. One US manufacturer advises taking mycophenolate 2 hours before sevelamer.

Mycophenolate + Vaccines ✗

The body's immune response is suppressed by mycophenolate. The antibody response to vaccines may be reduced. The use of live attenuated vaccines may result in generalised infection.

For many inactivated vaccines even the reduced response seen is considered clinically useful and, in the case of renal transplant patients, influenza vaccination is actively recommended. If a vaccine is given, it may be prudent to monitor the response, so that alternative prophylactic measures can be considered where the response is inadequate. Note that even where effective antibody titres are produced, these may not persist as long as in healthy subjects, and more frequent booster doses may be required. The use of live vaccines is generally considered to be contraindicated. Ideally vaccines should take place before immunosuppressive treatment is started, and live vaccines should not be given for up to 6 months after treatment has stopped.

M

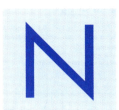

Nasal decongestants

Nasal decongestants + **Sibutramine**

There do not appear to be any studies on the use of sibutramine with decongestants, cough and cold medications, but the manufacturers predict that a rise in blood pressure and/or heart rate could occur. Ephedrine, pseudoephedrine, and xylometazoline (all indirect-acting sympathomimetics) have been specifically named. It would also seem prudent to apply this caution to the related drug, oxymetazoline.

Monitor the outcome of concurrent use carefully.

Nasal decongestants + **Theophylline**

There is some information suggesting an increased frequency of adverse effects when ephedrine is used with theophylline.

Note that ephedrine is an ingredient of a number of cough and cold remedies. It may be prudent to use an alternative. Patients taking theophylline requiring ephedrine should be advised to report any adverse effects.

Neomycin

Neomycin + **Penicillins**

The serum levels of oral phenoxymethylpenicillin can be halved by oral neomycin.

The clinical significance of this interaction is unclear. Monitor concurrent use to ensure phenoxymethylpenicillin is effective.

Neomycin + Vitamin A ❓

Neomycin can markedly reduce the absorption of vitamin A (retinol). The extent to which chronic treatment with neomycin would impair the treatment of vitamin A deficiency has not been determined.

> The general importance of this interaction is unknown, but bear it in mind in case of an unexpected response to treatment.

Neomycin + Warfarin and other oral anticoagulants ✔

Normally no interaction occurs, but in rare cases neomycin can cause a malabsorption syndrome, which may reduce vitamin K absorption and lead to over-anticoagulation.

> This interaction seems rare, and only likely to occur in those with totally inadequate diets, starvation or some other condition in which the intake of vitamin K is very limited and who are given long-term antibacterial treatment.

Nicorandil

Nicorandil + Phosphodiesterase type-5 inhibitors ✖

When sildenafil, tadalafil or vardenafil are given with *nitrates* potentially serious hypotension can occur, and myocardial infarction may possibly be precipitated. A number of fatalities have occurred as a result of this interaction. Nicorandil is expected to interact in the same way as the nitrates.

> The concurrent use of these phosphodiesterase inhibitors and nicorandil is contraindicated. Sildenafil should not be used within 24 hours of a *nitrate*, and some evidence suggests this is also a suitable separation for vardenafil. *Nitrates* should not be given for at least 48 hours after the last dose of tadalafil. Similar cautions would seem to apply to nicorandil.

Nicotinic acid (Niacin)

Nicotinic acid (Niacin) + Statins ⚠

The risk of muscle toxicity, such as rhabdomyolysis, may possibly be increased in patients taking a statin with nicotinic acid. In particular, a higher than expected incidence of myopathy has been reported in Chinese patients.

> This interaction has been disputed. Nevertheless, if the decision is made to use nicotinic acid with a statin the outcome should be closely monitored. All patients

should be warned to report promptly any unexplained muscle aches, tenderness, cramps, stiffness or weakness. The manufacturers of simvastatin state that the dose should not exceed 10 mg daily in patients taking nicotinic acid in doses of at least 1 g daily. It is also advised that Chinese patients taking simvastatin 80 mg should not take nicotinic acid. The manufacturer of lovastatin recommends a maximum dose of 20 mg daily in patients taking nicotinic acid in doses of 1 g or more daily. The manufacturers of atorvastatin and rosuvastatin suggest that the lowest statin dose should be used or a statin dose reduction considered.

Nitrates

Nitrates + Phosphodiesterase type-5 inhibitors ⊗

If sildenafil, tadalafil or vardenafil are given with organic nitrates (e.g. glyceryl trinitrate (nitroglycerin), isosorbide dinitrate, isosorbide mononitrate) potentially serious hypotension can occur, and myocardial infarction may possibly be precipitated. A number of fatalities have occurred as a result of this interaction.

The concurrent use of these phosphodiesterase inhibitors and all organic nitrates is contraindicated. Sildenafil should not be used within 24 hours of a nitrate, and some evidence suggests this is also a suitable separation for vardenafil. Nitrates should not be given for at least 48 hours after the last dose of tadalafil.

NNRTIs

The NNRTIs are extensively metabolised by cytochrome P450, particularly by CYP3A4. They are also inducers (nevirapine, efavirenz, and etravirine to a lesser degree) or inhibitors (delavirdine) of CYP3A4. The NNRTIs therefore have the potential to interact with drugs metabolised by CYP3A4, and may also be affected by CYP3A4 inhibitors and inducers. Delavirdine, efavirenz and etravirine may also inhibit some other cytochrome P450 isoenzymes and therefore the interaction profile varies between members of this drug group.

NNRTIs + Opioids

Buprenorphine

Delavirdine may markedly increase buprenorphine exposure more than 4-fold, and efavirenz may decrease buprenorphine exposure (by 50%).

One manufacturer states that the starting dose of sublingual buprenorphine (when used as a substitute for opioid dependence) should be halved; however, other manufacturers state that concurrent use should be avoided when buprenorphine is given parenterally or sublingually as a strong analgesic. One manufacturer states that no precaution is necessary in patients using transdermal buprenorphine. Be aware that buprenorphine may be less effective in patients also taking efavirenz.

Methadone ⚠

Methadone levels can be markedly reduced by efavirenz or nevirapine, and methadone withdrawal symptoms have been seen.

If efavirenz or nevirapine are added to established treatment with methadone, be alert for evidence of opiate withdrawal, and raise the methadone dose accordingly. Some patients may require an increase in the methadone dose frequency to twice daily. In patients who subsequently discontinue the NNRTI, the methadone dose should be gradually reduced over 1 to 2 weeks.

NNRTIs + Phenobarbital ⚠

The concurrent use of *carbamazepine* and efavirenz leads to a modest reduction in the plasma levels of both drugs; similar effects are predicted to occur with phenobarbital (and therefore primidone). Nevirapine would be expected to interact similarly. Phenobarbital may reduce the levels of delavirdine by up to 90%. The levels of etravirine are predicted to be reduced by phenobarbital. Note that primidone is metabolised to phenobarbital, and would therefore be expected to interact similarly.

The manufacturers state that when efavirenz is given with phenobarbital, there is a potential for reduction or increase in the levels of each drug: they therefore recommend periodic drug level monitoring. Note that efavirenz may cause seizures and caution is recommended in patients with a history of convulsions. Although evidence for an interaction with nevirapine is lacking, it would seem prudent to follow the monitoring suggested for efavirenz. The manufacturers of delavirdine and etravirine advise against their concurrent use with phenobarbital.

NNRTIs + Phenytoin ⚠

The concurrent use of *carbamazepine* and efavirenz leads to a modest reduction in the levels of both drugs; similar effects are predicted to occur with phenytoin (and therefore possibly fosphenytoin) Two cases of low or undetectable efavirenz levels have been reported with concurrent use phenytoin. Phenytoin may reduce the levels of delavirdine by up to 90% and limited evidence suggests that nevirapine levels are also reduced by phenytoin. The levels of etravirine are predicted to be reduced by phenytoin.

The manufacturers state that when efavirenz is given with phenytoin, there is a potential for a reduction or an increase in the levels of each drug: they therefore recommend periodic drug level monitoring of both drugs. Note that efavirenz may cause seizures and caution is recommended in patients with a history of convulsions. Although evidence for nevirapine is sparse it may be prudent to follow the same precautions given for efavirenz. The manufacturers of delavirdine and etravirine advise against concurrent use with phenytoin.

NNRTIs + **Phosphodiesterase type-5 inhibitors**

Delavirdine ⚠

Delavirdine is predicted to significantly increase sildenafil levels. Vardenafil and tadalafil are likely to interact similarly.

> Monitor the outcome of concurrent use, and decrease the dose of the phosphodiesterase type-5 inhibitor if adverse effects become troublesome. It may be prudent to consider a lower starting dose of sildenafil, tadalafil or vardenafil in patients taking delavirdine.

Other NNRTIs ⚠

Etravirine halves sildenafil levels; vardenafil and tadalafil may be similarly affected. Although evidence appears to be lacking, it would be reasonable to assume that efavirenz and nevirapine may interact similarly.

> If these phosphodiesterase type-5 inhibitors are not effective in patients taking efavirenz, etravirine or nevirapine, it would seem sensible to try a higher dose with close monitoring.

NNRTIs + **Prasugrel**

Prasugrel may slightly inhibit the metabolism of *bupropion* by CYP2B6 and decrease the levels of its metabolite by 23%. The manufacturers suggest that the metabolism of other substrates of CYP2B6 with a narrow therapeutic margin, such as efavirenz, may also be affected.

> A clinically significant interaction would seem unlikely. Consider an interaction if efavirenz adverse effects (such as rash, dizziness and headache) are troublesome.

NNRTIs + **Proton pump inhibitors**

Delavirdine

Antacids roughly halve the AUC of delavirdine, and proton pump inhibitors are predicted to interact similarly.

> Long-term concurrent use is not recommended.

Etravirine

Omeprazole modestly increases the AUC of etravirine by about 40%; however, the maximum concentration was not significantly affected.

> This modest increase is not considered clinically relevant. The manufacturer recommends that no dose adjustment is needed if etravirine is taken with a proton pump inhibitor.

NNRTIs + Rifabutin

Delavirdine ✖

Rifabutin causes a 5-fold increase in delavirdine clearance, and an 84% fall in its steady-state levels. Rifabutin levels may be raised up to 5-fold if the delavirdine dose is increased to compensate for this.

> The manufacturers and the Center for Disease Control (CDC) in the US recommend that rifabutin should not be used with delavirdine.

Efavirenz ⚠

Rifabutin does not affect efavirenz levels, but efavirenz may decrease rifabutin levels: a case of treatment failure has been reported.

> The Center for Disease Control (CDC) in the US states that the combination is probably clinically useful, and they suggest increasing the dose of rifabutin to 450 mg or 600 mg (taken daily or intermittently). The British HIV Association (BHIVA) also recommend increasing the rifabutin dose to 450 mg daily in patients taking efavirenz. Monitor the outcome of concurrent use carefully.

Etravirine or Nevirapine ⚠

Only minor increases in the AUC of nevirapine seem to occur with rifabutin; however, some patients may be more susceptible to adverse effects due to raised rifabutin levels. No significant pharmacokinetic interaction appears to occur between rifabutin and etravirine.

> In the UK, the use of rifabutin in patients taking nevirapine is not recommended. The Center for Disease Control (CDC) in the US and the British HIV Association (BHIVA) advise caution on the concurrent use of rifabutin and etravirine. They state that no dose adjustment of either drug is required on concurrent use, although the manufacturer of etravirine advises caution with rifabutin due to the theoretical risk of reduced levels of both drugs.

NNRTIs + Rifampicin (Rifampin)

Delavirdine ✖

Rifampicin causes a 27-fold increase in clearance of delavirdine, and the steady-state levels become almost undetectable.

> The Center for Disease Control (CDC) in the US and the manufacturer recommend that rifampicin should not be used with delavirdine.

Efavirenz ⚠

Rifampicin modestly reduces the AUC and levels of efavirenz, although there is debate about whether this requires a dose increase of efavirenz.

> The manufacturers advise that the dose of efavirenz should be raised to 800 mg daily when it is taken with rifampicin, whereas the British HIV Association (BHIVA) recommend this dose increase only in patients weighing more than 50 kg. The Center for Disease Control (CDC) in the US state that no dose alteration of efavirenz is usually needed, but note that some experts recommend increasing the

efavirenz dose to 800 mg daily in patients weighing more than 60 kg. Monitor closely for efavirenz efficacy and adverse effects, adjusting the efavirenz dose accordingly.

Etravirine

Rifampicin is predicted to significantly reduce etravirine levels and possibly lead to therapeutic failure.

The CDC in the US and the manufacturer contraindicate concurrent use of etravirine with rifampicin.

Nevirapine

A clinical study showed that the AUC of nevirapine was reduced by 31% in patients given rifampicin. Other information suggests that rifampicin reduces the AUC of nevirapine by 58%.

In the UK concurrent use is not generally advised but if both drugs are necessary, standard doses and monitoring of nevirapine is advised. The Center for Disease Control (CDC) in the US state that rifampicin no dose alteration is needed for either nevirapine or rifampicin on concurrent use.

NNRTIs + SSRIs

A case of serotonin syndrome, page 454, occurred in a woman taking fluoxetine when efavirenz was added; this resolved when the dose of fluoxetine was halved. Efavirenz decreases sertraline levels, and nevirapine decreases fluoxetine levels, whereas fluvoxamine modestly increases nevirapine levels.

Monitor for fluoxetine efficacy if nevirapine is given, and sertraline efficacy if efavirenz is given: adjust the SSRI dose as required. Monitor for signs of nevirapine adverse effects in patients also taking fluvoxamine. Bear the case of serotonin syndrome in mind if efavirenz and fluoxetine are both given.

NNRTIs + Statins

Delavirdine

Delavirdine is expected to raise the levels of atorvastatin, fluvastatin, simvastatin and lovastatin. This expectation is supported by a case of rhabdomyolysis, which developed in a patient taking atorvastatin and delavirdine.

The US manufacturer of delavirdine advises against the use of either simvastatin or lovastatin. Caution is advised with concurrent use of atorvastatin or fluvastatin, and the lowest possible statin dose should be used. Patients should be made aware of the risks of myopathy and rhabdomyolysis, and asked to promptly report muscle pain, tenderness or weakness, especially if accompanied by malaise, fever or dark urine.

Efavirenz, Etravirine or Nevirapine

Efavirenz (and possibly nevirapine) lowers the levels of atorvastatin, simvastatin, and

N

pravastatin. Etravirine modestly reduces the levels of atorvastatin and its active metabolites, and is predicted to have a similar effect on lovastatin and simvastatin. Etravirine is also predicted to *increase* the levels of fluvastatin.

> It would seem prudent to monitor the lipid profile of patients taking efavirenz and any of these statins, adjusting the dose as necessary, although bear in mind that NNRTIs are often used with protease inhibitors, page 438, which dramatically *increase* the levels of some statins.

NNRTIs + Tacrolimus

Limited evidence suggests that efavirenz may increase the clearance of tacrolimus resulting in reduced levels. Nevirapine and etravirine may interact similarly. Delavirdine is predicted to increase the levels of tacrolimus.

> Tacrolimus levels should be monitored as a matter of routine but it would seem prudent to increase monitoring if any of these NNRTIs is started, adjusting the tacrolimus dose as necessary.

NNRTIs + Warfarin and other oral anticoagulants

Three cases suggest that warfarin requirements are approximately doubled by nevirapine. One case of an unusually low warfarin dose requirement has been reported in a patient taking an efavirenz-based regimen. Etravirine appears to increase the exposure to warfarin; delavirdine is predicted to interact similarly.

> Monitor the effect of concurrent use of these NNRTIs on the anticoagulant response and adjust the coumarin dose as necessary.

NRTIs

The NRTIs are prodrugs, which need to be activated by phosphorylation within cells. Drugs may therefore interact with NRTIs by increasing or decreasing intracellular activation. NRTIs are water soluble, and are mainly eliminated by the kidneys (didanosine, lamivudine, stavudine, and zalcitabine) or undergo hepatic glucuronidation (abacavir, zidovudine). The few important interactions with these drugs primarily involve altered renal clearance. For zidovudine (and possibly abacavir) some interactions occur via altered glucuronidation, but the clinical relevance of these are less clear. Cytochrome P450-mediated interactions are not important for this class of drugs. Didanosine chewable tablets are formulated with antacid buffers that are intended to facilitate didanosine absorption by minimising acid-induced hydrolysis in the stomach. These preparations can therefore alter the absorption of other drugs that are affected by antacids (e.g. azoles, quinolones, tetracyclines). This interaction may be minimised by separating administration by at least 2 hours. Alternatively, the enteric-coated preparation of didanosine (gastro-resistant capsules) may be used.

NRTIs + Opioids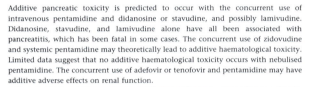

Zidovudine had no effect on methadone levels in one study, but there is one report of a patient requiring a modest increase in his methadone dose after starting zidovudine. Similarly, small changes in the pharmacokinetics of abacavir and methadone may occur on concurrent use, and there is a report of 2 patients requiring increases in their methadone doses. Methadone can increase zidovudine levels, and reduce the levels of abacavir, stavudine; and didanosine from the tablet formulation.

The clinical relevance of the changes in methadone levels is unclear. It may be prudent to monitor methadone dose requirements until more is known. The reduction in didanosine levels may be clinically relevant, and it would seem prudent to monitor virological response, adjusting the dose of the tablet formulation, or swapping to the enteric-coated preparation (which is not affected), if needed. The reduction in abacavir and stavudine levels with methadone is probably not clinically relevant, but this needs confirmation.

NRTIs + Pentamidine

Additive pancreatic toxicity is predicted to occur with the concurrent use of intravenous pentamidine and didanosine or stavudine, and possibly lamivudine. Didanosine, stavudine, and lamivudine alone have all been associated with pancreatitis, which has been fatal in some cases. The concurrent use of zidovudine and systemic pentamidine may theoretically lead to additive haematological toxicity. Limited data suggest that no additive haematological toxicity occurs with nebulised pentamidine. The concurrent use of adefovir or tenofovir and pentamidine may have additive adverse effects on renal function.

The manufacturers of didanosine advise that if pentamidine is needed, didanosine should be stopped, although if concurrent use is unavoidable, patients should be closely monitored. Similar precautions are advised with lamivudine. Careful monitoring is also recommended if pentamidine is given with stavudine. Monitor full blood count in patients given systemic pentamidine with zidovudine. If pentamidine is given with adefovir or tenofovir increase the frequency of renal function monitoring (the manufacturers of tenofovir advise at least weekly).

NRTIs + Phenobarbital

The UK manufacturer of abacavir says that potent enzyme inducers such as phenobarbital (and therefore probably primidone) may slightly decrease abacavir concentrations.

The clinical significance of this prediction is unclear but it may be prudent to monitor to ensure abacavir is effective.

NRTIs + Phenytoin

Phenytoin is predicted to decrease abacavir levels. Zidovudine may alter the pharmacokinetics of phenytoin, although this may be due to HIV infection itself. Fosphenytoin, a prodrug of phenytoin, may interact similarly.

The clinical significance of these interactions is unclear. However, it may be prudent to monitor the concurrent use of these NRTIs with phenytoin, and adjust the NRTI or phenytoin dose as necessary.

NRTIs + Probenecid ⚠️

Probenecid reduces the clearance of zidovudine, increasing its levels. The incidence of adverse effects is reported to be very much increased.

Concurrent use need not be avoided, but monitor carefully for zidovudine toxicity.

NRTIs + Rifabutin ⚠️

Studies suggest that rifabutin may increase the clearance of zidovudine by up to 50%, whereas other studies have found no interaction.

The clinical implications of this interaction are unknown. Be alert for any evidence of a reduced response to zidovudine if rifabutin is given.

NRTIs + Rifampicin (Rifampin) ⚠️

Several studies suggest that rifampicin more than doubles the clearance of zidovudine. In some subjects increased haematological toxicity was also seen. Rifampicin is predicted to interact similarly with abacavir.

Be alert for any evidence of a reduced response to these antivirals and monitor for haematological toxicity with zidovudine.

NRTIs + Valproate ⚠️

Valproate increases the AUC of zidovudine by 80%. In one case valproate increased zidovudine levels up to 3-fold, and increased the CSF levels of zidovudine by 74%. Cases of severe anaemia and liver toxicity have been attributed to this interaction.

It would seem prudent to monitor for zidovudine adverse effects and possible toxicity.

NSAIDs

NSAIDs + NSAIDs ❌

The combined use of two or more NSAIDs increases the risk of gastrointestinal damage.

As there is no clear clinical rationale for the combined use of different NSAIDs, such use should be avoided.

NSAIDs + Opioids

NSAIDs, general ✔

On the whole the concurrent use of NSAIDs and opioids is successful and without incident; however, see the specific instances discussed below.

No action needed.

Diclofenac ❓

An isolated report describes grand mal seizures in a patient given diclofenac and pentazocine. Diclofenac did not alter morphine pharmacokinetics in one study. However, in another, diclofenac slightly increased respiratory depression despite a reduction in morphine use, possibly because of persistent levels of an active metabolite of morphine.

These interactions are not established and they seem unlikely to be of general significance, but be alert to the possibility of increased sedation, or, with pentazocine, use with caution in patients who are known to be seizure-prone.

Ketorolac ⚠

A single case report describes marked respiratory depression in a man taking buprenorphine with ketorolac.

This seems unlikely to be of general significance but be alert to the possibility of increased sedation.

NSAIDs + Paracetamol (Acetaminophen) ✔

On the whole the concurrent use of NSAIDs with paracetamol is beneficial and without serious adverse effects. One epidemiological study found that paracetamol alone, and particularly when given with an NSAID, was associated with an increased risk of gastrointestinal bleeding, but other studies have not found such an effect. Diflunisal raises paracetamol levels by 50% but does not alter its total bioavailability.

The interaction with diflunisal has not been shown to be clinically significant but the manufacturers advise caution because of the risks of increased paracetamol levels. Paracetamol is not usually considered to increase the risk of upper gastrointestinal adverse effects and there is insufficient evidence to suggest that the concurrent use of paracetamol and any NSAID should be avoided.

NSAIDs + Penicillamine ❓

Indometacin has been found to increase the peak levels of penicillamine by about 22%. The manufacturers warn that the concurrent use of NSAIDs and penicillamine may increase the risk of nephrotoxicity.

The US manufacturer specifically recommends avoiding oxyphenbutazone or phenylbutazone because these drugs are also associated with serious haematological and renal effects. There seems to be no reason to avoid other NSAIDs and penicillamine, but if problems occur bear the possibility of a drug interaction in mind.

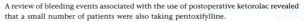

NSAIDs + Pentoxifylline ✖

A review of bleeding events associated with the use of postoperative ketorolac revealed that a small number of patients were also taking pentoxifylline.

The UK manufacturer of ketorolac, rather cautiously, contraindicates concurrent use, whereas the US manufacturer makes no mention of an interaction. There seems to be no evidence regarding this interaction with other NSAIDs; however, as both pentoxifylline and the non-selective NSAIDs may cause bleeding it would be prudent to be alert for this possible interaction.

NSAIDs + Phenytoin ✖

Phenytoin levels can be markedly increased by azapropazone, and toxicity can develop rapidly. A similar interaction has been seen with phenylbutazone, and it seems likely that oxyphenbutazone will interact similarly. Fosphenytoin, a prodrug of phenytoin, may interact similarly with these NSAIDs.

The concurrent use of phenytoin and azapropazone is contraindicated. Monitor the outcome of adding phenylbutazone or oxyphenbutazone and reduce the phenytoin dose as necessary. Warn the patient to monitor for indicators of phenytoin toxicity (blurred vision, nystagmus, ataxia or drowsiness).

NSAIDs + Prasugrel ❓

The concurrent use of prasugrel with chronic NSAID treatment has not been studied. The manufacturer notes that there is a potential increased risk of bleeding.

If concurrent use is necessary, patients should be monitored for signs of excessive bleeding and advised to report any unusual bleeding. Consider giving additional gastrointestinal prophylaxis (e.g. an H_2-receptor antagonists or a proton pump inhibitor) in patients at risk of gastrointestinal ulceration and bleeding. Note that some NSAIDs (particularly coxibs but also non-selective NSAIDs) are associated with an increased thrombotic/cardiovascular risk, particularly when used at high doses and for long-term treatment. Therefore coxibs are contraindicated, and NSAIDs should generally be avoided, in those with ischaemic heart disease, cerebrovascular disease, and peripheral artery disease.

NSAIDs + Probenecid ❓

Probenecid reduces the clearance of dexketoprofen, diflunisal, ketoprofen, ketorolac, indometacin, meclofenamate, naproxen, tenoxicam and tiaprofenic acid, and raises their levels. Increased clinical effects have been seen for indometacin, but indometacin toxicity has also occurred.

Increased levels do occur, which could reasonably be expected to result in increased beneficial and adverse effects. However, the clinical outcome of this interaction is uncertain and so action (e.g. dose adjustments) should be based on the response of the patient. Reduce the NSAID dose if necessary. Note that probenecid is specifically contraindicated by the manufacturers of ketorolac.

NSAIDs + Propafenone

Because valdecoxib (the metabolite of parecoxib) increases *dextromethorphan* levels about 3-fold and celecoxib increases *dextromethorphan* levels about 2.4-fold, the manufacturers predict that the levels of flecainide (which is similarly metabolised) will also be raised by these coxibs.

> The general importance of this interaction is unclear. Monitor concurrent use for adverse effects, and consider reducing the dose of the antiarrhythmic if these become troublesome.

NSAIDs + Quinolones

Convulsions have been seen in patients given fenbufen with enoxacin, and several NSAIDs with ofloxacin or ciprofloxacin. The CSM in the UK warns that this interaction could occur with any combination of an NSAID and a quinolone.

> Convulsions are rare, so in the majority of patients concurrent use should be without problem. Patients with epilepsy, or those predisposed to convulsions, seem to be at greater risk, so avoid concurrent use in these patients or monitor very closely.

NSAIDs + Rifampicin (Rifampin)

The levels of celecoxib, diclofenac, and etoricoxib are reduced by rifampicin.

> The clinical relevance of these interactions is unclear, but it seems likely that the efficacy of these NSAIDs will be reduced by rifampicin. Concurrent use should be well monitored, and the NSAID dose increased if necessary.

NSAIDs + SSRIs ❓

The SSRIs may increase the risk of upper gastrointestinal bleeding and the risk appears to be further increased by the concurrent use of NSAIDs.

> The manufacturers of the SSRIs state that patients should be warned that the concurrent use of NSAIDs should be undertaken with caution. Alternatives such as paracetamol (acetaminophen) or less gastrotoxic NSAIDs such as ibuprofen may be considered, but if the combination of an SSRI and NSAID cannot be avoided, prescribing of gastroprotective drugs such as proton pump inhibitors, or H_2-receptor antagonists should be considered, especially in elderly patients or those with a history of gastrointestinal bleeding.

NSAIDs + Tacrolimus

The UK manufacturers of tacrolimus suggest that all NSAIDs may have additive nephrotoxic effects with tacrolimus. Cases of renal failure have been reported in patients receiving the combination. However, a study in rheumatoid arthritis patients found no increased risk.

> Tacrolimus levels and/or effects (e.g. on renal function) should be monitored as a

matter of routine, but it may be prudent to increase monitoring if NSAIDs are started.

NSAIDs + Ticlopidine ❓

The risk of faecal blood loss, gastrointestinal haemorrhage and other bleeding is increased by concurrent use of *clopidogrel* and NSAIDs. Ticlopidine is expected to interact similarly.

The manufacturers advise caution if NSAIDs and ticlopidine are given together. Consider giving additional gastrointestinal prophylaxis such as a proton pump inhibitor in patients at risk of gastrointestinal ulceration and bleeding. Note that giving NSAIDs to patients with ischaemic heart disease may increase the risk of thrombotic events.

NSAIDs + Tricyclics ⚠

The manufacturers of celecoxib (a CYP2D6 inhibitor) predict that it will raise the levels of the tricyclics (CYP2D6 substrates). The levels of other CYP2D6 substrates have been more than doubled by celecoxib.

Monitor concurrent use for tricyclic adverse effects (such as nausea, dry mouth, palpitations), and consider reducing the dose if these become troublesome.

NSAIDs + Vancomycin ⚠

Indometacin reduces the renal clearance of vancomycin in premature neonates. This interaction appears not to have been studied in adults.

The effect in adults is unclear, but in neonates be prepared to reduce the dose of vancomycin in the presence of indometacin.

NSAIDs + Warfarin and other oral anticoagulants

Azapropazone, Ketorolac, Oxyphenbutazone, Phenylbutazone ✖

The anticoagulant effects of warfarin are markedly increased by azapropazone, ketorolac, oxyphenbutazone and phenylbutazone. Bleeding has been reported in patients taking phenindione or phenprocoumon when given phenylbutazone.

Concurrent use is contraindicated.

Coxibs ❓

There is some evidence to suggest that celecoxib and parecoxib do not normally interact with warfarin. However, raised INRs accompanied by bleeding, particularly in

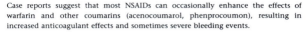

the elderly, have been attributed to the use of warfarin and celecoxib. Etoricoxib causes a small increase in INR when it is taken with warfarin.

> Monitor the anticoagulant effect if these NSAIDs are added to or withdrawn from the treatment of patients taking anticoagulants.

Other NSAIDs ❓

Case reports suggest that most NSAIDs can occasionally enhance the effects of warfarin and other coumarins (acenocoumarol, phenprocoumon), resulting in increased anticoagulant effects and sometimes severe bleeding events.

> Monitor the anticoagulant effect if NSAIDs are added to or withdrawn from the treatment of patients taking anticoagulants. Note that since NSAIDs reduce platelet aggregation and cause gastrointestinal irritation they can prolong and worsen any bleeding events.

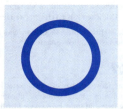

Opioids

Opioids with mixed agonist/antagonist properties (e.g. buprenorphine, butorphanol, nalbuphine, pentazocine) may precipitate opioid withdrawal symptoms in patients taking pure opioid agonists such as fentanyl, methadone, morphine and tramadol.

Opioids + Phenobarbital

Buprenorphine, Fentanyl, Methadone or Pethidine (Meperidine) ⚠

Phenobarbital and primidone appear to increase fentanyl and methadone requirements, and methadone withdrawal reactions have been seen. The analgesic effects of pethidine can be reduced by barbiturates, but in one study, increased sedation was seen with phenobarbital. The manufacturers predict that phenobarbital and primidone will reduce the levels of buprenorphine.

Anticipate the need to increase the dose of these opioids in patients taking phenobarbital or primidone. Monitor concurrent use to ensure the opioid effects are adequate. It may be necessary to give the methadone twice daily, remembering to reduce the methadone dose if phenobarbital is stopped. One manufacturer of sublingual buprenorphine advises avoiding the concurrent use of phenobarbital, and one manufacturer of methadone advises against concurrent use with CNS depressants including barbiturates.

Opioids, general ❓

The concurrent use of opioids (including weak opioids such as codeine) and barbiturates appears to increase sedation and respiratory depression.

Concurrent use need not be avoided, but be aware of the potential for respiratory depression, especially in patients with a restricted respiratory capacity. Note that tramadol should be avoided if possible as it may increase the risk of seizures.

Opioids + **Phenytoin**

Phenytoin appears to increase fentanyl and methadone requirements and methadone withdrawal reactions have been seen. The manufacturers predict that phenytoin will decrease buprenorphine levels. Phenytoin increases the production of the toxic metabolite of pethidine (meperidine), which resulted in pethidine toxicity in one case. Fosphenytoin, a prodrug of phenytoin, may interact similarly with these opioids.

0

> Anticipate the need to increase the dose of these opioids in patients taking phenytoin and monitor concurrent use to ensure the opioid effects are adequate. It may be necessary to give the methadone twice daily. Remember to reduce the opioid dose if phenytoin is stopped. Note that one manufacturer of sublingual buprenorphine advises avoiding concurrent use.

Opioids + **Pregabalin**

The manufacturer of pregabalin notes that there was no clinically relevant pharmacokinetic interaction between pregabalin and oxycodone, and that there was no clinically important effect on respiration. However, pregabalin appeared to cause an additive impairment in cognitive and gross motor function when given with oxycodone. It seems possible that all opioids may have this effect.

> The degree of impairment will depend on the individual patient. However, warn all patients of the potential effects, and counsel against driving or undertaking other skilled tasks.

Opioids + **Protease inhibitors**

Alfentanil and Fentanyl

Ritonavir markedly increases the levels of fentanyl, and markedly increases alfentanil-induced miosis. Concurrent use is expected to increase the risk of prolonged or delayed respiratory depression. Other protease inhibitors may also be expected to interact similarly but there seems little documented about these effects in practice. Care should also be taken if ritonavir is used with other protease inhibitors as a pharmacokinetic enhancer.

> Concurrent use should be monitored. Dose reductions of fentanyl (given by any route) or alfentanil are likely to be required, particularly with long-term use.

Buprenorphine

Ritonavir increases the levels of buprenorphine and increase its adverse effects such as sedation. Other protease inhibitors may also be expected to interact similarly.

> Some suggest halving the starting dose of buprenorphine when it is used for opioid dependence, although note that the interaction may not be of significance with low-dose ritonavir alone in patients who are opioid-tolerant. If buprenorphine is given with any protease inhibitor it would seem prudent to monitor the outcome of concurrent use and adjust the dose of buprenorphine accordingly. Note that one manufacturer of sublingual and injectable buprenorphine states that concurrent use should be avoided. There appears to be less likelihood of an interaction with buprenorphine used transdermally.

Dextropropoxyphene (Propoxyphene)

Ritonavir is predicted to increase the effects of dextropropoxyphene. Other protease inhibitors may also be expected to interact similarly but there seems little documented about these effects in practice.

0

The UK manufacturer of ritonavir contraindicates its use with dextropropoxyphene as extremely raised dextropropoxyphene levels may occur, which would increase the risk of serious adverse events (e.g. respiratory depression). However, the US manufacturer only suggests that a dose decrease may be needed.

Methadone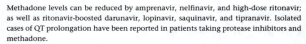

Methadone levels can be reduced by amprenavir, nelfinavir, and high-dose ritonavir; as well as ritonavir-boosted darunavir, lopinavir, saquinavir, and tipranavir. Isolated cases of QT prolongation have been reported in patients taking protease inhibitors and methadone.

An increased methadone dose may be needed in some patients to prevent opiate withdrawal. Patients taking methadone in doses greater than 100 mg and with additional risk factors for QT prolongation should be carefully monitored, see also Drugs that prolong the QT interval, page 277.

Morphine

Ritonavir is predicted to decrease the levels of morphine.

The clinical significance of this prediction is unclear however it would be prudent to monitor concurrent use to ensure morphine is effective and pain control is adequate.

Pethidine (Meperidine)

Ritonavir decreased pethidine levels but increased norpethidine levels, which may possibly increase toxicity on long-term use.

The manufacturers of pethidine oral preparations and injection contraindicate or advise against its use with ritonavir because of the risk of norpethidine toxicity. Long-term use of pethidine with other protease inhibitors that are given with low-dose ritonavir is also not recommended.

Other opioids ❓

Ritonavir is predicted to increase the effects of dihydrocodeine, oxycodone, and tramadol. Although, there is no clinical evidence that this occurs it is in line with the known metabolism of these drugs. Ritonavir may also *decrease* the effects of codeine by inhibiting its metabolism to an active metabolite.

Caution and careful monitoring of effects is warranted with dihydrocodeine, oxycodone, and tramadol as high levels may lead to CNS depression. Smaller initial doses may be appropriate. In contrast, codeine may be less effective than expected. Low-dose ritonavir would be expected to have a less potent effect on the metabolism of these opioids and dose adjustments would not generally be required.

Opioids + Quinidine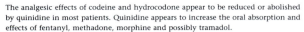

The analgesic effects of codeine and hydrocodone appear to be reduced or abolished by quinidine in most patients. Quinidine appears to increase the oral absorption and effects of fentanyl, methadone, morphine and possibly tramadol.

> The interaction with codeine, and hydrocodone is possible in the majority of patients. Consider the use of an alternative analgesic. The pharmacokinetics of dihydrocodeine, hydromorphone and oxycodone do not appear to be affected to a clinically significant extent. Monitor for increased opioid effects after the oral administration of fentanyl, methadone, and morphine. Note that quinidine and high-dose methadone may prolong the QT interval, see drugs that prolong the QT interval, page 277.

Opioids + Quinolones

It has been suggested that opioids decrease oral ciprofloxacin levels, but good evidence for this appears to be lacking.

> Based on this rather slim evidence, some have suggested that the concurrent use of opioids and ciprofloxacin as pre-medication should be avoided. Note that both high-dose methadone and some quinolones (gatifloxacin, levofloxacin, moxifloxacin and in particular sparfloxacin) may prolong the QT interval, see drugs that prolong the QT interval, page 277.

Opioids + Rifampicin (Rifampin)

Methadone levels can be markedly reduced by rifampicin, and withdrawal symptoms have occurred in some patients. Similarly, rifampicin markedly increases the metabolism of alfentanil, codeine, fentanyl, morphine and possibly oxycodone, and reduces their effects.

> Monitor concurrent use for reduced opioid effects and adjust the dose accordingly.

Opioids + Sibutramine ❌

The concurrent use of serotonergic drugs and sibutramine may theoretically lead to the potentially fatal serotonin syndrome, page 454.

> The manufacturers of sibutramine state that it should not be taken with any serotonergic drugs and specifically name fentanyl, pentazocine and pethidine (meperidine).

Opioids + SSRIs

Tramadol

Several case reports describe the development of serotonin syndrome, page 454, in patients taking citalopram, fluoxetine, paroxetine or sertraline with tramadol. Another patient developed hallucinations when taking tramadol with paroxetine.

> There would seem to be little reason for totally avoiding the concurrent use of the

SSRIs and tramadol but it would clearly be prudent to use the combination cautiously and monitor the outcome closely. Tramadol should be used with caution with SSRIs because of the possible increased risk of seizures.

Other opioids 🔞

In isolated cases the concurrent use of SSRIs and opioids (including fentanyl, hydromorphone, oxycodone, pentazocine, pethidine (meperidine), and possibly morphine) has resulted in the serotonin syndrome. Methadone levels are modestly increased by fluvoxamine, paroxetine and sertraline, and possibly fluoxetine.

Serotonin syndrome, page 454, seems to be a rare occurrence, but the possibility should be borne in mind if an SSRI is given with one of these opioids. Be aware that the use of fluvoxamine, paroxetine, sertraline or fluoxetine may alter the response to methadone. Monitor the outcome of concurrent use for methadone adverse effects.

Opioids + Tricyclics

Opioids, general 🔞

In general, the concurrent use of most opioids and tricyclics is uneventful, although lethargy, sedation, and respiratory depression have been reported. In addition, the incidence of myoclonus (muscle twitching or spasm) in patients on high doses of morphine appeared to be increased by tricyclic antidepressants in one study.

Serious adverse interactions seem rare and concurrent use may be beneficial in pain management. Be alert for any evidence of increased CNS depression and warn patients that sedation can occur. Respiratory depression is more likely to be of significance in those who already have respiratory impairment. Note that some tricyclics and high-dose methadone may prolong the QT interval, see drugs that prolong the QT interval, page 277.

Tramadol ⚠️

The CSM in the UK recommends caution if tramadol is used with a tricyclic antidepressant as both drugs may reduce the seizure threshold. There have been reports of seizures on concurrent use. In addition, concurrent use may lead to the development of serotonin syndrome, page 454.

Consider an alternative analgesic or antidepressant if possible, or use with caution, particularly in epileptic patients or those taking other drugs that affect serotonin.

Opioids + Triptans ⚠️

Sumatriptan given by injection appears not to interact with butorphanol nasal spray, but if both drugs are given by nasal spray a significant interaction may occur, resulting in a modest reduction in butorphanol levels.

When butorphanol was given 30 minutes after sumatriptan no significant pharmacokinetic interaction was noted. It would therefore seem prudent to separate administration to ensure the full effects of butorphanol are achieved.

Opioids + **Warfarin and other oral anticoagulants**

Tramadol has been reported to increase the anticoagulant effects of acenocoumarol, fluindione, warfarin and phenprocoumon in a few patients and a retrospective cohort study also found an increased risk of bleeding when acenocoumarol or phenprocoumon was given with tramadol. Several patients taking warfarin have shown a marked increase in prothrombin times and/or bleeding when given co-proxamol (which contains dextropropoxyphene (propoxyphene)), but the interaction seems to be uncommon.

> It would be prudent to consider monitoring prothrombin times in any patient taking anticoagulants when tramadol is first added, being alert for the need to reduce the anticoagulant dose. An interaction with dextropropoxyphene seems rare, but bear it in mind in case of an excessive response to anticoagulant treatment.

0

Orlistat

Orlistat + **Vitamins**

Orlistat decreases the absorption of supplemental betacarotene and vitamin E. There is some evidence to suggest that some patients may have low vitamin D levels while taking orlistat, even if they are also taking multivitamins.

> It is recommended that multivitamin preparations should be taken at least 2 hours after orlistat, such as at bedtime. The US manufacturers suggest that patients taking orlistat should be advised to take multivitamins, because of the possibility of reduced vitamin levels. Note that it has been suggested that monitoring of vitamin D may be required, even if multivitamins are given.

Orlistat + **Warfarin and other oral anticoagulants**

Orlistat does not appear to affect the pharmacokinetics of warfarin, however it reduces fat absorption, and might therefore reduce vitamin K absorption and affect coagulation. Several cases of increased INR have been reported in patients taking either warfarin or acenocoumarol after also taking orlistat.

> Close monitoring for changes in coagulation parameters is recommended in patients taking orlistat with a coumarin or indanedione. As changes in diet are known to affect anticoagulant effects this seems prudent.

Oxcarbazepine

Oxcarbazepine is a derivative of carbamazepine, but appears to have a lesser effect on CYP3A4. Oxcarbazepine can also act as an inhibitor of CYP2C19.

Oxcarbazepine + Phenytoin ❓

High doses of oxcarbazepine increase phenytoin levels. Elevations in phenytoin levels of up to 40% have been seen in retrospective studies. Fosphenytoin, a prodrug of phenytoin, may interact similarly.

> Bear this interaction in mind on concurrent use, and with high oxcarbazepine doses consider monitoring phenytoin levels; decrease the dose as necessary. Indicators of phenytoin toxicity include blurred vision, nystagmus, ataxia or drowsiness.

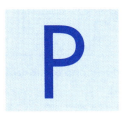

Paracetamol (Acetaminophen)

Paracetamol (Acetaminophen) + Rifampicin (Rifampin)

Rifampicin induces the glucuronidation of paracetamol and increases its clearance, but does not increase the formation of hepatotoxic metabolites of paracetamol.

The clinical importance of these findings awaits further study.

Paracetamol (Acetaminophen) + Warfarin and other oral anticoagulants

An equal number of randomised studies have found a modest increase in the anticoagulant effect (e.g. an increase in INR of 1) of coumarins as have reported no effect. Other cohort studies found no evidence of a change in anticoagulant effect. There are isolated case reports of an increase in anticoagulant effects in patients taking warfarin or acenocoumarol and paracetamol.

On the basis of the available data, it is not possible to firmly recommend increased monitoring, or dismiss its advisability. Further study is clearly needed. Note that paracetamol is still considered to be safer than aspirin or NSAIDs as an analgesic in the presence of an anticoagulant because it does not affect platelets or cause gastric bleeding.

Penicillins

Penicillins + Probenecid

Probenecid reduces the excretion of the penicillins, and usually raises their levels.

This is generally considered to be a beneficial interaction, but bear in mind that, in some cases, such as in patients with renal impairment, the increase in penicillin levels may be undesirably large.

Penicillins + **Warfarin and other oral anticoagulants** ⚠

Isolated cases of increased prothrombin times and/or bleeding in patients taking coumarins have been seen in patients given amoxicillin (with or without clavulanic acid) or intravenous benzylpenicillin. There is also some evidence that phenoxymethylpenicillin (penicillin V) does not increase the risk of bleeding in patients taking coumarins. In contrast, dicloxacillin may cause a modest reduction in warfarin effects, and an isolated case of thrombosis has been reported.

Even though the general picture is of no interaction, factors associated with infection, such as fever, can also affect anticoagulant response. Therefore, if a patient is unwell enough to require an antibacterial, it may be prudent to increase monitoring of coagulation status. Monitor within 3 days of starting the antibacterial.

Pentoxifylline

Pentoxifylline + **Quinolones** ⚠

Evidence from one study suggests that ciprofloxacin increases the peak serum levels of pentoxifylline by 60%, and may increase the incidence of adverse effects. In some clinical studies ciprofloxacin has been used to boost the levels of pentoxifylline.

It has been suggested that the dose of pentoxifylline should be halved if ciprofloxacin is also given, which may be a sensible precaution. Alternatively, it may be sufficient to recommend a reduction in pentoxifylline dose only in those who experience adverse effects (e.g. nausea, headache). Note that other quinolones may also interact, see quinolones, page 444.

Pentoxifylline + **Theophylline** ⚠

Pentoxifylline can raise serum theophylline serum levels by about 30%. Aminophylline is expected to be similarly affected.

Patients should be well monitored for theophylline adverse effects (headache, nausea, palpitations) while taking both drugs and it may be necessary to decrease the theophylline dose in some cases. Note that one manufacturer of intravenous aminophylline contraindicates concurrent use.

Pentoxifylline + **Warfarin and other oral anticoagulants**

Some studies have found that pentoxifylline does not alter the anticoagulant effects of phenprocoumon or acenocoumarol; however, one study suggests that there might be an increased risk of serious bleeding if pentoxifylline is given with acenocoumarol. Pentoxifylline alone has rarely been associated with bleeding.

> It may be prudent to increase the frequency of INR monitoring on the concurrent use of pentoxifylline and warfarin. This would seem sensible with any coumarin or indanedione.

Phenobarbital

Studies in man and *animals* clearly show that the barbiturates are potent liver enzyme inducers. The most commonly used barbiturate is phenobarbital, which is known to induce CYP3A4, amongst other isoenzymes. Most of the interaction information concerns phenobarbital, but all barbiturates would be expected to share its interactions to a greater or lesser extent. Note that primidone is metabolised to phenobarbital, and so would therefore also be expected to share many of its interactions.

Phenobarbital + **Phenytoin** ⚠

The concurrent use of phenytoin and phenobarbital is normally uneventful. However, changes in phenytoin levels (often decreases but sometimes increases) can occur if phenobarbital is added, but seizure control is not usually affected by this pharmacokinetic interaction. Phenytoin toxicity following barbiturate withdrawal has been seen. Increased phenobarbital levels and possibly toxicity may occur as a result of the addition of phenytoin to phenobarbital. Similar interactions may occur with primidone and fosphenytoin.

> Given the unpredictable outcome of concurrent use it would seem prudent to monitor levels if one drug is added to the other or if a dose is changed. Indicators of phenobarbital toxicity include drowsiness, ataxia or dysarthria.

Phenobarbital + **Phosphodiesterase type-5 inhibitors** ❓

Phenobarbital (and therefore probably primidone) are expected to reduce the levels of phosphodiesterase type-5 inhibitors, because other inducers of CYP3A4 have been shown to do so. For example, sildenafil levels are reduced by 70% by *bosentan* and tadalafil levels are reduced by 88% by *rifampicin*. Vardenafil is also metabolised by CYP3A4, and therefore its levels may possibly be lowered by phenobarbital and primidone.

> If these phosphodiesterase type-5 inhibitors are not effective in patients taking

phenobarbital or primidone, it would seem sensible to try a higher dose with close monitoring.

Phenobarbital + Praziquantel

Phenobarbital (and therefore probably primidone) markedly reduces praziquantel levels, but whether this results in neurocysticercosis treatment failures is unclear.

When treating systemic worm infections such as neurocysticercosis some authors have advised increasing the praziquantel dose from 25 to 50 mg/kg if phenobarbital is being used; however, note that the manufacturers recommended dose of praziquantel for neurocysticercosis is 50 mg/kg daily in three divided doses. The interaction with antiepileptics is of no importance when praziquantel is used for intestinal worm infections (where its action is a local effect on the worms in the gut).

Phenobarbital + Propafenone

Phenobarbital reduces propafenone levels by 26 to 87%. Primidone is metabolised to phenobarbital and may therefore interact similarly.

The clinical importance of this interaction awaits assessment but check that propafenone remains effective if phenobarbital is added, and that toxicity does not occur if it is stopped.

Phenobarbital + Protease inhibitors

Phenobarbital and other barbiturates are predicted to increase the metabolism of the protease inhibitors, thereby reducing their levels and possibly resulting in therapeutic failure. However, one case suggested that this may not have occurred when primidone was given with ritonavir-boosted saquinavir.

The combination of protease inhibitors and barbiturates should be used with caution. Monitor for antiviral efficacy. Note that some manufacturers contraindicate or advise against concurrent use.

Phenobarbital + Pyridoxine

Daily doses of pyridoxine 200 mg can cause reductions of 40 to 50% in phenobarbital levels in some patients. Primidone is metabolised to phenobarbital and may therefore be affected similarly, although this does not appear to have been studied.

Concurrent use should be monitored if large doses of pyridoxine are used, being alert for the need to increase the phenobarbital dose. It seems unlikely that small doses (as in multivitamin preparations) will interact to any great extent.

Phenobarbital + Quinidine

Quinidine levels can be reduced by the concurrent use of phenobarbital or primidone. Loss of arrhythmia control is possible if the quinidine dose is not increased.

Concurrent use need not be avoided, but be alert for the need to increase the quinidine dose. If phenobarbital or primidone are withdrawn the quinidine dose may need to be reduced to avoid quinidine toxicity. Quinidine levels should be monitored if possible.

Phenobarbital + Ranolazine

Rifampicin (*rifampin*) reduces ranolazine levels by 95%, and loss of efficacy is expected. Phenobarbital (and therefore probably primidone, which is metabolised to phenobarbital) are predicted to interact in the same way as rifampicin.

The manufacturers recommend avoiding concurrent use. In the absence of any information on the magnitude of the effect of phenobarbital on ranolazine levels, this seems prudent.

Phenobarbital + Rifampicin (Rifampin)

Phenobarbital possibly modestly increases the clearance of rifampicin (up to a 40% reduction in rifampicin levels in one study). The effect of rifampicin on phenobarbital levels is unknown, but note that rifampicin markedly increases the clearance of hexobarbital. Primidone is metabolised to phenobarbital and may therefore interact similarly with rifampicin.

The outcome of concurrent use is unclear but a reduction in the levels of both rifampicin and the barbiturate seems possible. Concurrent use need not be avoided, but be alert for a reduced response to both drugs.

Phenobarbital + Sirolimus

The manufacturers of sirolimus predict that phenobarbital (and therefore probably primidone) may lower the serum levels of sirolimus, probably because rifampicin (rifampin), another CYP3A4 inducer, has been shown to do so.

The extent of any change in sirolimus levels is uncertain, but it would seem prudent to increase the frequency of monitoring of sirolimus levels during concurrent use. The manufacturers state that concurrent use should be avoided.

Phenobarbital + Solifenacin

Ketoconazole increases solifenacin levels 2- to 3-fold by *inhibiting* CYP3A4. The manufacturers predict that potent CYP3A4 *inducers* (e.g. phenobarbital, and therefore probably primidone) will decrease solifenacin levels.

Be alert for a reduction in the efficacy of solifenacin in patients taking phenobarbital or primidone.

Phenobarbital + SSRIs

In one study in 6 subjects phenobarbital caused reductions of 10 to 86% in the AUC of paroxetine, but the mean values were not altered to a statistically significant extent. One subject showed an *increase* of about 60% in their AUC. Primidone is metabolised to phenobarbital and may therefore interact similarly with paroxetine.

Although there seems to be little correlation between plasma paroxetine levels and its efficacy, be alert for the need to increase its dose if phenobarbital is given. Note that SSRIs can decrease the seizure threshold and so they should be used with caution in patients given barbiturates for epilepsy.

Phenobarbital + Tacrolimus

Phenobarbital (and therefore probably primidone) is predicted to reduce tacrolimus levels (this effect has been used therapeutically).

Based on the known metabolism of these drugs it would be prudent to monitor tacrolimus levels in a patient given phenobarbital or primidone.

Phenobarbital + Tetracyclines

The serum levels of doxycycline are reduced and may fall below the accepted minimum inhibitory concentration in patients receiving long-term treatment with barbiturates.

It has been suggested that the doxycycline dose could be doubled to overcome this reaction. Alternatively, tetracycline, oxytetracycline, and chlortetracycline appear not to interact and may therefore be suitable alternatives.

Phenobarbital + Theophylline

Theophylline serum levels can be reduced by phenobarbital or pentobarbital (clearance increased by roughly one-third). A single report describes a similar interaction with secobarbital, and an interaction would be expected to occur with other barbiturates.

It would be prudent to monitor theophylline levels if a barbiturate is added to or withdrawn from theophylline treatment.

Phenobarbital + Tiagabine

Tiagabine levels may be reduced 1.5- to 3-fold by both phenobarbital and primidone.

The manufacturers recommend that tiagabine 30 to 45 mg (in divided doses) should be given to patients taking enzyme-inducing antiepileptics.

Phenobarbital + **Topiramate**

Phenobarbital and primidone can reduce topiramate levels by about 30%.

> When topiramate is given with phenobarbital or primidone, its dose should be titrated to effect. If phenobarbital or primidone are added or withdrawn be aware that the dose of topiramate may be need adjustment.

Phenobarbital + **Toremifene**

Phenobarbital can reduce toremifene levels. Primidone is metabolised to phenobarbital and may therefore interact similarly.

> The manufacturers of toremifene suggest that its dose may need to be doubled in the presence of phenobarbital.

Phenobarbital + **Tricyclics**

Barbiturates reduce the levels of the tricyclic antidepressants, which has been associated with the re-emergence of depression. Although not all combinations have been studied, they would all be expected to interact similarly.

> Monitor the outcome of concurrent use anticipating reduced tricyclic antidepressant effects. Consider an alternative to the barbiturate, or raise the tricyclic dose if problems occur. Note that tricyclics lower the seizure threshold and so they should be used with caution in patients given barbiturates for epilepsy.

Phenobarbital + **Vaccines**

Influenza vaccine can cause a transient moderate (30%) rise in phenobarbital levels. Primidone is metabolised to phenobarbital and may therefore interact similarly.

> Warn the patient to monitor for indicators of phenobarbital toxicity (drowsiness, ataxia or dysarthria), and take levels if necessary. Levels may still be moderately raised after 28 days. However, most patients seem unlikely to require dose adjustments.

Phenobarbital + **Valproate**

Phenobarbital levels (including those derived from primidone) can be increased by sodium valproate whereas the effect of valproate on primidone levels is variable (increases, decreases, and no change reported). Phenobarbital may cause small reductions in sodium valproate. The concurrent use of phenobarbital and valproate may cause an increase in serum liver enzymes.

> Use of this combination may result in excessive sedation and lethargy. To control this interaction the dose of phenobarbital has been reduced by up to about 50%, without loss of seizure control. Indicators of phenobarbital toxicity include drowsiness, ataxia or dysarthria. Monitor levels as necessary. Valproate has been associated with serious hepatotoxicity, especially in children aged less than 3 years, and this has been more common in those receiving other antiepileptics. Valproate monotherapy is to be preferred in this group.

Phenobarbital + **Vigabatrin**

Vigabatrin causes a small decrease in phenobarbital and primidone levels. There is some evidence that phenobarbital may reduce the efficacy of vigabatrin in infantile spasms.

> Generally no action seems necessary, but bear the possibility of reduced efficacy in mind.

Phenobarbital + **Vitamin D** ⚠

The long-term use of phenobarbital can disturb vitamin D and calcium metabolism, which may result in osteomalacia. There are a few reports of patients taking vitamin D supplements as replacement therapy who responded poorly while taking phenobarbital or primidone.

> Monitor the outcome of concurrent use. Larger doses of vitamin D may be needed.

Phenobarbital + **Warfarin and other oral anticoagulants** ⚠

The effects of the coumarins (acenocoumarol, phenprocoumon and warfarin) are reduced by the barbiturates.

> Reduced anticoagulant effects may occur within 2 to 4 days (maximum effect after about 3 weeks). Monitor the INR closely until stable and be aware that dose increases of 30 to 60% are likely to be needed. Also monitor if the barbiturate is stopped (note that the interaction may persist for up to several weeks after concurrent use is stopped). The benzodiazepines do not usually interact with anticoagulants, and may therefore be a suitable alternative in some circumstances.

Phenobarbital + **Zonisamide**

Phenobarbital (and therefore probably primidone) can cause a small to moderate reduction in zonisamide levels, but zonisamide appears not to affect phenobarbital or primidone levels.

> The clinical importance of this interaction is unknown, but bear the possibility of reduced zonisamide levels in mind if either of these barbiturates is given.

Phenytoin

Phenytoin is extensively metabolised by hydroxylation, principally by CYP2C9, although CYP2C19 plays a role. These isoenzymes show genetic polymorphism, and CYP2C19 may assume a greater role in individuals who have a poor metaboliser phenotype of CYP2C9. The concurrent use of inhibitors of CYP2C9, and sometimes also CYP2C19, can lead to phenytoin toxicity. In addition, phenytoin metabolism is saturable (it shows nonlinear pharmacokinetics), therefore, small changes in metabolism or phenytoin dose can result in marked changes in plasma levels. Fosphenytoin is a prodrug of phenytoin, which is rapidly and completely hydrolysed to phenytoin in the body. It is predicted to interact with other drugs in the same way as phenytoin. No drugs are known to interfere with the conversion of fosphenytoin to phenytoin.

Phenytoin + Phosphodiesterase type-5 inhibitors

Phenytoin is predicted to reduce the levels of phosphodiesterase type-5 inhibitors, because other inducers of CYP3A4 have been shown to do so. For example, sildenafil levels are reduced by 70% by *bosentan* and tadalafil levels are reduced by 88% by *rifampicin*. Vardenafil is also metabolised by CYP3A4, and therefore its levels may possibly be lowered by phenytoin.

> If these phosphodiesterase type-5 inhibitors are not effective in patients taking phenytoin, it would seem sensible to try a higher dose with close monitoring. Note that fosphenytoin, a prodrug of phenytoin, may interact similarly.

Phenytoin + Praziquantel

Phenytoin markedly reduces praziquantel levels, but whether this results in neurocysticercosis treatment failures is unclear. Fosphenytoin, a prodrug of phenytoin, may interact similarly.

> When treating systemic worm infections such as neurocysticercosis some authors have advised increasing the praziquantel dose from 25 to 50 mg/kg if phenytoin is being used, but in one case this dose was not effective. Furthermore, note that the manufacturers recommended dose for praziquantel for neurocysticercosis is 50 mg/kg daily in 3 divided doses. The interaction with antiepileptics is of no importance when praziquantel is used for intestinal worm infections (where its action is a local effect on the worms in the gut).

Phenytoin + Protease inhibitors

Nelfinavir, and ritonavir-boosted fosamprenavir and lopinavir appear to modestly reduce phenytoin levels. In case reports, ritonavir has decreased, increased or not altered phenytoin levels. Phenytoin decreased lopinavir levels, and possibly also indinavir and ritonavir levels, had only had a minor effect on the levels of amprenavir (given as ritonavir-boosted fosamprenavir), but did not alter nelfinavir levels. Phenytoin is predicted to reduce the levels of atazanavir, darunavir, saquinavir, and tipranavir.

> Phenytoin should be used with caution in combination with any protease inhibitor, with close monitoring of antiviral efficacy and phenytoin levels. Consider using an alternative antiepileptic where possible. Some manufacturers advise against concurrent use. Note that fosphenytoin, a prodrug of phenytoin, may interact similarly.

Phenytoin + Proton pump inhibitors

A study found that omeprazole 20 mg daily did not affect phenytoin levels, whereas

P

earlier studies suggested that phenytoin levels might be modestly raised by omeprazole 40 mg daily. A study with esomeprazole also suggests that it may cause a minor rise in phenytoin levels. Lansoprazole does not normally interact with phenytoin, but an isolated case report of toxicity is tentatively attributed to an interaction. Fosphenytoin, a prodrug of phenytoin, may interact similarly with these proton pump inhibitors.

> This interaction is unlikely to be generally significant, but bear it in mind in case of an unexpected response to treatment. Indicators of phenytoin toxicity include blurred vision, nystagmus, ataxia or drowsiness. However, note that the manu-facturers of esomeprazole recommend monitoring phenytoin levels.

Phenytoin + Pyridoxine

Daily doses of pyridoxine 80 to 400 mg can cause reductions of about 35% in phenytoin levels in some patients. The effect on fosphenytoin, a prodrug of phenytoin, does not appear to have been studied, but it may be prudent to assume it may interact similarly.

> Concurrent use should be monitored if large doses of pyridoxine are used, being alert for the need to increase the phenytoin dose. It seems unlikely that small doses (as in multivitamin preparations) will interact to any great extent.

Phenytoin + Quinidine

Quinidine levels can be reduced by phenytoin. Loss of arrhythmia control is possible if the quinidine dose is not increased. Fosphenytoin, a prodrug of phenytoin, may interact similarly.

> Concurrent use need not be avoided, but be alert for the need to increase the quinidine dose. If phenytoin is withdrawn the quinidine dose may need to be reduced to avoid quinidine toxicity. Quinidine levels should be monitored if possible.

Phenytoin + Quinolones

Studies suggest that ciprofloxacin does not usually have a clinically significant effect on phenytoin levels. However, case reports describe both a rise and a fall in phenytoin levels in patients given ciprofloxacin. Fosphenytoin, a prodrug of phenytoin, may interact similarly.

> It has been suggested that it may be prudent to monitor phenytoin levels in those given ciprofloxacin. Quinolones alone very occasionally cause convulsions, therefore they should be used with caution in patients with epilepsy.

Phenytoin + Ranolazine

Rifampicin (*rifampin*) reduces ranolazine levels by 95%, and loss of efficacy is expected. Phenytoin (and therefore probably its prodrug, fosphenytoin) are predicted to interact in the same way as rifampicin.

> The manufacturers recommend avoiding concurrent use. In the absence of any

information on the magnitude of the effect of phenytoin on ranolazine levels, this seems prudent.

Phenytoin + Rifampicin (Rifampin)

Phenytoin levels can be markedly reduced by rifampicin (clearance doubled in one study). If rifampicin is given with isoniazid, phenytoin levels may fall in patients who are fast acetylators of isoniazid, but may occasionally rise in those who are slow acetylators. Fosphenytoin, a prodrug of phenytoin, may interact similarly.

It is unlikely that the acetylator status of the patient will be known. Therefore monitor phenytoin levels and adjust the dose accordingly.

P

Phenytoin + Sirolimus

The manufacturers predict that phenytoin (and therefore possibly fosphenytoin) may lower the serum levels of sirolimus, probably because rifampicin (rifampin), another CYP3A4 inducer, has been shown to do so. This prediction seems to be confirmed by 2 patients who needed an increase in their sirolimus doses when they were given phenytoin.

The extent of any change in sirolimus levels is uncertain, but it would seem prudent to increase the frequency of monitoring sirolimus levels, both during concurrent use and also if phenytoin is withdrawn. The manufacturers state that concurrent use should be avoided.

Phenytoin + Solifenacin

Ketoconazole increases solifenacin levels 2- to 3-fold by *inhibiting* CYP3A4. The manufacturers predict that potent CYP3A4 *inducers* (e.g. phenytoin, and therefore probably fosphenytoin) will decrease solifenacin levels.

Be alert for a reduction in the efficacy of solifenacin in patients taking phenytoin or fosphenytoin.

Phenytoin + SSRIs ❓

Phenytoin levels can be increased by fluoxetine and fluvoxamine in some patients and toxicity may occur. Phenytoin and sertraline do not normally interact, but 2 patients have had increased phenytoin levels while taking sertraline. Fosphenytoin, a prodrug of phenytoin, may interact similarly with these SSRIs.

Monitor patients for signs of phenytoin toxicity, such as blurred vision, nystagmus, ataxia or drowsiness. Consider monitoring phenytoin levels and adjust the dose accordingly. Note that SSRIs should be avoided in unstable epilepsy and used with care in patients with controlled epilepsy.

Phenytoin + Statins ❓

A number of isolated case reports describe a reduced cholesterol-lowering effect of simvastatin, fluvastatin and atorvastatin in patients taking phenytoin. In a study, the concurrent use of phenytoin and fluvastatin modestly raises the levels of both drugs.

The change in phenytoin levels with fluvastatin seems unlikely to be significant. There is a small risk that the concurrent use of fluvastatin and phenytoin could result in myopathy. Patients should be counselled regarding myopathy (e.g. report any unexplained muscle pain, tenderness or weakness). The general importance of these case reports is unknown, but bear them in mind if lipid levels are not satisfactorily controlled.

Phenytoin + Sulfinpyrazone

Some limited evidence indicates that phenytoin levels may be markedly increased by sulfinpyrazone. Fosphenytoin, a prodrug of phenytoin, may interact similarly.

Warn the patient to monitor for indicators of phenytoin toxicity (blurred vision, nystagmus, ataxia or drowsiness). It would seem advisable to monitor phenytoin levels and adjust the dose accordingly.

Phenytoin + Sulfonamides

Phenytoin levels can be raised by co-trimoxazole (which contains sulfamethoxazole), sulfamethizole, sulfamethoxazole, and sulfadiazine. Phenytoin toxicity may develop in some cases. Fosphenytoin, a prodrug of phenytoin, may interact similarly.

The risk of toxicity is small and is most likely in those with phenytoin levels at the top end of the range. Monitor phenytoin levels and adjust the dose accordingly. Indicators of phenytoin toxicity include blurred vision, nystagmus, ataxia or drowsiness.

Phenytoin + Tacrolimus

An isolated report describes an increase in phenytoin levels, which was attributed to the use of tacrolimus. Phenytoin decreased tacrolimus levels in several cases. Fosphenytoin, a prodrug of phenytoin, may interact similarly.

Based on the known metabolism of these drugs it would be prudent to monitor tacrolimus levels in a patient given phenytoin. Similarly, based on the single case of phenytoin toxicity, it may also be advisable to monitor for indicators of phenytoin toxicity (blurred vision, nystagmus, ataxia or drowsiness) and take phenytoin levels as necessary.

Phenytoin + Tetracyclines

The serum levels of doxycycline are reduced and may fall below the accepted minimum inhibitory concentration in patients receiving long-term treatment with phenytoin. Fosphenytoin, a prodrug of phenytoin, may interact similarly.

It has been suggested that the doxycycline dose could be doubled to overcome this interaction. Tetracycline, oxytetracycline and chlortetracycline appear not to interact and may therefore be suitable alternatives.

Phenytoin + **Theophylline**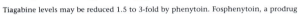

Theophylline levels can be markedly reduced by phenytoin. Some limited evidence suggests that theophylline may also reduce phenytoin levels. Fosphenytoin, a prodrug of phenytoin, may interact similarly.

Ideally theophylline levels should be measured to confirm that they remain within the therapeutic range. Dose increases of theophylline of up to 50% or more may be required. The effect of theophylline on phenytoin is not established, but it may be prudent to monitor phenytoin levels as well. Separating the oral dose by 1 to 2 hours appears to minimise the effects of theophylline on phenytoin.

P

Phenytoin + **Tiagabine**

Tiagabine levels may be reduced 1.5 to 3-fold by phenytoin. Fosphenytoin, a prodrug of phenytoin, may interact similarly.

The manufacturers recommend that tiagabine 30 to 45 mg (in divided doses) should be given to patients taking enzyme-inducing antiepileptics.

Phenytoin + **Ticlopidine**

There are a number of case reports of patients taking phenytoin who developed toxicity when ticlopidine was added. Ticlopidine appears to inhibit phenytoin metabolism. Fosphenytoin, a prodrug of phenytoin, may interact similarly.

It would be prudent to monitor phenytoin levels if ticlopidine is added. Warn the patient to monitor for indicators of phenytoin toxicity (blurred vision, nystagmus, ataxia or drowsiness).

Phenytoin + **Topiramate**

Phenytoin increases the clearance of topiramate 2- to 3-fold, which appears to result in topiramate levels that are up to 50% lower. Topiramate slightly increases the phenytoin AUC by up to about 55% but this is said not to be clinically significant based on several other analyses showing no interaction. Fosphenytoin, a prodrug of phenytoin, may interact similarly.

Topiramate dose adjustments may be required if phenytoin is added or discontinued. Be aware that a few patients may have increased phenytoin levels, particularly at high topiramate doses. Warn the patient to monitor for indicators of phenytoin toxicity (blurred vision, nystagmus, ataxia or drowsiness). Consider monitoring phenytoin levels.

Phenytoin + **Toremifene**

Phenytoin can reduce toremifene levels. Fosphenytoin, a prodrug of phenytoin, may interact similarly.

The manufacturers of toremifene suggest that the dose may need to be doubled in the presence of phenytoin.

Phenytoin + Tricyclics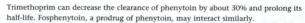

Some very limited evidence suggests that imipramine can raise phenytoin levels. Phenytoin possibly reduces desipramine levels. Fosphenytoin, a prodrug of phenytoin, may interact similarly.

None of these interactions is established. Note that the tricyclic antidepressants as a group lower the seizure threshold, which suggests that extra care should be taken if deciding to use them in patients with epilepsy.

Phenytoin + Trimethoprim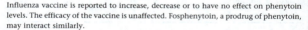

Trimethoprim can decrease the clearance of phenytoin by about 30% and prolong its half-life. Fosphenytoin, a prodrug of phenytoin, may interact similarly.

The risk of toxicity is small and is most likely in those with phenytoin levels at the top end of the range. Monitor phenytoin levels and adjust the dose accordingly. Indicators of phenytoin toxicity include blurred vision, nystagmus, ataxia or drowsiness.

Phenytoin + Vaccines ✅

Influenza vaccine is reported to increase, decrease or to have no effect on phenytoin levels. The efficacy of the vaccine is unaffected. Fosphenytoin, a prodrug of phenytoin, may interact similarly.

Phenytoin levels appear to return to normal after about 14 days. Warn the patient to monitor for indicators of phenytoin toxicity (blurred vision, nystagmus, ataxia or drowsiness). However, be aware that any alteration in levels may take a couple of weeks to develop and usually resolves spontaneously.

Phenytoin + Valproate ⚠️

The concurrent use of phenytoin and valproate is usually uneventful. Initially total phenytoin levels may fall by 20 to 50% but this is offset by a rise in the levels of free (and active) phenytoin, which may very occasionally cause some toxicity. After continued use total phenytoin levels rise once again. Phenytoin also reduces valproate levels. Fosphenytoin, a prodrug of phenytoin, may interact similarly.

Monitor phenytoin levels and adjust the dose accordingly. When monitoring concurrent use it is important to understand fully the implications of changes in 'total', and 'free' or 'unbound' phenytoin levels. Where monitoring of free phenytoin levels is not available, various nomograms have been designed for predicting unbound phenytoin levels during the use of sodium valproate. Consider monitoring valproate levels for an indication of toxicity if phenytoin is stopped.

Phenytoin + Vigabatrin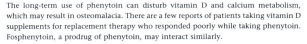

Vigabatrin causes a small to moderate 20 to 30% reduction in phenytoin levels. Fosphenytoin, a prodrug of phenytoin, may interact similarly

Occasional patients may require a small adjustment in dose. Note that this interaction can take several weeks to develop.

Phenytoin + Vitamin D

The long-term use of phenytoin can disturb vitamin D and calcium metabolism, which may result in osteomalacia. There are a few reports of patients taking vitamin D supplements for replacement therapy who responded poorly while taking phenytoin. Fosphenytoin, a prodrug of phenytoin, may interact similarly.

Monitor the outcome of concurrent use. Larger doses of vitamin D may be needed.

Phenytoin + Warfarin and other oral anticoagulants

Phenytoin would be expected to reduce the anticoagulant effects of the coumarins and this has been seen with warfarin. However, cases where the effects of warfarin were *increased* have been reported, and one study found that the effects of phenprocoumon were generally unaltered by phenytoin. Limited evidence suggests that phenytoin levels may rise in patients taking phenprocoumon or, more rarely, warfarin. Fosphenytoin, a prodrug of phenytoin, may interact similarly.

None of these interactions have been extensively studied nor are they well established. Warn patients to monitor for indicators of phenytoin toxicity (blurred vision, nystagmus, ataxia or drowsiness) and to report any increased bruising or bleeding. Consider monitoring phenytoin levels and anticoagulant control if acenocoumarol, phenprocoumon or warfarin is given with phenytoin.

Phenytoin + Zonisamide

Phenytoin can cause a small to moderate reduction in zonisamide levels. Zonisamide appears not to affect phenytoin levels in most studies, although two studies suggest a modest rise of about 20% may occur. Fosphenytoin, a prodrug of phenytoin, may interact similarly.

The general importance of this interaction is unknown although a serious interaction is unlikely. Consider the importance of a possible reduction in zonisamide levels. Bear the potential for a modest increase in phenytoin levels in mind should a patient taking zonisamide develop signs of phenytoin toxicity (blurred vision, nystagmus, ataxia or drowsiness).

Phosphodiesterase type-5 inhibitors

Phosphodiesterase type-5 inhibitors + Protease inhibitors

P

Ritonavir ❌

Ritonavir can cause marked rises in sildenafil levels; tadalafil and vardenafil interact similarly. A fatal heart attack occurred in a man taking ritonavir and saquinavir when he also took sildenafil.

The concurrent use of ritonavir with sildenafil for pulmonary hypertension is not advised, or in the UK, contraindicated. When single doses of sildenafil are used for erectile dysfunction, the UK manufacturer also says concurrent use with ritonavir is not advised, but if sildenafil is given, the dose should not exceed 25 mg in 48 hours. The US manufacturer advises that, for erectile dysfunction, the 'as needed' tadalafil dose should not exceed 10 mg every 72 hours and the daily dose should not exceed 2.5 mg, whereas the UK manufacturer simply advises caution. For pulmonary hypertension, the US manufacturer advises that if the protease inhibitor is boosted with ritonavir, tadalafil should only be given if ritonavir has been taken for at least 7 days. Start at a dose of tadalafil 20 mg daily and increase to 40 mg daily, if tolerated. The UK manufacturer of vardenafil contraindicates concurrent use, whereas the US manufacturer recommends that the dose of vardenafil should not exceed 2.5 mg in 72 hours when used with ritonavir.

Saquinavir ❌

Saquinavir causes a marked rise in sildenafil levels; it seems likely tadalafil and vardenafil will be similarly affected. Ritonavir-boosted saquinavir prolongs the QT interval and the manufacturers of saquinavir suggest that this effect may be potentiated in the presence of sildenafil.

The UK manufacturers contraindicate concurrent use. If both drugs are given sildenafil dose reductions will be necessary. If sildenafil is given for erectile dysfunction, use a maximum dose of 25 mg every 48 hours. If sildenafil is given for pulmonary hypertension avoid concurrent use, or reduce the sildenafil dose to 20 mg once or twice daily (oral) or 10 mg once or twice daily (intravenous). Monitor the outcome of concurrent use closely. No specific advice is given for tadalafil, but if both drugs are given, it may be prudent to use the precautions advised for ritonavir (see above) and titrate to effect. If both drugs are given, the US manufacturer recommends that the dose of vardenafil should not exceed 2.5 mg in 24 hours. For ritonavir-boosted protease inhibitors, it may be prudent to also consider the dosing advice under Ritonavir, above.

Other protease inhibitors ⚠

Indinavir can cause a marked rise in sildenafil and vardenafil levels; tadalafil would be expected to be similarly affected. It seems likely that all protease inhibitors will interact with these phosphodiesterase inhibitors.

If sildenafil is given for erectile dysfunction a low starting dose (25 mg) should be considered, although some suggest that a starting dose of 12.5 mg may be more appropriate in those taking indinavir, with a maximum dose frequency of once or twice weekly. If sildenafil is given for pulmonary hypertension, consider reducing the sildenafil dose to 20 mg twice daily. No specific advice is given for tadalafil, but, until more is known, it may be prudent to use the precautions advised for ritonavir (see above) and titrate to effect. The UK manufacturer of vardenafil contraindicates the concurrent use of indinavir, whereas the US manufacturer recommends that the dose of vardenafil should not exceed 2.5 mg in 24 hours. The US manufacturer of vardenafil also recommends the same dose restriction for atazanavir, whereas the manufacturer of tipranavir advises that the maximum dose of vardenafil should not exceed 2.5 mg in 72 hours. For other protease inhibitors, it would seem prudent to start with a low dose and titrate to effect. For ritonavir-boosted protease inhibitors, it may be prudent to also consider the dosing advice under Ritonavir, above.

Phosphodiesterase type-5 inhibitors + Rifabutin ⚠️

Rifabutin is predicted to reduce the levels of phosphodiesterase type-5 inhibitors, because other inducers of CYP3A4 have been shown to do so. For example, sildenafil levels are reduced by 70% by *bosentan* and tadalafil levels are reduced by 88% by *rifampicin*. Vardenafil is also metabolised by CYP3A4, and therefore its levels may possibly be lowered by rifabutin.

If these phosphodiesterase type-5 inhibitors are not effective in patients taking rifabutin, it would seem sensible to try a higher dose with close monitoring.

Phosphodiesterase type-5 inhibitors + Rifampicin (Rifampin) ❓

Tadalafil levels are reduced by 88% by rifampicin, by inhibiting CYP3A4. Rifampicin is predicted to reduce the levels of other phosphodiesterase type-5 inhibitors, which are also metabolised by CYP3A4.

If these phosphodiesterase type-5 inhibitors are not effective in patients taking rifampicin, it would seem sensible to try a higher dose with close monitoring.

Prasugrel

Prasugrel + Warfarin and other oral anticoagulants ⚠️

Prasugrel has no effect on the metabolism of warfarin. However, the manufacturer recommends caution due to the theoretical increased risk of bleeding.

If the concurrent use of prasugrel and a coumarin or indanedione is necessary, the patient should be monitored for signs of increased bleeding, and told to report any unexplained bruising or bleeding.

Praziquantel

Praziquantel + Rifampicin (Rifampin)

Plasma levels of praziquantel are markedly reduced by rifampicin pretreatment, to undetectable levels in half of the subjects in one study.

It is predicted that rifampicin will reduce the efficacy of praziquantel, and therefore the combination should be avoided.

Probenecid

Probenecid + Pyrazinamide

The interactions of probenecid and pyrazinamide and their effects on the excretion of uric acid are complex. The overall effect is that if probenecid were to be used to treat the hyperuricaemia caused by pyrazinamide, the normal uricosuric effects of probenecid would be diminished and larger doses would be required.

Note that pyrazinamide should be used with caution or is contraindicated in patients with a history of gout. If hyperuricaemia accompanied by gouty arthritis occurs, pyrazinamide should be stopped.

Probenecid + Quinolones

Probenecid increases the serum levels and/or decreases the urinary excretion of cinoxacin, ciprofloxacin, clinafloxacin, enoxacin, fleroxacin, levofloxacin, nalidixic acid and norfloxacin.

This is unlikely to be of clinical significance unless other drugs that affect renal clearance (such as some penicillins or cephalosporins) are taken concurrently, or in the presence of renal impairment. Moxifloxacin, sparfloxacin, and probably ofloxacin, appear not to interact with probenecid.

Procainamide

Procainamide + Trimethoprim ⚠

Trimethoprim causes a marked increase in the plasma levels of procainamide and its active metabolite, *N*-acetylprocainamide.

The need to reduce the procainamide dose should be anticipated if trimethoprim is given to patients already taking stable doses of procainamide.

Proguanil

Proguanil + Warfarin and other oral anticoagulants

An isolated report describes bleeding in a patient taking warfarin after she took proguanil for about 5 weeks.

> The general importance of this interaction is uncertain, as factors related to travel (such as a changing diet and changing dose times in different time zones) may have had a part to play.

Propafenone

Propafenone + Protease inhibitors ✖

Ritonavir is expected to produce large elevations in the plasma levels of propafenone, which may lead to life-threatening arrhythmias. Ritonavir-boosted protease inhibitors are expected to interact similarly.

> It would seem prudent to avoid the concurrent use of propafenone with ritonavir-boosted protease inhibitors if possible. However if concurrent use is necessary, closely monitor for an increase in propafenone adverse effects. Note that some manufacturers contraindicate concurrent use.

Propafenone + Quinidine ⚠

Quinidine doubles the plasma levels of propafenone and halves the levels of its active metabolite, but the antiarrhythmic effects appear to be unaffected.

> Anticipate the need to reduce the propafenone dose (maybe by as much as half) if the combination is used. Monitor well.

Propafenone + Ranolazine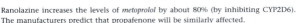

Ranolazine increases the levels of *metoprolol* by about 80% (by inhibiting CYP2D6). The manufacturers predict that propafenone will be similarly affected.

> Be aware of a possible interaction if propafenone adverse effects e.g. hypotension, bradycardia, dizziness, dry mouth) occur. The manufacturer of ranolazine suggests a dose reduction of propafenone may be needed.

Propafenone + **Rifampicin (Rifampin)**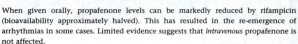

When given orally, propafenone levels can be markedly reduced by rifampicin (bioavailability approximately halved). This has resulted in the re-emergence of arrhythmias in some cases. Limited evidence suggests that *intravenous* propafenone is not affected.

> The dose of oral propafenone will probably need increasing if rifampicin is given. Alternatively, if possible, it has been advised that another antibacterial be used because of the probable difficulty in adjusting the propafenone dose.

Propafenone + **SSRIs**

Fluoxetine markedly inhibits the metabolism (5-hydroxylation) of propafenone, and paroxetine would also be expected to behave similarly, but the clinical consequences of this are unknown. Fluvoxamine would be expected to inhibit the metabolism of propafenone by *N*-dealkylation, but in most patients this is only expected to have a small effect.

> Until more is known, it would be prudent to use caution when giving any of these SSRIs with propafenone, monitoring for an increase in propafenone adverse effects (e.g. hypotension, bradycardia, dizziness, dry mouth) and consider decreasing the dose of propafenone if these become troublesome.

Propafenone + **Terbinafine**

In vitro studies suggest that terbinafine is an inhibitor of CYP2D6. It may therefore be expected to increase the plasma levels of other drugs that are substrates of this enzyme, such as propafenone.

> Until more is known it would seem wise to be aware of the possibility of an increase in adverse effects (e.g. hypotension, bradycardia, dizziness, dry mouth) if propafenone is given with terbinafine and consider a dose reduction if necessary.

Propafenone + **Warfarin and other oral anticoagulants**

The anticoagulant effects of warfarin are increased by propafenone. Case reports suggest that phenprocoumon and fluindione interact similarly.

> Monitor the anticoagulant effect if propafenone is added or withdrawn. This interaction appears to start in the first week of concurrent use.

Protease inhibitors

The protease inhibitors are extensively metabolised by cytochrome P450, particularly CYP3A4. All of the protease inhibitors inhibit CYP3A4, with ritonavir being the most potent inhibitor, followed by indinavir, nelfinavir, amprenavir, and saquinavir. The protease inhibitors therefore have the potential to interact with other drugs metabolised by CYP3A4, and may also be affected by CYP3A4 inhibitors and inducers. Ritonavir and tipranavir also affect some other cytochrome P450 isoenzymes, particularly CYP2D6. In addition, protease inhibitors are substrates as well as inhibitors of P-glycoprotein. The plasma level of protease inhibitors is thought to be critical in maintaining efficacy and minimising the potential for development of viral resistance. Therefore even modest reductions in levels are potentially clinically important.

Protease inhibitors + **Proton pump inhibitors**

Atazanavir, Nelfinavir or Saquinavir

Omeprazole reduced ritonavir-boosted atazanavir levels by almost 80% in some patients. Similarly, omeprazole reduced nelfinavir levels by almost 40% (although some patients had *increased* levels) and decreased the levels of its active metabolite by about 90%. In contrast, ritonavir-boosted saquinavir levels are increased by about 80% by omeprazole.

Atazanavir or ritonavir-boosted atazanavir should not be given with omeprazole or other proton pump inhibitors. One UK manufacturer states that if concurrent use is necessary, the dose of ritonavir-boosted atazanavir should be increased to 400 mg daily, and both UK and US manufacturers advise that a maximum dose of 20 mg of omeprazole (or the equivalent in other proton pump inhibitors). The US manufacturers limit this advice to treatment-naive patients, and advise that the dose of the proton pump inhibitor should be taken 12 hours before atazanavir. In general, the concurrent use of nelfinavir and a proton pump inhibitor is contraindicated. If omeprazole or other proton pump inhibitors are taken with ritonavir-boosted saquinavir, monitor for potential saquinavir toxicity. However, the UK manufacturers note that because saquinavir may prolong the QT interval this increase is clinically important, and concurrent use is not recommended.

Indinavir or Tipranavir

Omeprazole appears to reduce indinavir levels (by about 50% in one study) but not all patients seem to be affected. Ritonavir appears to negate the effects of any interaction. Omeprazole does not appear to affect the levels of ritonavir-boosted tipranavir, whereas ritonavir-boosted tipranavir reduces omeprazole levels by about 70%. Esomeprazole is similarly affected.

Omeprazole should probably not be used with indinavir unless ritonavir is also given. This would be likely to apply to other proton pump inhibitors given with indinavir. The use of tipranavir with omeprazole or esomeprazole is not recommended, but if both drugs are given consider increasing the dose of the proton pump inhibitor, according to response.

Protease inhibitors + **Quinidine**

The protease inhibitors are generally expected to increase quinidine levels, which may increase the risk of arrhythmias and other adverse effects such as nausea, diarrhoea, and tinnitus.

The manufacturers of ritonavir contraindicate concurrent use with quinidine. In general, the UK manufacturers of the protease inhibitors contraindicate concurrent use, the exceptions being lopinavir and saquinavir, where caution is advised: quinidine levels should be monitored, where possible. In contrast, in the US, most manufacturers advise caution and close monitoring of quinidine levels, with the exception of the manufacturers of nelfinavir, saquinavir and tipranavir, who contraindicate the concurrent use of quinidine.

Protease inhibitors + Quinine

Ritonavir increases the levels of quinine about 4-fold: this may lead to an increase in quinine adverse effects, including QT prolongation. Single-dose quinine appears to have only modest effects on ritonavir pharmacokinetics.

Avoid concurrent use, if possible. If concurrent use is essential, monitor for increased quinine adverse effects (e.g. tinnitus, headache, vomiting and vertigo); reduce the dose of quinine as necessary. However, note that increased quinine levels are likely to increase the risk of QT prolongation, see Drugs that prolong the QT interval, page 277 for more information.

Protease inhibitors + Ranolazine

Ketoconazole increases the AUC, peak and trough levels, and half-life of ranolazine 2.5- to 4.5-fold. The dose-related adverse effects of ranolazine such as nausea and dizziness were increased by *ketoconazole*. Further, increases in plasma levels of ranolazine may cause significant QT prolongation and increase the risk of arrhythmias. The protease inhibitors are expected to interact in the same way as ketoconazole.

The manufacturers of ranolazine contraindicate its use with potent CYP3A4 inhibitors. They specifically name indinavir, nelfinavir, ritonavir and saquinavir.

Protease inhibitors + Rifabutin

Rifabutin bioavailability is significantly increased by the protease inhibitors, in particular ritonavir, and this is associated with an increased risk of toxicity. Rifabutin modestly decreases the bioavailability of indinavir, nelfinavir, and particularly saquinavir (with an increased risk of therapeutic failure), and appears to increase the bioavailability of ritonavir-boosted darunavir.

The combination of rifabutin with protease inhibitors may be used, but large dose reductions of rifabutin and/or increases in the doses of the protease inhibitors are often necessary. The treatment of tuberculosis in patients taking antiretrovirals is complex and up-to-date guidelines should be consulted.

Protease inhibitors + Rifampicin (Rifampin)

Rifampicin markedly reduces the bioavailability of amprenavir, atazanavir, indinavir, ritonavir-boosted lopinavir, nelfinavir, ritonavir-boosted saquinavir and saquinavir, but only modestly reduces that of ritonavir. It is also predicted to reduce the levels of ritonavir-boosted darunavir and tipranavir. Some protease inhibitors increase the levels of rifampicin.

> The use of many of the protease inhibitors with rifampicin is contraindicated. The treatment of tuberculosis in patients taking antiretrovirals is complex and up-to-date guidelines should be consulted.

Protease inhibitors + **Salbutamol (Albuterol) and related bronchodilators**

Ketoconazole increases the AUC of inhaled salmeterol 16-fold, which may result in systemic adverse effects of salmeterol. Although, clinically significant effects were not seen on blood pressure, heart rate, blood glucose and blood potassium levels, this increase in the exposure to salmeterol increases the risk of QT prolongation. A number of the protease inhibitors (the manufacturers name ritonavir, atazanavir, indinavir, nelfinavir, and saquinavir) are expected to interact in the same way as *ketoconazole*.

> Avoid unless the benefits outweigh the risks. If a protease inhibitor and salmeterol are given be alert for salmeterol adverse effects such as hypokalaemia and tachycardia.

Protease inhibitors + **Sirolimus**

Nelfinavir increased the levels of sirolimus in one patient. Other protease inhibitors are predicted to raise sirolimus levels.

> Sirolimus levels and effects (e.g. on renal function) should be monitored as a matter of routine, but it would be prudent to increase monitoring if protease inhibitors are given. Note that the manufacturers advise against the use of potent inhibitors of CYP3A4 with sirolimus.

Protease inhibitors + **Solifenacin**

Ketoconazole increases solifenacin levels 2- to 3-fold by inhibiting CYP3A4. The manufacturers state that other potent CYP3A4 inhibitors (such as the protease inhibitors) will have the same effect.

> It is recommended that the daily dose of solifenacin is limited to 5 mg daily in patients taking potent CYP3A4 inhibitors. The concurrent use of solifenacin is contraindicated in patients with severe renal impairment or moderate hepatic impairment who are taking potent CYP3A4 inhibitors.

Protease inhibitors + **SSRIs**

Ritonavir-boosted protease inhibitors appear to reduce paroxetine and sertraline levels. Fluoxetine would be expected to be similarly affected. However, the US manufacturer of tipranavir predicts that ritonavir-boosted tipranavir will result in an *increase* in the levels of fluoxetine, paroxetine and sertraline, presumably because tipranavir, unlike some of the other protease inhibitors, may also inhibit CYP2D6.

Two cases of serotonin syndrome have been attributed to the use of fluoxetine and ritonavir.

It would be prudent to anticipate some reduction in efficacy when starting these protease inhibitors (and probably any ritonavir-boosted protease inhibitors) in patients taking fluoxetine, sertraline or paroxetine. Monitor the clinical effect and increase the SSRI dose as necessary. The general relevance of the few cases of serotonin syndrome, page 454 is uncertain.

P

Protease inhibitors + **Statins**

Atorvastatin

The levels of atorvastatin appear to be markedly increased by ritonavir-boosted darunavir, lopinavir, saquinavir and tipranavir; and nelfinavir. Other protease inhibitors seem likely to interact similarly. Several cases of rhabdomyolysis have been attributed to this interaction.

It is generally recommended that atorvastatin is used at low doses (i.e. 10 mg) and with care in patients taking protease inhibitors. The US manufacturer says that in the presence of a ritonavir-boosted protease inhibitor, for doses of atorvastatin exceeding 20 mg, appropriate clinical assessment is recommended to ensure the lowest dose necessary is used. Patients should be counselled regarding myopathy (e.g. report any unexplained muscle pain, tenderness or weakness).

Rosuvastatin

Ritonavir-boosted tipranavir and lopinavir increase rosuvastatin levels. Until more is known it would seem prudent to consider this interaction with all protease inhibitors.

The US manufacturer of rosuvastatin states that the dose should be limited to 10 mg daily in patients taking ritonavir-boosted lopinavir: it may be prudent to apply this restriction to any ritonavir-boosted protease inhibitor. However, the UK manufacturer of rosuvastatin says that the concurrent use of protease inhibitors is not recommended.

Simvastatin or Lovastatin

The levels of simvastatin appear to be markedly increased by nelfinavir, ritonavir and ritonavir-boosted saquinavir. Other protease inhibitors seem likely to interact similarly. Several cases of rhabdomyolysis have been attributed to this interaction. Lovastatin is metabolised in the same way as simvastatin, and is therefore likely to be similarly affected.

It is generally recommended that simvastatin and lovastatin should be avoided in patients taking any protease inhibitor.

Other statins

Pravastatin pharmacokinetics are usually only modestly affected by the protease inhibitors, although there can be large interindividual variations in effect. There do not appear to be any reports of interactions with fluvastatin and protease inhibitors.

Pravastatin and fluvastatin can probably be used without dose adjustments with most protease inhibitors, but monitoring is needed to confirm this. Until more is known, it would seem prudent to initiate the concurrent use of pravastatin and a protease inhibitor at the lowest dose of pravastatin. Patients should be counselled regarding myopathy (e.g. report any unexplained muscle pain, tenderness or weakness).

Protease inhibitors + **Tacrolimus**

Protease inhibitors including ritonavir-boosted lopinavir and saquinavir; and nelfinavir very markedly inhibit the metabolism of tacrolimus and increase its levels. All ritonavir-boosted protease inhibitors are expected to interact similarly.

When protease inhibitors are given to patients taking tacrolimus, careful monitoring and probably a marked reduction in the dose of tacrolimus is required. Note that in some cases tacrolimus was dosed just once weekly to achieve appropriate levels.

Protease inhibitors + **Theophylline**

Ritonavir can reduce the minimum levels of theophylline by up to 57%.

Monitor the effect of concurrent use on theophylline levels. It may be necessary to increase the theophylline dose. Note that the interaction may take a week to fully develop.

Protease inhibitors + **Tolterodine**

Ketoconazole raises the AUC of tolterodine by more than 2-fold in some patients. Other potent inhibitors of CYP3A4, such as the protease inhibitors, are predicted to interact similarly.

The UK manufacturers advise avoiding concurrent use. The US manufacturers suggest reducing the tolterodine dose to 1 mg twice daily, which seems practical. It may be prudent to assess experience of adverse effects in these patients, and to reduce the dose further or withdraw the drug if it is not tolerated.

Protease inhibitors + **Trazodone**

Ritonavir increases the AUC of trazodone more than 2-fold and sedation and fatigue were increased. Cases of serotonin syndrome, page 454 have been reported in patients taking trazodone and ritonavir or indinavir. Other protease inhibitors may interact similarly.

A lower dose of trazodone should be considered if it is given with potent CYP3A4 inhibitors such as ritonavir and indinavir, although note that in the UK it has been suggested that the combination should be avoided where possible. Note that, because saquinavir may prolong the QT interval, in the UK, its concurrent use with trazodone is contraindicated.

Protease inhibitors + Tricyclics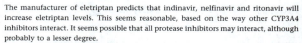

Ritonavir raises desipramine levels and is predicted to also raise the levels of other tricyclic antidepressants. Theoretically, tipranavir may interact similarly.

> Monitor for increased tricyclic adverse effects (e.g. dry mouth, urinary retention, constipation). Consider starting desipramine at a low dose in patients taking ritonavir 500 mg twice daily, increasing the dose slowly. When ritonavir is given as a pharmacokinetic enhancer (i.e. at a dose of 100 mg twice daily) a dose adjustment of the tricyclic is unlikely to be necessary. There seems to be little information regarding other tricyclics, but similar precautions to those suggested for desipramine would seem prudent. Note that, because saquinavir (with ritonavir) may prolong the QT interval, in the UK, its concurrent use with tricyclics is contraindicated.

Protease inhibitors + Triptans

The manufacturer of eletriptan predicts that indinavir, nelfinavir and ritonavir will increase eletriptan levels. This seems reasonable, based on the way other CYP3A4 inhibitors interact. It seems possible that all protease inhibitors may interact, although probably to a lesser degree.

> The manufacturers of eletriptan say that the concurrent use of indinavir, nelfinavir and ritonavir should be avoided. In addition, the US manufacturer recommends that eletriptan should not be given within 72 hours of ritonavir and nelfinavir.

Protease inhibitors + Venlafaxine

In a single-dose study venlafaxine lowered indinavir levels by about 35%.

> Monitor concurrent use to confirm that the effects of indinavir remain adequate.

Protease inhibitors + Warfarin and other oral anticoagulants

In pharmacokinetic studies, ritonavir slightly raised *S*-warfarin levels and modestly decreased *R*-warfarin levels, while ritonavir-boosted lopinavir decreased *R*- and *S*-warfarin levels. A number of case reports describe a decrease in warfarin or acenocoumarol effects (with indinavir, ritonavir-boosted lopinavir, nelfinavir, ritonavir or ritonavir-boosted saquinavir). In contrast, a couple of case reports describe an increase in warfarin effects (with nelfinavir and ritonavir, or saquinavir).

> It would seem prudent to monitor the use of any coumarin and protease inhibitor for an alteration in anticoagulant effect.

Proton pump inhibitors

Proton pump inhibitors + **SSRIs**

Fluvoxamine

Fluvoxamine inhibits the metabolism of lansoprazole, omeprazole and rabeprazole in some patients. Theoretically other proton pump inhibitors may be similarly affected.

> The proton pump inhibitors have a wide therapeutic margin and therefore the clinical significance of this interaction is unknown. Bear it in mind in case of increased proton pump inhibitors adverse effects and consider reducing the dose if necessary.

Other SSRIs

Omeprazole (and therefore probably esomeprazole) increases escitalopram (and therefore probably citalopram) levels by 50%.

> Monitor concurrent use for SSRI adverse effects (such as nausea, diarrhoea, dry mouth, palpitations). The manufacturers of escitalopram say that dose adjustments may be necessary, but this would seem unlikely in most patients.

Proton pump inhibitors + **Tacrolimus**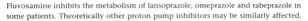

Lansoprazole may increase tacrolimus levels in some patients. Pantoprazole and omeprazole are predicted to interact similarly, although there is some evidence of a lack of interaction for both these drugs. Rabeprazole appeared less likely to interact on the basis of one pharmacokinetic study and case reports, but not from another clinical study.

> Until more is known, it might be prudent to be alert for the possibility of an interaction with any proton pump inhibitor, and consider increasing monitoring (e.g. tacrolimus levels).

Proton pump inhibitors + **Warfarin and other oral anticoagulants**

Isolated reports describe raised INRs and/or bleeding in patients taking warfarin with esomeprazole, lansoprazole, omeprazole, pantoprazole or rabeprazole, and acenocoumarol or phenprocoumon with omeprazole, but on the whole the proton pump inhibitors do not appear to have any clinically significant pharmacokinetic interactions with these anticoagulants.

> It is possible that the isolated cases of interactions with proton pump inhibitors just represent idiosyncratic effects attributable to other factors, and not to any interaction. Nevertheless, it would seem prudent to bear in mind that rarely bleeding can occur. Note that most manufacturers of the proton pump inhibitors recommend monitoring the INR in all patients.

Pyrimethamine

Pyrimethamine + Sulfonamides

Serious pancytopenia and megaloblastic anaemia have been described in patients given pyrimethamine and either co-trimoxazole (which contains sulfamethoxazole) or other sulfonamides.

Pyrimethamine is usually given with a sulfonamide for toxoplasmosis and malaria. Nevertheless, caution should be used, especially in the presence of other drugs (e.g. methotrexate) or disease states that may predispose to folate deficiency. When high-dose pyrimethamine is used for the treatment of toxoplasmosis, the manufacturer recommends that all patients should receive a folate supplement. Note that the manufacturer of sulfadoxine/pyrimethamine recommends that the concurrent use of sulfonamides (including co-trimoxazole) should be avoided.

Pyrimethamine + Trimethoprim

Serious pancytopenia and megaloblastic anaemia have been described in patients given pyrimethamine and co-trimoxazole (which contains trimethoprim).

Caution should be used, especially in the presence of other drugs (e.g. methotrexate) or disease states that may also affect folate metabolism. When high-dose pyrimethamine is used for the treatment of toxoplasmosis, the manufacturer recommends that all patients should receive a folate supplement.

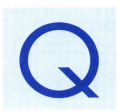

Quinidine

Quinidine + Rifabutin

The levels of quinidine and its therapeutic effects can be markedly reduced by *rifampicin*. In one case quinidine levels were reduced from 4 to 0.5 micrograms/mL. Rifabutin is predicted to interact similarly, but probably to a lesser extent.

A quinidine dose increase may be necessary if rifabutin is given. Monitor concurrent use (including quinidine levels, where possible) and adjust the dose as necessary.

Quinidine + Rifampicin (Rifampin)

The levels of quinidine and its therapeutic effects can be markedly reduced by rifampicin. In one case quinidine levels were reduced from 4 to 0.5 micrograms/mL.

The dose of quinidine will need to be increased (possibly more than doubled in some patients) if rifampicin is given concurrently. The quinidine dose will need to be reduced when the rifampicin is stopped. Monitor quinidine levels where possible.

Quinidine + Tricyclics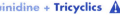

Quinidine can significantly reduce the clearance of some tricyclics (desipramine, imipramine, nortriptyline and trimipramine), thereby increasing their levels, to varying degrees.

This interaction is expected to be clinically relevant with nortriptyline, and possibly desipramine, but probably not with imipramine. Monitor for signs of tricyclic adverse effects (dry mouth, urinary retention, constipation) on concurrent use. Additive QT-prolonging effects are also possible, see drugs that prolong the QT interval, page 277.

Quinidine + **Warfarin and other oral anticoagulants**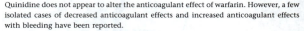

Quinidine does not appear to alter the anticoagulant effect of warfarin. However, a few isolated cases of decreased anticoagulant effects and increased anticoagulant effects with bleeding have been reported.

No interaction would normally be anticipated.

Quinine

Quinine + **Rifampicin (Rifampin)**

Rifampicin increases the clearance of quinine 6-fold.

It has been suggested that rifampicin should not be given with quinine for the treatment of malaria. Increased quinine doses should be considered if the concurrent use of rifampicin is essential: monitor concurrent use carefully to assess efficacy.

Quinine + **Warfarin and other oral anticoagulants**

Normally no significant interaction occurs between warfarin and quinine but two women required warfarin dose reductions and one man taking phenprocoumon developed extensive haematuria after drinking large amounts of quinine-containing tonic water.

Any interaction seems rare, but bear it in mind in case of unexpected bleeding.

Quinolones

The quinolones are generally considered to be inhibitors of CYP1A2; however, it should be noted that they vary in the strength of this effect. Quinolones that are more potent inhibitors of CYP1A2 are likely to have greater effects on substrates of this isoenzyme, and therefore their use seems more likely to be associated with greater clinical consequences. Caffeine is used as a probe substrate for CYP1A2. Therefore the magnitude of the effect the quinolones have on caffeine can be used as a guide to the strength of their effect on CYP1A2. The interactions of the quinolones with caffeine suggests that enoxacin has the greatest effects, ciprofloxacin and pipemidic acid have moderate effects, while gatifloxacin, levofloxacin, lomefloxacin, moxifloxacin, nalidixic acid, norfloxacin, ofloxacin, pefloxacin, rufloxacin and sparfloxacin only inhibit CYP1A2 to a small or clinically irrelevant extent.

Quinolones + Sevelamer

Sevelamer reduced the bioavailability of ciprofloxacin by 48% in one study.

> The manufacturers advise that ciprofloxacin should be taken at least 1 hour before or 3 hours after sevelamer. It seems possible that other quinolones could be similarly affected.

Quinolones + Strontium

The manufacturer of strontium predicts that it will form a complex with quinolones, and therefore prevent their absorption.

> It is recommended that when treatment with a quinolone is required, strontium ranelate should be temporarily suspended.

Q

Quinolones + Sucralfate

Sucralfate causes a marked reduction in the absorption of ciprofloxacin, enoxacin, gemifloxacin, lomefloxacin, moxifloxacin, ofloxacin, norfloxacin, and sparfloxacin, which may lead to therapeutic failure. It seems possible that other quinolones could be similarly affected.

> Separate the doses as much as possible, giving the quinolone first. The manufacturer advises that ciprofloxacin should be given 1 to 2 hours before or 4 hours after sucralfate. The UK manufacturer of moxifloxacin advises separating administration by 6 hours, whilst the US manufacturer recommends that moxifloxacin is taken at least 4 hours before or 8 hours after sucralfate. Proton pump inhibitors and H$_2$-receptor antagonists do not normally interact with the quinolones and may therefore be possible alternatives in some patients.

Quinolones + Theophylline

Theophylline levels can be markedly increased in most patients by enoxacin. Pipemidic acid is likely to interact similarly. Theophylline levels can be markedly increased in some patients by ciprofloxacin, and possibly pefloxacin. Norfloxacin and ofloxacin normally cause a much smaller rise in theophylline levels, although serious toxicity has been seen in a few patients taking norfloxacin. Convulsions have been reported with theophylline and ciprofloxacin, norfloxacin, or pefloxacin. With some of these cases it is difficult to know if this was due to increased theophylline levels, to patient predisposition, to potential additive effects on the seizure threshold, or to all three factors combined.

> Monitor theophylline levels closely. The theophylline dose should be modified based on the theophylline level on day 2 of quinolone use. Theophylline dose reductions of 50 to 75% have been suggested for enoxacin, and 30 to 50% for ciprofloxacin, although this is not always needed. It may be prudent to follow similar precautions with ofloxacin, pipemidic acid and norfloxacin. Seizures resulting from concurrent use are relatively rare. Gatifloxacin, levofloxacin, lomefloxacin, moxifloxacin, nalidixic acid and sparfloxacin appear not to significantly affect theophylline levels and may therefore be suitable alternatives in some cases.

Quinolones + Tizanidine

Ciprofloxacin increases the AUC of tizanidine tenfold, which increases the hypotensive and sedative effects of tizanidine. Other quinolones may also interact, see quinolones, page 444.

Concurrent use of ciprofloxacin with tizanidine is contraindicated, and the manufacturers state that concurrent use of enoxacin and norfloxacin should generally be avoided, or undertaken with caution. If concurrent use is necessary, anticipate the need to reduce the tizanidine dose before starting ciprofloxacin, and if starting tizanidine, start with the lowest dose, increasing gradually according to clinical response. Closely monitor for adverse effects such as marked hypotension, bradycardia, and sedation.

Quinolones + Triptans ⚠

Quinolones are predicted to raise zolmitriptan levels.

The manufacturer recommends a dose reduction of zolmitriptan to a maximum of 5 mg in 24 hours in patients taking quinolones such as ciprofloxacin. Other quinolones may interact to varying extents, see quinolones, page 444.

Quinolones + Warfarin and other oral anticoagulants ⚠

The quinolones do not normally alter the effects of the coumarins in most patients, but increased effects and even bleeding have been seen in some patients.

It would be prudent to monitor the effects of concurrent use. Monitor the INR within 3 to 5 days of starting the quinolone.

Quinolones + Zinc ⚠

Limited evidence suggests zinc interacts like iron, page 340 to reduce quinolone levels.

As the quinolones are rapidly absorbed, taking them 2 hours before the zinc should minimise the risk of admixture in the gut and largely avoid this interaction.

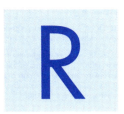

Raloxifene

Raloxifene + Warfarin and other oral anticoagulants ⚠

Raloxifene may cause a minor increase in warfarin levels. However, a 10% decrease in prothrombin time may also occur. The manufacturers report that modest changes in prothrombin times may occur over a period of several weeks. Other coumarins would be expected to be similarly affected.

The manufacturers recommend that prothrombin times should be monitored on the concurrent use of coumarin anticoagulants.

Ranolazine

Ranolazine + Rifabutin ✗

Rifampicin (rifampin) reduces ranolazine levels by 95%, and loss of efficacy is expected. Rifabutin is predicted to interact in the same way as rifampicin.

The manufacturers recommend avoiding concurrent use. In the absence of any information on the magnitude of the effect of rifabutin on ranolazine levels, this seems prudent.

Ranolazine + Rifampicin (Rifampin) ✗

Rifampicin reduces ranolazine levels by 95%, and loss of efficacy is expected.

The manufacturers contraindicate concurrent use.

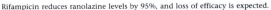

Ranolazine + **Statins** ❓

Ranolazine may increase the levels of simvastatin. Other statins that are similarly metabolised (lovastatin and to a lesser extent, atorvastatin) may also be affected.

> The increased simvastatin levels seen appear to be modest; however, they may be clinically significant in some patients. All patients taking statins should be warned about the symptoms of myopathy and told to report muscle pain or weakness. It would be prudent to reinforce this advice if patients given simvastatin, lovastatin, and possibly atorvastatin, are also given ranolazine.

Ranolazine + **Tricyclics** ❓

Ranolazine increases the levels of *metoprolol* by about 80% (by inhibiting CYP2D6). The manufacturers predict that the tricyclics, which are metabolised, at least in part, by CYP2D6 will be similarly affected.

> Be aware of a possible interaction if tricyclic adverse effects (nausea, dry mouth, urinary retention) increase. The manufacturer of ranolazine suggests a dose reduction of the tricyclic may be needed. Note that ranolazine prolongs the QT interval, and effect that may be additive with some tricyclics, see drugs that prolong the QT interval, page 277.

Reboxetine

Reboxetine + **SSRIs** ✖

The manufacturers of reboxetine predict that potent inhibitors of CYP3A4 will reduce its metabolism. They name fluvoxamine, but note that fluvoxamine is more usually considered a potent inhibitor of CYP1A2 and is generally considered a weak inhibitor of CYP3A4.

> The manufacturers say that concurrent use of fluvoxamine should be avoided, although this appears to be over-cautious.

Rifabutin

Rifabutin + **Sirolimus** ✖

Rifampicin (*rifampin*) greatly decreases sirolimus levels. Rifabutin is predicted to interact similarly.

> The manufacturers state that concurrent use is not recommended.

Rifabutin + Tacrolimus

Rifampicin (rifampin) increases the clearance and decreases the bioavailability of tacrolimus; rifabutin is expected to interact similarly, although to a lesser extent. This is supported by the findings of a case report.

> Tacrolimus levels and effects (e.g. on renal function) should be monitored as a matter of routine, but it is advisable to increase monitoring if rifabutin is started or stopped, adjusting the dose of tacrolimus as necessary.

Rifabutin + Warfarin and other oral anticoagulants

The anticoagulant effects of warfarin are markedly reduced by *rifampicin (rifampin)*. Other coumarins may be similarly affected. The manufacturers and the CSM in the UK therefore warn that rifabutin may reduce the effects of oral anticoagulants, although it is likely to interact to a lesser degree.

> Expect any interaction to occur within 7 days of starting rifabutin. It may persist for several weeks after the rifabutin is stopped. Monitor the INR closely.

R

Rifampicin (Rifampin)

Rifampicin (Rifampin) + Sirolimus

A clinical study found that multiple doses of rifampicin increased the clearance of sirolimus 5.5-fold, and reduced its maximum levels by 71%.

> The manufacturers state that concurrent use is not recommended.

Rifampicin (Rifampin) + Solifenacin

Ketoconazole increases solifenacin levels 2- to 3-fold by *inhibiting* CYP3A4. The manufacturers predict that potent CYP3A4 *inducers* (e.g. rifampicin) will decrease solifenacin levels.

> Be alert for a reduction in the efficacy of solifenacin in patients taking rifampicin and adjust the dose if necessary.

Rifampicin (Rifampin) + SSRIs

In two cases rifampicin decreased the efficacy of citalopram and sertraline. In theory rifampicin could similarly affect other SSRIs but there appear to be no reports of this.

> Information is limited. The dose adjustment of any SSRI on starting or stopping rifampicin should be guided by clinical effect. Be alert for evidence of SSRI withdrawal symptoms of loss of effect.

Rifampicin (Rifampin) + **Statins**

Limited evidence suggests that rifampicin may reduce atorvastatin, fluvastatin, pravastatin, and simvastatin levels, and may increase or decrease the levels of rosuvastatin in some subjects.

The general significance of this interaction is unclear but it would be prudent to monitor the outcome of concurrent use to ensure that the statin remains effective. Additionally, be aware of the possibility of an increase in rosuvastatin adverse effects on the concurrent use of rifampicin.

Rifampicin (Rifampin) + **Sulfonamides**

Rifampicin modestly reduces the AUC of sulfamethoxazole (given as co-trimoxazole) by 28% in HIV-positive subjects.

This would not be expected to be clinically relevant with sulfamethoxazole alone; however a greater effect is seen on trimethoprim levels, which may affect the efficacy when sulfamethoxazole is given as co-trimoxazole. Consider also co-trimoxazole, page 249. The effect of rifampicin on other sulfonamides does not appear to have been studied..

Rifampicin (Rifampin) + **Tacrolimus**

Rifampicin increases the clearance and decreases the bioavailability of tacrolimus.

Anticipate the need to raise the dose of tacrolimus if rifampicin is added in any patient. In some cases a 10-fold increase in the tacrolimus dose has been needed to manage this interaction. Tacrolimus levels and effects (e.g. on renal function) should be monitored as a matter of routine, but it is essential to increase monitoring if rifampicin is started or stopped.

Rifampicin (Rifampin) + **Terbinafine**

Rifampicin doubles the clearance of terbinafine and halves its AUC.

Terbinafine seems likely to be less effective in the presence of rifampicin. Monitor carefully and consider increasing the terbinafine dose.

Rifampicin (Rifampin) + **Tetracyclines**

Rifampicin may cause a marked reduction in doxycycline exposure (AUC reported to be reduced by 60% in one study), which has led to treatment failures in some cases.

Monitor the effects of concurrent use and increase the doxycycline dose as necessary.

Rifampicin (Rifampin) + **Theophylline**

Rifampicin increases the clearance of theophylline by up to about 85%. In one study rifampicin (with isoniazid) increased theophylline clearance during the initial few days of treatment, but another study suggested that these antimycobacterials decreased theophylline clearance within 4 weeks.

> Monitor theophylline levels. An effect has been seen within 36 hours of starting rifampicin. Expect to need to increase the theophylline dose. The picture is less clear when isoniazid is also taken. In this situation it would seem prudent to monitor theophylline levels closely for the first month of treatment.

Rifampicin (Rifampin) + **Toremifene**

Rifampicin increases the metabolism of toremifene (peak levels more than halved), and might be expected to reduce its efficacy.

> Monitor the outcome of concurrent use to ensure the effects of toremifene are adequate. The manufacturers of toremifene suggest that the toremifene dose may need to be doubled.

R

Rifampicin (Rifampin) + **Trimethoprim**

Rifampicin reduces the AUC of trimethoprim (given as co-trimoxazole) by 56% in HIV-positive subjects, but apparently has no effect on trimethoprim alone in healthy subjects.

> The interaction between rifampicin and trimethoprim seems unlikely to be relevant in subjects who are not infected with HIV. Consider also co-trimoxazole, page 249.

Rifampicin (Rifampin) + **Warfarin and other oral anticoagulants**

The anticoagulant effects of acenocoumarol, phenprocoumon and warfarin are markedly reduced by rifampicin.

> A marked reduction occurs within 5 to 7 days of starting rifampicin, persisting for up to 5 weeks after the rifampicin is stopped. Monitor the INR closely. The warfarin dose may need to be markedly increased (2- to 5-fold) over a number of weeks. Remember to re-adjust the coumarin dose when rifampicin is stopped.

S

Salbutamol (Albuterol) and related bronchodilators

Salbutamol (Albuterol) and related bronchodilators + Theophylline ❓

The concurrent use of theophylline and beta$_2$ agonist bronchodilators such as salbutamol is a useful option in the management of asthma and chronic obstructive pulmonary disease, but potentiation of some adverse reactions can occur. The most serious of these are hypokalaemia and tachycardia, particularly with high-dose theophylline. Some patients may show a significant fall in theophylline levels if given oral or intravenous salbutamol or intravenous isoprenaline (isoproterenol).

> Potassium should be monitored, particularly in acutely unwell patients receiving high-dose intravenous treatment. The CSM in the UK particularly recommends monitoring potassium levels in those with severe asthma as the hypokalaemic effects of beta$_2$ agonists can be potentiated by concurrent use of theophylline, corticosteroids, diuretics and hypoxia.

Sevelamer

Sevelamer + Tacrolimus

Sevelamer reduced the absorption of tacrolimus in one patient (AUC *increased* 2.4-fold when sevelamer *stopped*).

> Tacrolimus levels should be closely monitored as a matter of routine; however, it may be prudent to increase monitoring when sevelamer is started or stopped, adjusting the tacrolimus dose as needed. The manufacturers advise that tacrolimus should be taken at least 1 hour before or 3 hours after sevelamer.

Sibutramine

Sibutramine + SSRIs

Serotonin syndrome has been seen in 2 cases when sibutramine was taken with SSRIs.

The manufacturers advise that concurrent use should be avoided, or only undertaken with appropriate monitoring, see serotonin syndrome, page 454.

Sibutramine + Triptans

Sibutramine inhibits serotonin uptake. The serious serotonin syndrome, page 454, has, rarely, been seen when sibutramine has been taken with serotonergic drugs. The manufacturers therefore say that sibutramine should not be taken with any serotonergic drugs and specifically name sumatriptan.

Concurrent use should be avoided.

Sibutramine + Tryptophan

Central and peripheral toxicity developed in a number of patients taking *fluoxetine* with tryptophan. On theoretical grounds an adverse reaction (such as serotonin syndrome, page 454) seems possible between any serotonergic drug (such as sibutramine) and tryptophan.

Avoid concurrent use.

Sibutramine + Venlafaxine

Serotonin syndrome developed in a woman given venlafaxine and sibutramine.

In general the concurrent use of two serotonergic drugs should be undertaken with caution because of the risks of serotonin syndrome, page 454. However, one UK manufacturer of venlafaxine specifically advises against its use with weight loss drugs.

Sirolimus

Sirolimus + Vaccines

The body's immune response is suppressed by sirolimus. The antibody response to vaccines may be reduced and the use of live attenuated vaccines may result in generalised infection.

For many inactivated vaccines even the reduced response seen is considered clinically useful and, in the case of renal transplant patients, influenza vaccination is actively recommended. If a vaccine is given, it may be prudent to monitor the response, so that alternative prophylactic measures can be considered where the response is inadequate. Note that even where effective antibody titres are produced, these may not persist as long as in healthy subjects, and more frequent booster doses may be required. The use of live vaccines is generally considered to be contraindicated. Ideally vaccines should take place before immunosuppressive treatment is started, and live vaccines should not be given for up to 6 months after treatment has stopped.

SSRIs

Although the SSRIs are likely to share pharmacodynamic interactions (for example development of serotonin syndrome with other serotonergic drugs) they do have differing effects on cytochrome P450, which leads to different metabolic actions. Fluvoxamine is a potent inhibitor of CYP1A2, whereas fluoxetine and paroxetine have moderate inhibitory effects on CYP2D6. Citalopram (and therefore probably escitalopram) and sertraline only weakly inhibit this isoenzyme. Serotonin syndrome is thought to result from the over-stimulation of the 5-HT$_{1A}$ and 5-HT$_{2A}$ receptors and possibly other serotonin receptors in the central nervous system. It can, exceptionally, occur with the use of one drug, but much more usually it develops when two or more drugs with serotonergic actions are given together. The characteristic symptoms fall into three main areas, namely altered mental status (agitation, confusion, mania), autonomic dysfunction (diaphoresis, diarrhoea, fever, shivering) and neuromuscular abnormalities (hyperreflexia, incoordination, myoclonus, tremor). Serotonin syndrome usually resolves within about 24 hours if the offending drugs are withdrawn and supportive measures given. Most patients recover uneventfully, but there have been a few fatalities. Many drugs have serotonergic actions, but the advice on concurrent use of these drugs varies greatly between manufacturers. The SSRIs are amongst the most commonly implicated drugs, and it is generally advised that the concurrent use of serotonergic drugs with SSRIs should be undertaken with caution. The most practical approach therefore seems to be to monitor for potential symptoms, and to seek medical advice should they occur.

SSRIs + Tacrine ⚠

Fluvoxamine can increase the AUC of tacrine by up to 8-fold. Tacrine adverse effects (nausea, vomiting, diarrhoea, sweating) are increased.

It is likely that standard tacrine doses will be poorly tolerated and a decrease in the tacrine dose will probably be needed. Other SSRIs such as fluoxetine, paroxetine, or sertraline, may theoretically be suitable alternatives, as these are unlikely to inhibit tacrine metabolism.

SSRIs + Tamoxifen

Paroxetine, a CYP2D6 inhibitor, reduces the metabolism of tamoxifen to one of its active metabolites and it has been suggested that this may decrease the efficacy of tamoxifen. Several case-control studies and one retrospective cohort study investigating the effects of SSRIs on tamoxifen have not found an increase in breast cancer recurrence, although one case-control study with CYP2D6 inhibitors did suggest an increased recurrence. In addition, one retrospective cohort study reported an increased risk of breast cancer recurrence in patients taking paroxetine with tamoxifen.

Many commentators suggest that paroxetine (and therefore probably fluoxetine, which has similar CYP2D6 inhibitory potential) should be avoided. Given that alternatives to these SSRIs are available, and given the potential seriousness of the proposed interaction, until the risks are established, it would seem prudent to use an alternative SSRI (such as citalopram) or perhaps the SNRI, venlafaxine, which have a low potential for affecting CYP2D6.

SSRIs + Terbinafine

Terbinafine modestly increased paroxetine levels in one study. Other SSRIs may interact similarly.

The clinical relevance of this interaction is unclear; increases of the magnitude seen would seem likely to increase adverse effects, although this was not seen in one study. Nevertheless be alert for an increase in SSRI adverse effects, and consider reducing the dose if these become troublesome.

SSRIs + Theophylline

Theophylline levels can be markedly and rapidly increased by the concurrent use of fluvoxamine. Toxicity has occurred.

Ideally concurrent use should be avoided. If this is not possible, reduce the theophylline dose and monitor theophylline levels. Some preliminary clinical evidence suggests that fluoxetine and citalopram (and therefore probably escitalopram) may not interact with theophylline, and *in vitro* evidence suggests that paroxetine and sertraline are also unlikely to interact. They may therefore be suitable alternatives.

SSRIs + Tizanidine

Fluvoxamine causes a very marked 12-fold increase in tizanidine levels with a consequent increase in its adverse effects such as hypotension, bradycardia and sedation.

Concurrent use is contraindicated. Consider changing fluvoxamine to another SSRI as they are not expected to significantly affect tizanidine metabolism.

SSRIs + Trazodone

Trazodone and fluoxetine have been used concurrently with advantage, although fluoxetine may modestly increase the levels of trazodone and some patients may develop increased adverse effects. Additive adverse effects such as sedation are predicted to possibly occur with other SSRIs.

It may be prudent to monitor for an increase in adverse effects (such as dysarthria, tremor and sedation) when trazodone is used with any SSRI.

SSRIs + Tricyclics ⚠

The levels of the tricyclic antidepressants can be raised by the SSRIs, but the extent varies greatly, from 20% to 10-fold: fluvoxamine, fluoxetine and paroxetine appear to cause the greatest increase. Tricyclic toxicity has been seen in a number of cases. Tricyclics may increase the levels of citalopram and possibly fluvoxamine, but the significance of this is unclear. There are several case reports of the serotonin syndrome, page 454, following concurrent and even sequential use of the SSRIs and tricyclics.

The increased tricyclic antidepressant levels can be beneficial. However, it has been suggested that patients given fluoxetine should have their tricyclic dose reduced to a quarter. Similar recommendations have been made with fluvoxamine (reduction in tricyclic dose to one-third) and sertraline. It would also seem prudent to consider a dose reduction of the tricyclic if paroxetine is added. Some suggest that a small initial dose of the SSRI should also be used. Patients taking any combination of tricyclic and SSRI should be monitored for adverse effects (e.g. dry mouth, sedation, confusion) with tricyclic levels monitored where possible. Note that the active metabolite of fluoxetine has a half-life of 7 to 15 days, and so any interaction may persist for some time after the fluoxetine is withdrawn, and may therefore occur on sequential use. The manufacturer of clomipramine advises a washout period of 2 to 3 weeks before and after treatment with fluoxetine.

SSRIs + Triptans ⚠

The concurrent use of a triptan and an SSRI is normally uneventful, but adverse reactions (such as serotonin syndrome, page 454, reported with sumatriptan and some SSRIs) do occasionally occur. Fluvoxamine has been shown to increase the blood levels of frovatriptan by 27 to 49%, and is predicted to increase the levels of zolmitriptan.

The combination need not be avoided, but monitor carefully, especially if other serotonergic drugs are also used. The manufacturers of zolmitriptan recommend a dose reduction to a maximum of 5 mg in 24 hours in the presence of fluvoxamine.

SSRIs + Tryptophan ⚠

Central and peripheral toxicity developed in a number of patients taking fluoxetine with tryptophan and adverse effects (headache, nausea, sweating, and dizziness) have been reported with concurrent use of paroxetine. On theoretical grounds, an adverse reaction (such as serotonin syndrome, page 454) seems possible between any SSRI and tryptophan.

The combination is probably best avoided; however, if tryptophan is given with an SSRI, the SSRI should be started at a low dose and tryptophan gradually introduced, starting with a low dose. Patients should be closely monitored for adverse effects.

SSRIs + Venlafaxine ⚠

The manufacturer of venlafaxine cautions its use with SSRIs because of the potential risks of serotonin syndrome. Cases of this reaction have been reported. Additive antimuscarinic effects have also been seen.

Monitor concurrent use carefully. Patients should told to report any symptoms of serotonin syndrome, page 454 and antimuscarinic adverse effects (such as dry mouth, blurred vision and urinary retention).

SSRIs + Warfarin and other oral anticoagulants

Warfarin levels can be increased by fluvoxamine and raised INRs have been seen in several cases. Isolated reports describe raised INRs and/or haemorrhage in patients taking acenocoumarol with citalopram or paroxetine, and warfarin with fluoxetine or paroxetine, although no pharmacokinetic interaction appears to occur. SSRIs alone have, rarely, been associated with bleeding.

Studies have not demonstrated a consistent interaction, with the exception of fluvoxamine and warfarin. It may be prudent to monitor the INR when fluvoxamine is first added, being alert for the need to decrease the anticoagulant dose. As SSRIs alone can rarely cause bleeding, caution is advised with the concurrent use of oral anticoagulants and SSRIs; consider monitoring with other SSRIs, but note only a few patients appear to have demonstrated this interaction. Any interaction appears to occur in about the first 2 weeks of treatment.

S

Statins

Lovastatin and simvastatin are extensively metabolised by CYP3A4 so that drugs that moderately or potently inhibit this enzyme can cause marked rises in statin levels. Atorvastatin is also metabolised by CYP3A4, but to a lesser extent than lovastatin or simvastatin. Fluvastatin is metabolised primarily by CYP2C9, rosuvastatin by CYP2C9 and CYP2C19, while the cytochrome P450 system does not appear to be involved in the metabolism of pravastatin. Therefore the statins tend to interact differently. In order to reduce the risk of myopathy the CSM in the UK advises that statins should be used with care in patients who are at increased risk of this adverse effect, such as those taking interacting drugs. They also recommend that patients should be made aware of the risks of myopathy and rhabdomyolysis, and asked to promptly report muscle pain, tenderness or weakness, especially if accompanied by malaise, fever or dark urine.

Statins + Warfarin and other oral anticoagulants

Fluvastatin and Rosuvastatin

Studies and case reports have suggested that fluvastatin can increase warfarin levels and/or effects. Rosuvastatin can increase the anticoagulant effects of warfarin but does not alter warfarin levels. Not all patients are affected.

Increased monitoring is required when starting or stopping fluvastatin or rosuvastatin, or changing the statin dose.

Other statins

Studies with atorvastatin, lovastatin, pravastatin, and simvastatin suggest that they do not usually significantly alter the effects of warfarin, although cases of bleeding have been seen when these statins were given with coumarins and fluindione.

> It has been suggested that it would be prudent to monitor the early stages of concurrent use of statins and anticoagulants in all patients, or if the dose of statin is changed, being alert for the need to adjust the anticoagulant dose. However, this interaction has only been clinically significant in a handful of patients, so monitoring every patient may be over-cautious.

Strontium

Strontium + Tetracyclines ✖

The manufacturer of strontium ranelate predicts that it will complex with tetracyclines, and therefore prevent their absorption.

> It is recommended that when treatment with a tetracycline is required, strontium ranelate should be temporarily suspended.

Sucralfate

Sucralfate + Tetracyclines ⚠

On theoretical grounds the absorption of tetracycline may possibly be reduced by sucralfate, but clinical confirmation of this appears to be lacking.

> The manufacturers suggest that they should be given 2 hours apart to minimise their admixture in the gut.

Sucralfate + Warfarin and other oral anticoagulants ❓

Case reports describe a marked reduction in the effects of warfarin in patients given sucralfate. Other evidence suggests that this interaction is uncommon.

> Concurrent use need not be avoided but bear this interaction in mind if a patient has a reduced anticoagulant response to warfarin. Information about other anticoagulants is lacking, but be aware that a similar interaction is possible.

Sulfinpyrazone

Sulfinpyrazone + Theophylline ✅

Sulfinpyrazone causes a small 22% increase in the clearance of theophylline.

This small reduction is unlikely to be clinically relevant.

Sulfinpyrazone + Warfarin and other oral anticoagulants ⚠

The anticoagulant effects of warfarin and acenocoumarol are increased by sulfinpyrazone and serious bleeding has occurred.

The INR should be well monitored and suitable anticoagulant dose reductions made. Halving the dose of warfarin and reducing the acenocoumarol dose by 20% has proven to be adequate in some patients. Bear in mind that the antiplatelet effects of sulfinpyrazone might increase the risk of bleeding with oral anticoagulants.

Sulfonamides

Sulfonamides + Warfarin and other oral anticoagulants ⚠

The anticoagulant effects of warfarin, acenocoumarol, and phenprocoumon are increased by co-trimoxazole (sulfamethoxazole with trimethoprim). Bleeding may occur if the anticoagulant dosage is not reduced appropriately. There is also evidence that sulfaphenazole, sulfafurazole (sulfisoxazole) and sulfamethizole may interact like co-trimoxazole. Anecdotal evidence suggests that phenindione might not interact with co-trimoxazole, but sulfaphenazole has been reported to increase the effects of phenindione.

The incidence of the interaction with co-trimoxazole appears to be high. If bleeding is to be avoided the INR should be well monitored and the coumarin dose should be reduced. Some suggest avoiding concurrent use because of the difficulties with re-establishing anticoagulation. Phenindione is said not to interact; however, bear the case report of an interaction with sulfaphenazole in mind. The other interactions are poorly documented. However, it would seem prudent to follow the precautions suggested for co-trimoxazole if any sulfonamide is given with a coumarin or indanedione.

S

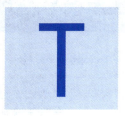

Tacrine

Tacrine + Theophylline ⚠

Limited evidence suggests that tacrine reduces the clearance of theophylline by 50%. It seems possible that aminophylline may be similarly affected.

> Until more is known it may be prudent to monitor theophylline levels if tacrine is started or stopped.

Tacrolimus

Tacrolimus + Vaccines ✖

The body's immune response is suppressed by tacrolimus. The antibody response to vaccines may be reduced and the use of live attenuated vaccines may result in generalised infection.

> For many inactivated vaccines even the reduced response seen is considered clinically useful and, in the case of renal transplant patients, influenza vaccination is actively recommended. If a vaccine is given, it may be prudent to monitor the response, so that alternative prophylactic measures can be considered where the response is inadequate. Note that even where effective antibody titres are produced, these may not persist as long as in healthy subjects, and more frequent booster doses may be required. The use of live vaccines is generally considered to be contraindicated. Ideally vaccines should take place before immunosuppressive treatment is started, and live vaccines should not be given for up to 6 months after treatment has stopped.

Tamoxifen

Tamoxifen + Warfarin and other oral anticoagulants

Tamoxifen may increase the effects of warfarin and cases of serious bleeding, in one case fatal, have been reported. A case report describes a similar effect with acenocoumarol.

> Monitor the effects closely if tamoxifen is added to treatment with warfarin or acenocoumarol and reduce the dose as necessary. Reports indicate that, generally, a reduction of between one-half to two-thirds may be needed for warfarin. Consider also that, from a disease perspective, when treating venous thromboembolic disease in patients with cancer, warfarin is generally inferior (higher risk of major bleeds and recurrent thrombosis) to low-molecular-weight heparins.

Terbinafine

Terbinafine + Tricyclics

Terbinafine markedly increased the AUC of desipramine in one study. Case reports describe increases in the serum levels of amitriptyline, desipramine, imipramine, and nortriptyline, with associated toxicity, in patients given oral terbinafine.

> Monitor for any increase in the adverse effects of the tricyclic (e.g. dry mouth, blurred vision, constipation), and be aware that the dose may need to be decreased, sometimes substantially. Note that an interaction may occur for a number of weeks after stopping terbinafine, because it has a long half-life.

Terbinafine + Venlafaxine

The metabolism of venlafaxine to its active metabolite O-desmethylvenlafaxine is reduced in the presence of terbinafine. However, the combined AUC of venlafaxine and its metabolite is only raised by a modest 22%.

> Until more is known, it may be prudent to be alert for any indication of increased venlafaxine adverse effects (e.g. nausea, insomnia, dry mouth) in patients also taking terbinafine.

Tetracyclines

Tetracyclines + **Warfarin and other oral anticoagulants** ⚠

Isolated cases suggest that doxycycline and tetracycline can increase the effects of coumarins. Similarly, some small studies (none controlled) suggest that chlortetracycline (alone or with oxytetracycline), doxycycline, or the tetracyclines as a class may increase the risks of over-anticoagulation.

> The clinical importance of this interaction is unknown, but bear it in mind in case of an excessive response to anticoagulant treatment. If a patient is unwell enough to require an antibacterial, it may be prudent to increase monitoring of coagulation status even if no specific drug interaction is expected. Monitor within 3 days of starting the antibacterial.

Tetracyclines + **Zinc** ⚠

The absorption of tetracycline is reduced by up to 50% by zinc. All tetracyclines (with perhaps the exception of doxycycline) are expected to interact similarly.

> Separate administration. In the case of *iron*, which interacts by the same mechanism, 2 to 3 hours is sufficient. Doxycycline may be a useful non-interacting alternative.

Theophylline

Theophylline is metabolised by cytochrome P450 in the liver, principally by CYP1A2. Many drugs interact with theophylline by inhibition or potentiation of its metabolism. Theophylline has a narrow therapeutic range, and small increases in serum levels can result in toxicity. Moreover, symptoms of serious toxicity such as convulsions and arrhythmias can occur before minor symptoms suggestive of toxicity. Furthermore, age, cigarette smoking, chronic obstructive airways disease, congestive heart failure, and liver disease (cirrhosis, acute hepatitis) can also affect theophylline clearance. Within the context of interactions, aminophylline is expected to behave like theophylline, because it is a complex of theophylline with ethylenediamine.

Theophylline + **Ticlopidine** ⚠

Ticlopidine reduces the clearance of theophylline by about 40%, and is expected to raise its serum levels. Aminophylline seems likely to be similarly affected.

> Monitor concurrent use for theophylline toxicity (headache, nausea, palpitations), particularly when levels are already at the top end of the range.

Theophylline + **Vaccines** ❓

BCG vaccine appears to slightly increase the half-life of theophylline. Normally influenza vaccines (whole-virion, split-virion and surface antigen) do not interact with theophylline, but raised theophylline levels and toxicity have been seen in occasional cases.

> Problems are very unlikely to arise now that purer vaccines are available, but bear this interaction in mind in case of an unexpected response to treatment.

Theophylline + **Zafirlukast** ❓

A single unverified case report describes a rapid rise in theophylline levels after the addition of zafirlukast. Other similar unpublished reports have been made to the manufacturer. Zafirlukast levels are modestly reduced by theophylline, but this does not appear to be clinically important. However, a study found that theophylline levels were not affected by zafirlukast.

> No adverse interaction would normally seem to occur with zafirlukast and theophylline.

Ticlopidine

Ticlopidine + **Warfarin and other oral anticoagulants** ❌

The anticoagulant effects of acenocoumarol may be modestly reduced by ticlopidine. However, the anticoagulant effects of warfarin are unchanged by ticlopidine. As with other antiplatelet drugs, concurrent use with coumarins might possibly increase bleeding risk. Cholestatic hepatitis has been reported in some patients given warfarin and ticlopidine.

> The US manufacturer recommends that if a patient is switched from an anticoagulant to ticlopidine, the anticoagulant should be stopped before ticlopidine is started. As with other antiplatelet drugs, an increased risk of bleeding is anticipated if coumarins or indanediones are also given.

Toremifene

Toremifene + **Warfarin and other oral anticoagulants** ❌

The anticoagulant effects of acenocoumarol and warfarin are markedly increased by *tamoxifen* and bleeding has been seen. Toremifene is expected to interact similarly.

Monitor the effects closely if toremifene is added to treatment with any coumarin and reduce the dose as necessary. Consider also that, from a disease perspective, when treating venous thromboembolic disease in patients with cancer, warfarin is generally inferior (higher risk of major bleeds and recurrent thrombosis) to low-molecular-weight heparins.

Trazodone

Trazodone + **Venlafaxine** ⚠

Isolated cases of serotonin syndrome have been reported in patients taking venlafaxine with trazodone.

Concurrent use should be monitored carefully. For more information, see serotonin syndrome, page 454.

Trazodone + **Warfarin and other oral anticoagulants** ⚠

A handful of case reports describe a moderate reduction in the anticoagulant effects of warfarin caused by trazodone, and another case report describes a rise in INR.

It might be prudent to monitor the INR in all patients taking warfarin if trazodone is started or stopped, adjusting the warfarin dose if necessary.

Tricyclics

Tricyclics + **Valproate** ❓

Amitriptyline and nortriptyline plasma levels can be increased by sodium valproate and valpromide. Status epilepticus, tremulousness and/or sleep disturbances have been attributed to elevated clomipramine or nortriptyline levels in patients taking valproate or valproic acid.

It would seem prudent to monitor for tricyclic adverse effects (such as dry mouth, blurred vision and urinary retention) and reduce the dose of the tricyclic if necessary. Tricyclics can lower the convulsive threshold and should therefore be used with caution in patients with epilepsy.

Tricyclics + **Venlafaxine** ⚠

The use of venlafaxine with the tricyclics is expected to increase the risk of serotonin syndrome, page 454, and cases have been seen. Increased antimuscarinic adverse effects, movement disorders and seizures have also been reported. Venlafaxine appears to increase the levels of desipramine or its 2-hydroxydesipramine metabolite. Other tricyclics are expected to interact similarly.

Be alert for any evidence of increased antimuscarinic adverse effects. Although there appears to be only one report, the possibility of an increased risk of seizures with concurrent use should be borne in mind, especially in those already at risk of seizures. It may be necessary to withdraw one or both of the drugs. The reports of serotonin syndrome highlight the need for caution when one or more serotonergic drugs are given.

Tricyclics + **Warfarin and other oral anticoagulants** ❓

Limited evidence suggests that amitriptyline and possibly other tricyclics can cause unpredictable increases or decreases in prothrombin times in patients taking coumarins, which can make stable anticoagulation difficult.

There is insufficient evidence to recommend an increased frequency of INR monitoring, but it would at least seem prudent to bear this interaction in mind when prescribing a coumarin and a tricyclic.

Triptans

Triptans + **Venlafaxine** ⚠

The manufacturers of venlafaxine advise caution on the concurrent use of drugs that affect serotonergic transmission, such as the triptans. This is because of the possible risks of serotonin syndrome, page 454.

Monitor concurrent use carefully for symptoms including agitation, confusion and tremor.

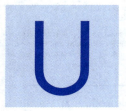

No interactions have been included for drugs beginning with the letter U.

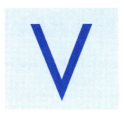

Vaccines

Vaccines + **Warfarin and other oral anticoagulants**

The concurrent use of warfarin and influenza vaccine is usually safe and uneventful, but there are reports of bleeding in a handful of patients (life-threatening in one case) attributed to an interaction. Acenocoumarol also does not normally interact.

> This interaction seems rare, but bear it in mind in case of unexpected bleeding. Note that, because of the theoretical risk of local muscle haematoma, it may be preferable to give influenza vaccines by deep subcutaneous injection in patients taking coumarins and related anticoagulants.

Venlafaxine

Venlafaxine + **Warfarin and other oral anticoagulants**

Unpublished cases of bleeding and raised prothrombin times have been reported with venlafaxine and warfarin. Note that venlafaxine alone has, rarely, been associated with bleeding, and there is the theoretical possibility that the risk might be increased when used with warfarin and related drugs.

> Consider increasing INR monitoring if venlafaxine is added or withdrawn from treatment with warfarin or any coumarin. Also bear in mind the possibility of increased bleeding risk in the absence of alterations in INR.

Vitamins

Vitamins + **Warfarin and other oral anticoagulants**

The effects of coumarins and indanediones can be reduced or abolished by vitamin K. This effect can be used to manage overdose, but unintentional and unwanted antagonism has occurred in patients after taking some proprietary chilblain preparations, health foods, food supplements, enteral feeds or exceptionally large amounts of some green vegetables, seaweed, or green tea, which can contain significant amounts of vitamin K. Giving 10 to 50 micrograms of vitamin K_1 (phytomenadione) generally will not significantly affect the INR in response to warfarin; however, patients with poor vitamin K status, even low vitamin K doses of 25 micrograms daily may have an important effect.

The drug intake and diet of any patient who shows warfarin resistance' should be investigated for the possibility of this interaction. It can be accommodated either by increasing the anticoagulant dose, or by reducing the intake of vitamin K. However, patients taking vitamin K-rich diets should not change their eating habits without at the same time reducing the anticoagulant dose, because excessive anticoagulation and bleeding may occur.

V

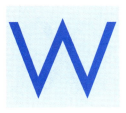

Warfarin and other oral anticoagulants

Warfarin, phenprocoumon and acenocoumarol are racemic mixtures of *S*- and *R*-enantiomers. The *S*-enantiomers of these coumarins have several times more anticoagulant activity than the *R*-enantiomers. The *S*-enantiomer of warfarin is metabolised primarily by CYP2C9. The metabolism of *R*-warfarin is more complex but this enantiomer is primarily metabolised by CYP1A2, CYP3A4, CYP2C19 and CYP2C8. There is much more known about the metabolism of warfarin compared to other anticoagulants but it is established that *S*-phenprocoumon and *S*-acenocoumarol are also substrates for CYP2C9. Whilst the metabolism of the coumarins, especially warfarin, is well known, the numerous interaction pathways and the variability in patient responses makes the clinical consequences of alterations in metabolism difficult to predict.

Warfarin and other oral anticoagulants + Zafirlukast ⚠

Zafirlukast increases the anticoagulant effects of warfarin and bleeding has been seen. Other coumarins may be expected to interact similarly.

> If zafirlukast is given to patients stable taking a coumarin, monitor prothrombin times closely and be alert for the need to reduce the coumarin dose to avoid over-anticoagulation.

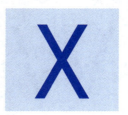

No interactions have been included for drugs beginning with the letter X.

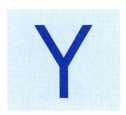

No interactions have been included for drugs beginning with the letter Y.

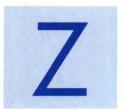

No interactions have been included for drugs beginning with the letter Z.

Index

Index

Index

Index